Community Health Care Nursing

Fourth Edition

Edited by

David Sines
Professor of Community Nursing and Executive Dean of the Faculty of Health and Social Care, London South Bank University

Mary Saunders
Head of Department of Primary and Social Care, London South Bank University

Janice Forbes-Burford
Operational & Service Planning Manager, NHS South West

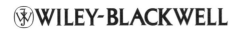

A John Wiley & Sons, Ltd., Publication

Library of Congress Cataloging-in-Publication Data
Community health care nursing / edited by David Sines, Mary Saunders, Janice Forbes-Burford. — 4th ed.
        p.   cm.
  Includes bibliographical references and index.
  ISBN 978-1-4051-8340-6 (pbk. : alk. paper)   1. Community health nursing—Great Britain.
2. Primary health care—Great Britain.   I. Sines, David. II. Saunders, Mary, 1955– III. Forbes-Burford, Janice.
  [DNLM: 1. Community Health Nursing—Great Britain. 2. Primary Health Care—Great Britain.
WY 106 C7342 2009]
  RT98.C6315   2009
  610.73'43—dc22

                                                                                        2009005452

A catalogue record for this book is available from the British Library.

Set in 9.5/12 Palatino Roman by Macmillan Publishing Solutions, Chennai, India
Printed and bound in Singapore by Fabulous Printers Pte Ltd

1   2009

Community I

Contents

Contributors

Dr Jaya Ahuja *Senior Lecturer in Non-Medical Prescribing/Pharmacology, Faculty of Health & Social Care, London South Bank University, London, UK*

Owen Barr *Head of School and Senior Lecturer in Nursing, University of Ulster, Northland Road, Londonderry, Northern Ireland, UK*

Sue Boran *Senior Lecturer in Community Health Care Nursing, Faculty of Health & Social Care, London South Bank University, London, UK*

Linda Burke *Reader and Associate Dean (Head of Nursing), Faculty of Health and Social Care, Kingston University and St George's, University of London, London, UK*

Pat Colliety *Director of Studies, Faculty of Health & Medical Sciences, University of Surrey, Surrey, UK*

Janice Forbes Burford *Operational & Service Planning Manager, NHS South West, Essex, UK*

Marion Frost *Previously Principal Lecturer, Surrey, UK*

Anne Harriss *Reader in Educational Development (Occupational Health Nursing), Faculty of Health & Social Care, London South Bank University, London, UK*

Sandra Horner *Senior Lecturer, Faculty of Health & Social Care, London South Bank University, London, UK*

Maxine Jameson *Senior Lecturer in Community Health Care Nursing (School Nursing), Faculty of Health & Social Care, London South Bank University, London, UK*

Dr Ann Long *Honorary Fellow of the University of Ulster, Belfast, Northern Ireland, UK*

Jane Lopez *Principal Lecturer, School of Nursing, Kingston on Thames, Surrey, UK*

Katrina Maclaine *Principal Lecturer in Advanced Nursing Practice, Faculty of Health & Social Care, London South Bank University, London, UK*

Derek McLaughlin *Lecturer in Community Mental Health Nursing, School of Health Sciences, University of Ulster at Jordanstown, Newtownabbey, Northern Ireland, UK*

Joan Myers *Consultant Nurse – Community Children's Nursing, NHS Islington, London, UK*

Liz Plastow *Independent Consultant in Primary Care and Public Health Nursing, Professional Advisor in Primary Care, Wilmington, Devon, UK*

Elizabeth Porter *Programme Leader, Specialist Practice, Nursing Department, Southampton University, Romsey, Hampshire, UK*

Professor Bob Sang *Professor of Patient and User Involvements, Faculty of Health & Social Care, London South Bank University, London, UK*

Mary Saunders *Head of Department, Primary and Social Care, Faculty of Health & Social Care, London South Bank University, London, UK*

Karol Selvey *Nurse Practitioner/Clinical Manager, Surrey, UK*

David Sines *Executive Dean, Faculty of Health & Social Care, London South Bank University, London, UK*

Professor Pam Smith *GNC Professor, Faculty of Health & Medical Sciences, University of Surrey, Surrey, UK*

Keiron Spires *Principal Lecturer, Faculty of Health & Social Care, London South Bank University, London, UK*

Karen Stubbs *Consultant Member of the Primary Care Changing Workforce Centre, Faculty of Health & Social Care, London South Bank University, London, UK*

Susie Sykes   *Senior Lecturer in Public Health and Health Promotion, Faculty of Health & Social Care, London South Bank University, London, UK*

Professor Ann Taket   *Head of School of Health and Social Development, School of Health and Social Development, Faculty of Health, Medicine, Nursing and Behavioural Sciences, Deakin University, Burwood, Victoria, Australia*

Val Thurtle *Programme Director, Public Health Nursing, School of Health and Social Care, University of Reading, Berkshire, UK*

Amanda Tragen   *Senior Lecturer in Non-Medical Prescribing/Pharmacology, Faculty of Health & Social Care, London South Bank University, London, UK*

Elizabeth Treadwell   *Senior Lecturer, School of Nursing, Kingston on Thames, Surrey, UK*

Dr Vasso Vydelingum   *Director of Studies-Doctorate Programmes, Faculty of Health & Medical Sciences, University of Surrey, Surrey, UK*

Helen Ward   *Principal Lecturer in Non-Medical Prescribing/Community Health Care Nursing, Faculty of Health & Social Care, London South Bank University, London, UK*

Mark Whiting   *Consultant Nurse, Children with Complex Health Needs, Hertfordshire Partnership NHS Trust, UK*

David Widdas   *Consultant Nurse, Children with Complex Health Care Needs, Coventry PCT and NHS Warwickshire, UK*

Jane Wills   *Professor of Health Promotion, Faculty of Health & Social Care, London South Bank University, London, UK*

Preface

Welcome to the fourth edition of *Community Health Care Nursing*. The past decade has witnessed unparalleled change and investment in the development of responsive services for patients and clients in the community, supported by new service commissioning strategies and significant advances in treatment modalities in the acute sector. Major investment has also been witnessed in the design and commissioning of new workforce solutions that have demanded major revision to the way in which we prepare nurses and specialist community public health nurses to work in primary care settings.

A key objective of proposed service reforms is to design a workforce that is both fit for practice and fit for purpose, equipped with competencies that will enable practitioners to function across a range of priority, inter-professional care pathways both within hospital and within primary care settings (including new polyclinics). This new edition takes account of the demand placed by service commissioners and providers to ensure flexibility in the workforce, irrespective of the location and focus of their present function. In so doing we have recognised that the demand for health care, influenced by changes in disease pattern and treatment response will change, based primarily on the co-delivery of health care in partnership between users, carers and professionals. The National Health Service (NHS) 'choice' agenda with emphasis being placed on home-based care (underpinned by an unmitigated resolve to engage service users as co-respondents to the health care agenda), has been a key driver for our revised text. Key tenets for health care modernisation and new models of delivery are also expounded following the emergence of an increasingly diverse range of providers, including the role of the third sector and reliance on the commercial sector to provide substantial elements of primary and secondary care provision in the UK.

The new edition also acknowledges the importance of providing a competent workforce that is prepared to confront challenges relating to inequalities in health and social care delivery. Standards of proficiency, the enhancement of clinical skill competence, and the acquisition of clinical judgement skills in decision-making and care planning have also been identified as key drivers for change, particularly in areas such as the emergence of advanced practice roles and the delivery of enhanced clinical skills and needs assessment.

The key policy directives that have shaped our book have derived originally from *The NHS Plan* of 2000, which has been updated significantly on an annual basis by the Department of Health. For example, we have recognised the importance of supporting people with longer-term conditions, which has gained greater emphasis in the Department of Health's *Next Stage Review* (2007). Fundamental changes were also envisaged by the Department of Health in its 2006 publication *Our health, Our Care, Our Say: A New Direction for Community Services*. These values have been analysed and embedded throughout the new edition in various chapters.

Nurses continue to be central to government plans as identified in the Department of Health's *Modernising Nursing Careers* strategy (2006; www.dh.gov.uk/cno). For example, nurses play key roles in establishing new models of primary care and social enterprise and are integral to developing care pathways as part of the multidisciplinary team. Following the successful implementation of national service frameworks programmes, care policy has progressed to produce national competence standards identified by Skills for Health, demanding revisions to the way in which community health care nurses transact their roles and functions. The government is also clearly committed to the establishment of community health care/primary care nursing as the focus for promoting health gain for the population and its constituent neighbourhoods. Associated with these changes has been a major refocusing to 'shift' emphasis within the NHS to embrace a 'health-enabling' philosophy, rather than one that 'majors' on responding to illness. Thus this book aims to change the focus of practitioner responses from 'treatment' to 'prevention' and 'expert practice'.

Government investment in the design of new commissioning infrastructures to support primary care and public health initiatives has further strengthened the need for our professions to review the standard, kind and content of the education and practice base of community health care nursing. Other challenges have been the implementation of clinical governance, underpinned by the desire to promote clinical excellence and evidence-based practice, and the need to systematically measure and 'performance measure' the quality of service delivery. In addition priority has been given to the emergence of innovative solutions and practices designed to manage longer-term conditions and to enhance and promote public health. This text acknowledges the changing face of community health care nursing in the UK and firmly places its academic base within a scientific framework that is underpinned and influenced by contemporary changes in social and economic policy.

There is no doubt that the pace of change involved in designing and developing a new culture of community health care nursing has required a radical and sometimes traumatic revision of personal attitudes and customised care and managerial practices. In their place we are now witnessing the advent and creation of new structures, processes and service systems, many of which have been developed and implemented by nurses working in the many constituent parts of the family of 'community health care nursing'. This book considers some of the main issues to be addressed in the design and introduction of the profession of community health care nursing. Its roots are firmly established in the evolutionary nature of professional development and recognise the innovative, adaptable and flexible nature of the practitioners themselves. Consequently, the book contains examples of these changes and traces their origins and potential contribution to the implementation of community care and public health nursing. Lessons have been learnt from experimentation and research design and from experimental learning, and in so doing there will be, inevitably, some overlap between individual contributions and the solutions they propose for the delivery of effective community health care nursing care and specialist community public health nursing.

It is suggested that there is no one solution or 'blue-print' for local service design for any client group. The nature of our communities is as varied as the sub-cultural influences that shape them. No standard model has been prescribed and wherever possible contributors have deliberately avoided the inclusion of specific solutions. However, as with earlier editions, the book presents many ideas, examples and suggestions for the introduction and implementation of sound infrastructures for community health care nursing delivery that may be adapted to suit local conditions and requirements.

Within any attempt to describe the basis for comprehensive service design and implementation there will always be a temptation to capitalise on the experiences of others who have pioneered excellence in local services. This, in essence, is the business of community health care nursing. Contributors to this text have once again been selected for their own knowledge, experience and evidence of providing excellence in service delivery and education. Many who have realised the introduction of innovative practice in their localities will recognise common elements as they read this book that relate to their own experience, and this is of course the intention.

It is our contention that the realisation of excellence in the design and delivery of community health care nursing services relies on the principle that the public, service users, carers and community health care nurses require (and deserve) mutual recognition as key stakeholders in the development and implementation of future policy imperatives that aim to shape and influence the nature of our neighbourhood and nursing services. As such our practitioners need to be prepared to respond to an increasingly well-informed public, keen to have a bigger say in their care and treatment. Our new chapter on user involvement strategy, written by Professor Bob Sang, promotes the concept of including users as key co-designers and deliverers of health and social care. Some may challenge the 'realism' of our suggestions and recommendations, but there is one statement that cannot be challenged – they are all feasible – and evidence exists to suggest that further investment in the community nursing workforce will result in effective health gain for our population.

David Sines

References

Department of Health (2006) *Modernising Nursing Careers*. Department of Health, London. Available at: www.dh.gov.uk/cno.

Department of Health (2006) *Our Health, Our Care, Our Say: A New Direction for Community Services*. Department of Health, London.

NHS London (2007) *Healthcare for London – A Framework for Action*. Professor, Lord Ara Darzi, London.

Chapter 1 **The Context of Primary Health Care Nursing**

David Sines

The changing context of service provision

The population of the UK is projected to increase by approximately 7.2% over the period to 2016. The key drivers for population increase within the UK relate to greater life expectancy and migration, particularly from eastern Europe. Other key demographic challenges relate to an increasing older age population (over the age of 65), which will increase from 16% in 2006 to 22% by 2031 (Office for National Statistics 2007). The age of the working population will also increase during this period, demonstrating unforeseen lifestyle patterns, which in turn will impact on those people of state pensionable age.

According to Mathers & Loncar (2006) the ten leading causes of death by 2030 will be ischaemic heart disease, cerebrovascular disease, upper respiratory tract and lung cancers, diabetes mellitus and chronic obstructive pulmonary disease (COPD). Within the top ten leading causes of death will also rank dementias, unipolar depressive disorders, alcohol use disorders, stomach and colon cancers and osteoarthritis. The combination of longer-term physical disorders and psychosocial challenges will demonstrate the importance of integrated service provision and workforce capability and capacity to respond to presenting co-morbidities. Other worldwide challenges relating to infectious diseases, such as human immunodeficiency virus (HIV) infection and tuberculosis, will provide additional pressures on our health care systems.

Lord, Professor Ara Darzi, is his review of health care for London (NHS London 2007) identified the importance of promoting self-care and in encouraging patient and user involvement in health care prediction and co-treatment. In his report he noted the major challenges facing the health of the population regarding sexual health, obesity, smoking and alcohol/substance misuse, all of which place a heavy burden on the state health care system and contribute to the incidence of dual diagnoses and longer-term health care conditions.

The expectations of higher service response from the health service and its professional workforce also continue to rise, particularly as service users engage more fully in the determination of the shape and scope of local health care provision. Sang (2005), for example has written of the important role that members of the public are now making to the governance of the National Health Service (NHS), mainly through 'ownership' of NHS foundation trusts and through engagement with expert patient programmes. NHS trusts, in turn, are now responding more purposefully and seriously to user and patient expectations and are required to publish action plans in response to local and national patient satisfaction surveys and to demonstrate compliance with local service user requirements and feedback. Associated with the rise in consumerism and user engagement is a marked improvement in the capacity and capability of the NHS to respond to user complaints and to enhance governance procedures. Even more challenging to the NHS, however, is the increased number of litigation cases presented by patients seeking recompense for less than satisfactory care experiences.

So how does society and its associated health and social systems respond to such challenges? In the first place it can be assumed that societal change moulds the institutions that are created to respond to the needs of the population. Demands change over time and in so doing socio-demographic factors drive the process of change that in turn requires the NHS to adapt its operational base. Examples of such changes relate to the needs of an increasingly ageing population, a reduction in the number of available informal carers, advances in scientific knowledge and technological innovation, and a heightened awareness of ethical challenges (such as gene therapy, stem cell research, embryology and euthanasia).

The impact of change, stimulated by a growing demand for flexible, high-quality services provided within local communities will inevitably re-mould the NHS of the future. Resources are already being moved to the community at a rapid rate and health service commissioners and providers are now required to demonstrate that the care they purchase and deliver is effective and responsive to consumer need (Department of Health [DH] 2006b). It is perhaps in the primary and community care sectors that change has been most rapid, demanding the creation of innovative workforce solutions and service reconfigurations. Lord Darzi in his vision for the future of these services has recognised the challenge that these changes demand and has called for the implementation of a new national board that will include community nurses to 'drive the overall programme of work and ensure that we continue to engage staff in developing and implementing the vision' (DH 2008d).

Key features of our contemporary society suggest that a focus on health promotion and public health is required since:

- People are living longer and healthier lives and are better informed about their needs and expectations of the health service.
- Advising and supporting patients to make positive choices about their health status is prominent with particular regard to promoting self-management.
- Demand to enable people to remain at home is rising, thus placing emphasis on integrated care, self-management of longer-term

diseases and supporting healthy lifestyle choices and self-care in the community (supported by robust, integrated case management principles and social service direct care payments).
- Significant emphasis has been placed on increasing social inclusion and valuing diversity for socially excluded groups, i.e. those least likely to access health care, and on the reduction of health and social care inequalities experienced by significant groups within our population.
- Geographical diversity demands local adaptation of national health care solutions (particularly within the context of devolved government to the four countries of the UK).
- Consumers and practitioners are becoming increasingly dependent on new technological solutions, e.g. tele-medicine, advances in bio-engineering, NHS Direct and web-based information systems.

In 2008, the government outlined its most challenging reforms for the delivery of health care in England, since the publication of *The NHS Plan* in 2000, which at that time was supported by the introduction of new NHS structures, including the inauguration of primary care and foundation trusts. In 2008, Health Minister, Lord Ara Darzi, building on the principles of community/ primary care enshrined within the NHS and Community Care Act 1990, outlined a reformed strategic framework for the provision of all health services in England, focusing specifically on the major role that primary care trusts (PCTs) will play in the future as both commissioners and, where desirable, providers of local, innovative services (DH 2008a). Current frameworks for the design and delivery of responsive primary care services are built on the principle of ensuring the existence of clear, national standards, supported by consistent evidence-based guidance to raise the quality of care provided by the health and social care services. (DH 2000a, 2008b). Ara Darzi's new vision for the NHS (DH 2008a) sets out the rationale for the introduction of improvements in the way in which care is provided throughout the NHS and identifies the need for decisions relating to primary care to be made on the basis of the best evidence and research-based practice, interfacing appropriately with self-care and more specialist diagnostic and treatment provided by secondary and tertiary care providers. The details of the proposals for new locally designed services were previously outlined by the government in a major paper entitled *Our Health, Our Care, Our Say: A New Direction for Community Services* (DH 2006b), which included emphasis on the implementation of consultation with users of services and empowered frontline staff to identify robust indicators of personal performance while obtaining greater access to control over the allocation and management of the resources required to deliver services. Other critical issues raised in this paper were the concept of user/patient choice of clinician/source of advice, choice of care package, choice of appointment time and location. Associated with choice has been a major drive to reduce waiting times for outpatient appointments, emergency department triage and treatment, and hospital admission. New targets have also been set for cancer treatment and access to other diagnostic and clinical care services. Lord Darzi's review went one step further and outlined a new vision for the provision of primary and community care services (DH 2008c). The review confirmed the significant role that primary care and health promotion plays in the reformed health economy and emphasised that our focus should be on health outcomes, user engagement and in the design and implementation of healthy communities and lifestyles at school, at home and at work (DH 2008c).

These policies have pledged to 'break down' organisational barriers and to forge stronger links with local authorities, thus placing the needs of the patient/client at the centre of the care process. In so doing, a new foundation has been laid on which to unite the principles of seamless care delivery and in particular the provision of self-directed care/direct payment packages, based on case management principles (DH 2008e). In practice this will require the provision of new inter-sectoral solutions to ensure that care is delivered between health and social service agencies through the development of positive partnerships and integrated case assessments between statutory agencies, consumers, their representatives and with the voluntary and independent sectors to provide a positive choice in the provision of services. Emphasis on primary care has been reaffirmed in that, wherever possible, care should be provided as close to the person's home as possible.

The primary care vision for the next decade

At the heart of the government's reformed health care strategy is the greater focus placed on the delivery of services in primary care, underpinned by a new relationship between health care professionals and patients/clients though the promotion of supported self-care management. Accompanying this philosophy of care is the recognition that many patients present with complex conditions, arising from co-morbidity (DH 2008c). According to Labour Government (Brown 2008), the NHS of the future:

> 'will do more than just care for and treat patients who are ill – it will be an NHS offering prevention. It will not be the NHS of the passive patient – the NHS of the future will be one of patient power, patients engaged and taking greater control over their own health and their healthcare too.'

Among the key reforms resulting from Professor Ara Darzi's fundamental review for NHS are (DH 2008a, pp. 9–14):

- 'The creation of an NHS that "helps people to stay healthy"
- PCT requirements to commission comprehensive wellbeing and prevention services, in partnership with local authorities, with the services offered personalised to meet the specific needs of their local populations
- A coalition for Better Health, with a set of new voluntary agreements between the Government, private and third sector organisations on actions to improve health outcomes
- Support for people to stay healthy at work

- Support for GPs [general practitioners] to help individuals and their families stay healthy
- Extended choice of GP practice
- Piloting of personal health budgets
- Care plans to ensure that everyone with a long-term condition has a personalised care plan
- Introduction of a new right to choice in the first NHS Constitution
- Guaranteed patient access to the most clinically and cost effective drugs and treatments
- Measures to ensure continuous improvement in the quality of primary and community care
- The creation of new partnerships between the NHS, universities and industry
- The provision of strengthened arrangements to ensure staff have consistent and equitable opportunities to update and develop their skills'

The new health service reforms have been underpinned by greater investment in hospital building programmes and in target/standard setting accompanied by matching increased diversity of supply with an ability to respond to the new diversity of demand in preventive and curative medicine–tackling the underlying causes of health inequalities as well as providing the best care. Decreased tolerance of failing services will also be a core component of the government's strategic health care plan. A new quality commission will therefore be introduced with tougher powers to impose fines and close down services in the case of poor standards. Foundation hospitals will also be able to take over failing hospitals to turn around their performance and in the case of primary care, there will be greater diversity of supply and strengthening of the power of PCT commissioners to ensure that GP or community health care services can be improved or replaced where they fail to respond to local patient/user demand.

Major advances in technology and bioengineering have also brought about significant changes in treatment patterns and modes of delivery. For example with cutting-edge techniques – ranging from genetics to stem cell therapy – and life-saving drugs to prevent, alleviate or cure conditions such as Alzheimer's disease, it is likely that many of today's diseases will succumb to either eradication or amelioration. Investment in the implementation of world-class research programmes will accompany the government's health care investment plan and new academic health science centres will be sponsored for implementation within our most prestigious foundation trusts and their partner universities. These will facilitate the discovery of new technologies, which, in turn, will enable clinicians the ability to diagnose and intervene at the earliest possible opportunity.

Similarly new alliances will be developed with our emergency care services (e.g. the Ambulance Service) to equip paramedical staff with the requisite skills to treat people experiencing a heart attack with life-saving drugs in their own homes or to provide emergency interventions for longer-term conditions outwith hospital specialist treatment units. For others, attendance at specialist treatment centres will become the norm. One such example if of stroke patients who now receive immediate treatment with the latest anticoagulant drugs in specialist stroke centres, thus extending their lives and enabling many people to lead an independent life. Other patients will benefit from attendance at new trauma centres.

There will also be improvements in the way in which the 15 million people in England who present with longer-term diseases, such as asthma, heart failure, diabetes or psychosocial challenges. The people who care for these service users – the 'carers', also require additional support and 'seamless' access to services. In some cases personal budgets and direct payments will be made available to enable individuals and their families to purchase responsive care packages directly. The use of personal health and social care budgets will underpin reforms of our social care system.

Many of the people who will benefit most from new care packages will present with 'lifestyle'-related diseases such as diabetes, cardiovascular disease, stroke and some cancers. In order to combat the rising trend in such conditions, the health service will work in close partnership with patients and carers to co-design and co-deliver effective preventive and direct treatment services, aimed at encouraging the population to take their own health 'seriously'. In order to achieve this objective more patients will become engaged with their care by managing their own conditions, taking advantage of support offered by GPs and nurses in their home or on the high street, and by exercising more control over their life and care. Greater emphasis on what we eat, and participation in sports and leisure activities, will also be encouraged – presenting a significant challenge for the way in which primary care nurses discharge their role and responsibilities.

There will also be opportunities for the provision of extended screening services, for example for colon cancer and for breast cancer. An increasing number of patients will also access NHS direct, the internet and digital television to improve their access to evidence-based information about their health. Others, through the use of personalised budgets, will take control of their care packages and manage their care plan directly, rather than having to rely on others. By so doing, a greater range of patients will become increasingly empowered, giving them a greater say in their care, particularly in the later years of their lives.

Such fundamental changes in health care policy and process will require primary services to adopt new flexible and responsive approaches and to develop new partnerships with the voluntary and private sectors where they can contribute and innovate. Greater synergy will also be required between acute and primary care, and between health and social care. New and dynamic approaches to PCT commissioning will be needed to deliver such changes, focusing on patient choice, direct payments (DH 2007, 2008c), quality provision and market contestability.

The enactment of this policy has reduced patient/client dependency on inpatient or long-stay residential care in favour of seeking the development of a range of options based on local need, which will be flexible enough to meet the demands of service provision required by local people in their neighbourhoods. Clinicians are therefore encouraged to work in close partnership with their patients and clients with the aim of making them more accountable for their practice and interventions.

At a strategic level the NHS now requires all strategic health authorities to secure significant improvements in the way in which services are delivered to the population, emphasising the promotion of positive health and the promotion of high-quality care in the community. In order to provide these services, strategic health authorities must demonstrate that providers offer/commission a range of services for their clients and families as equal participants, whenever decisions that will affect their lives are involved. Such principles now underpin the NHS philosophy and form the basis of the government's 'reformed' health and social care strategy.

NHS providers must also determine the role that they are going to play, with local authority social service departments, in making their contribution to a range of comprehensive service developments for clients. The Health Act 1999 also demands that planning agreements should be reached between health and social service departments that identify clearly which services will be provided by each agency and which identify the processes to be adopted in assessing the needs of individuals in their care. The principle of effective alliance building between the NHS and social services has been further clarified by the role of workforce development directorates located within strategic health authorities in England. Such directorates outline requirements for health and social care services to work together to encourage the joint design, training and education of staff from both agencies in order to provide a workforce with the necessary capacity, skills and diversity to meet the needs of the local population. Alliance building is crucial if user needs are to be met within the context of an increasingly pluralistic health and social care economy, characterised by self-care and user choice and involvement.

The principles outlined in this chapter also require each government department to demonstrate emphasis on public health as a central concept within their business plan – a cornerstone of 'joined up government'. For the health service, charged with responsibility to enact national service frameworks and to produce integrated health improvement plans for local communities, a fundamental review is required to assess local public health capacity and capability, across sector boundaries.

In the future emphasis must also be placed on the promotion of health and alliance building between professionals and users of services. The focus of care is clearly placed within the community with an expectation that resources will be deployed to meet identified health and social care needs through the provision of integrated, peripatetic support from a range of professionals who will include doctors, community health care nurses, community specialist public health nurses, social workers, clinical psychologists, physiotherapists, speech therapists, radiographers and occupational therapists (supported by an efficient and appropriately funded intermediate/acute sector, inpatient service) (DH 2008d). The acute sector will complement the work of local primary health care workers who will continue to provide the first point of contact for clients and their families through the provision of effective intermediate and ambulatory treatment/assessment services. In turn, such services will be supported by the implementation of primary care-led emergency care walk-in centres, polyclinics and diagnostic and treatment centres, thus providing a range of 'seamless' assessment, diagnostic and treatment services for their local communities.

The next decade will therefore be characterised by the development of highly focused primary care services that will respond to the needs of local practice populations. In this model, much of the activity currently carried out by the local acute hospital will be transferred to general local primary services, some of them managed directly by local PCTs, others provided by independent or voluntary sector agencies. New polyclinics (DH 2007b) will also be introduced to provide an integrated, eclectic range of health and social care services, including diagnostic treatment services for the local population. Such local services will increasingly undertake minor and invasive surgery, routine diagnostic testing,

support for cases requiring observation and most outpatient activity. Centralised or specialist hospital facilities will continue to deal with severely ill people with complex therapeutic needs and provide for major surgery. Older people and those with mental health needs or learning disabilities will also continue to be cared for (almost exclusively) in community care settings.

From a practical perspective the way in which primary care services will be delivered in the future will be determined from both national and local demand perspectives. Nationally key priorities are been determined annually by the DH and outlined in an operating framework document (see for example, the DH's operating framework for the NHS in England for 2008/2009 (DH 2008b). Examples of key operating targets include:

- Listening and responding to patients, the public and staff and improving patient outcomes and experience
- Moving towards local targets while delivering on national priorities
- Developing world-class commissioning as a key agent for change
- Sustaining a financial regime that supports service reform goals incentivises service improvement
- An emphasis on partnership working between PCTs, local authorities and other partners to ensure local health needs are better understood and addressed

Other priorities include the need for PCTs to:

- Empower patients, clients and carers and ensure more choice in service selection and treatment response; elicit objective feedback on 'the patient experience' and respond accordingly
- Tackle lifestyle issues, such as obesity and alcohol misuse
- Close the gap in life expectancy between affluent and deprived areas of the population
- Work closely with local authorities to provide integrated and co-located services, including joint commissioning

- Redesign and implement care pathways that respond effectively to patient and service demand to support patients with longer-term conditions
- Reduce the rate of hospital acquired infection
- Management, leadership and clinical excellence in the workforce to enhance both capacity and capability
- Put in place and lead local information and management, and technology plans

A range of enabling strategies will also be put in place to support the implementation of these delivery plans including the empowerment of patients, the provision of choice, world-class commissioning capability and investment in workforce development, estate developments/ hospital building programmes, leadership, education and training. Alongside these 'enablers' will be further investment in the development of more effective and responsive systems, information management and provider functions within the NHS (DH 2008a).

There is little doubt that the introduction of these new service delivery imperatives will provide the primary care nursing profession with a range of major challenges that must be addressed if the balance of care is to shift, according to government policy, to the community. One specific question must relate to the future education and training that will be required to equip practitioners with the necessary skills, knowledge and value base to be able to function effectively in the community. In reality, there is also likely to be a reallocation of tasks between nurses and others, including informal carers and other professionals (many of whom work currently in acute hospital settings and who will be required to transfer into new primary care settings as the context of care changes). Primary care nurses must therefore be prepared to develop and change, drawing on the very best of their past experience and becoming increasingly reliant on the production of research evidence to inform their future practice.

This section has proposed that the most effective way to meet the health needs of the local population is to focus primary health care services within the very heart of naturally occurring communities

and neighbourhoods. In so doing (using the general practice population of the focus and locus for care) opportunities for the further improvement of multi-disciplinary teamwork and improved communication systems with clients (and others) will be provided. In order to transact effective care, the potential role that primary care nurses can undertake to fulfil the new NHS mandate must be acknowledged.

The impact of primary care policy changes on the role of the primary care nurse

In 2002, the DH published a major document entitled *Liberating the Talents*, which confirmed the role that primary care nurses are expected to play within the context of the, then 'modernised' health care service:

> 'Nurses, midwives and health visitors are the largest group of professionals involved and will therefore have a significant impact on patient-led and community centred services. Like any profession their role cannot be described in isolation, and as the environment becomes more complex and uncertain, they will rely increasingly on a combination of developing their core skills (both general and specialist) and membership of multidisciplinary teams and networks. Their key attribute will be their ability to fit their skills with a wide range of others in a way that best meets the needs of the individual patient or group. They will play to the strengths of their professional role in integrating the medical and social aspects of health care, promoting self-care and crossing organisational boundaries to maximize continuity of patient care and health improvement.'

(Preface)

The essence of this statement has not changed. However, the policy drivers outlined in this chapter will have significant impact on the status of the primary care nurse as the 'lynchpin' within the context of a multi-disciplinary team of specialist health care practitioners. Their work has also been directed by the advent of consumerism that has placed new demands for new competencies among the workforce with an emphasis on therapeutic skills, case management (this concept will be discussed later in this text), prescribing, clinical leadership and social enterprise skills. Further endorsement of the significance of the role that community and primary care nurses and health visitors will play within the reformed health services has been provided by the DH in the *Next Stage Review* of the NHS:

'Community nurses, health visitors, allied health professionals and other staff working in our community health services are central to our vision for the future of primary and community care. The staff who work in these services speak with passion about the potential for using their professional skills to transform services. A dual focus on personal health care and community health lies at the heart of community services and underlies their key position in delivering high quality services and improving health outcomes.'

(DH 2008d, p. 4)

In summary, this will require that community and primary care nurses must be able to respond to the health needs, health gain requirements and expressed demands of their clients and local population groups so as to:

- Stimulate healthy lifestyles and self-care opportunities
- Design and deliver cost-effective and evidence-based treatment and care responses (including efficient and effective prescribing practice)
- Further educate families, informal carers, the community and other care workers
- Solve or assist in the solution of both individual and community health problems
- Orient their own as well as community efforts for health promotion and for the prevention of diseases, unnecessary suffering, disability and death
- Lead, work within, and with inter-professional teams, and participate in the development and leadership of such teams

- Participate in the enhancement and delivery of primary health care in a multi-disciplinary care context
- Co-design and co-deliver innovative and responsive packages of care in partnership with service users and their carers (particularly in the effective management of longer-term conditions)
- Contribute to the effective commissioning of new services that are designed to meet the needs of the local population
- Create the requisite conditions to provide entrepreneurial services that respond to the actual needs of local service users and commissioners

Finally, in this section, the importance of public health is emphasised. (Nursing and Midwifery Council [NMC] 2004, p. 1). While it is postulated that public health is a key role for all primary health care nurses, it is of course a fundamental role for specialist community public health nurses. Such practitioners are normally engaged in:

- Monitoring and profiling the health of their community/practice area
- Ensuring that public health issues are identified and reported to managers and commissioners
- Monitoring health outcomes of their interventions
- Improving the effectiveness of their activities
- Developing local health strategies and building healthy alliances necessary to implement these
- Developing and maintaining partnerships with clients, informal carers, other community members, and other professionals
- Collaborating with local authorities and other agencies to monitor and control health-related issues considered to be hazardous to the well-being of the community
- Informing the public about public health issues; engaging in health promotion programmes
- Ensuring that members of the community have access to appropriate public health advice

The scope of primary care nursing practice within the context of a changing workforce

One key enabler of the proposed health care reforms will be the workforce and its ability to prepare itself for the new world of work, characterised by inter-professional teamwork and inter-sectoral care practice that follows the 'patient experience' (e.g. transitional care provision between the acute and primary care sectors). Flexible and adaptable career (and associated educational) pathways will be needed to support the new workforce once they are registered (DH 2006). One key example relates to the need to provide flexible career progression opportunities to enable nurses and allied health professional staff to move seamlessly between acute and primary care service settings and to reduce dependency on the actual care setting itself. Flexibility will also be needed to encourage staff to move between employers and between the health care, social care and voluntary/independent care sectors.

Current government policy provides considerable opportunities for the development of innovative care solutions within which nurses, often in partnership with social workers and other support staff, will be able to provide responsive services to clients in response to their identified needs. As agency boundaries break down between primary, intermediate, secondary and tertiary care sectors, and professional skills transcend previously defended frontiers, service users will have freer access to nursing skills. The way in which access is negotiated for nursing skills will, in the future, be through single case assessment and case management or contractual processes, which should make nursing skills more easily accessible to the general practice population. Their understanding (often acquired from many years of experience and proven competence in the delivery of care to their clients) has placed primary care nurses (and those acute sector nurses who are intending to transfer to the community) in an ideal position within the 'reformed' NHS to respond more flexibly to locally identified health and social care-related needs.

These principles were set down earlier by the Department of Health in a consultation paper entitled *A Health Service of All the Talents: Developing the NHS Workforce* (DH 2000b). The paper noted the need for 'transformation' within the NHS workforce in order to ensure that it was 'fit for purpose' in delivering the proposed health care agenda. The paper confirmed that emphasis should be placed on:

- Team working across professional and organisational boundaries
- Flexible working to make best use of the range of skills and knowledge that staff possess
- Streamlined workforce planning and development which stems from the needs of patients, not professionals
- Maximising the contribution of all staff to patient care, doing away with barriers that say only doctors or nurses can provide particular types of care
- Modernising education and training to ensure staff are equipped with the skills they need to work in a complex, changing NHS
- Developing new, more flexible, careers for staff of all professions and grades
- Expanding the workforce to meet future demands

These principles continue to remain relevant as we reach the end of the current decade. However, the consequence of such proposals for many primary care nurses has required them to engage in lifelong learning with the aim of continuously seeking to enhance their skills and knowledge in accordance with evidence-based practice for the benefit of their clients and patients. In addition, new flexible roles and responsibilities will demand that primary care nurses seek to validate their skills and practices through the process of peer review and to share learning/education with other professionals. Increased emphasis will also be placed on competence-based education and in the acquisition of enhanced skills in clinical leadership and commissioning.

In order to respond to the demands of the new flexible workforce, primary care services will need to create, implement, share and explore key issues in relation to the local distribution, sustainability and transferability of innovative 'new role' solutions in primary and intermediate care in order to inform the competencies, practice, education and learning requirements of such new roles (DH 2008d). This will include:

- Agreeing actions arising from local and national discussion relating to the key practice, education/training and regulation issues that need to be addressed to enable sustainability, and spread of new 'fit for purpose' primary care practitioners whose roles are designed to meet the demands of evolving and complex inter-professional health and social care work streams.
- Ensuring that universities and their associated partner trusts/social service departments, engage in the design and implementation of new education programmes that are informed by the standards of practice that will be identified through the national changing workforce programmes and other 'modernisation' imperatives.
- Agreeing a framework for the development of competencies and associated regulation for new emergent roles in order to maximise opportunities for new ways of working within the NHS career framework.
- Undertaking operational research and evaluation that is designed to measure the effectiveness and impact of such new roles and competencies.

If these aims are to be achieved then there is a need to ensure that the primary, social and intermediate care workforce is not developed in isolation, but set within the context of national and local workforce requirements, supported by education frameworks developed in partnership with local practitioners. A new workforce will also need to be prepared to meet the diverse needs of the new emergent polyclinics, underpinned by a new cadre of advanced practitioners (NMC 2007), who will be able to assess, diagnose, treat patients and prescribe. Additionally new associate, or assistant practitioner, roles will emerge to enhance the skill base of the support worker workforce. Such 'new ways of working' have highlighted the challenges that the introduction of new roles present to employees, employers, regulators and educationalists. One key lesson learned to date is that new roles must be well defined and underpinned by competence-based role descriptions, accompanied by customised educational programmes and supervisory arrangements. The programmes of education that will be required to support the emergent primary care workforce should reflect/include:

- Diversity to provide flexible entry and progression points for new roles
- Co-designing and co-delivering programmes in partnership with users and carers.
- Career/competence development within the context of *Agenda for Change* (DH 2003a), and competence mapping against the NHS *Knowledge and Skills Framework*
- Design and delivery of comprehensive educational packages to ensure coherent implementation of changing workforce requirements, e.g. The provision of professional development programmes for nurses undertaking specialist roles such as public health, heart failure/chronic obstructive pulmonary disease, reducing readmission, commissioning, social enterprise, case management, clinical leadership, etc.
- Development of key leadership skills in primary care-led services
- Embedding and mainstreaming new roles and new ways of working for a range of practitioners from assistant to advanced practitioners
- Designing innovative work-based practice assessment methods to ensure staff are 'fit for purpose' and safe and effective practitioners (thereby affording public protection)
- Design of e-based virtual learning environments/distance learning through the use of innovative learning and teaching methodologies
- Development of shared learning with GPs, social workers and other members of the health care team (including intermediate care professionals)

- Determining, 'piloting' and evaluating a range of new competencies for such new roles
- Development and implementation of a defined 'role map' for a new inter-professional and multi-agency workforce
- Ensuring that the introduction of these new roles is underpinned by short-, medium- and long-term strategic plans in order to ensure flexibility, transferability and sustainability, and to encourage recruitment and retention of staff working in these new evolving roles
- Recognition of key policy drivers impacting on service provision (particularly in relation to the management of longer-term conditions, integrated case assessment, care/case management, unscheduled emergency care/ out of hours provision and specialist care provision), which require expediency in the introduction of these roles
- Ensuring that local PCT delivery plans facilitate the ability to change workforce profiles; current and future workforce profiles should focus on matching local need with national policy
- Provision of flexible commissioning arrangements for education programmes in and across strategic health/social care economies
- Supporting effective educational provision through the creation of 'fit for purpose' learning/knowledge transfer environments in primary care service settings
- Celebrating, recognising and disseminating excellence in service design and delivery

In addition proficient primary care practitioners will need to ensure the following.

- They provide essential services to their local communities. These services are needed by a range of care groups with differing needs delivered in a variety of settings. Whatever the title, employer or setting, there are, among others, core functions that staff will need to provide: first contact, expert continuing care and the delivery of effective prevention/ public health programmes.
- Their services are based on robust assessment of needs of individuals and populations and the skills required to meet those needs. These functions should be provided across all age and social groups according to need and designed around the journey that the patient/ client takes. In order to safeguard vulnerable people the local population requires high-quality generalist as well as specialist service responses.
- Patients, clients, carers and communities are involved actively in service changes and provided with greater choice – services will therefore need to respond to the people who use and fund them.
- A significant number of primary care practitioners are supported to assume advanced and specialist roles across a range of core functions, but in particular to:
  — Improve access to general practice services, as the role of nurses in assessing and managing conditions (previously seen to be the remit of GPs) is increasingly recognised
  — Provide more secondary care in the community (including care of people with longer-term conditions, ambulatory and palliative care needs)
  — Lead and deliver priority public health interventions
  — Acquire and apply expert skills in clinical leadership, informed by a thorough understanding of service commissioning.
- They engage in partnership with the wider health and social care team. As such there will be more generic working with practitioners working across settings, providing a wider range of care to individuals, families and communities. Support workers and qualified staff will become more integrated within the primary/social care workforce.
- They will be more understanding of the commonality of roles across health and social care and hospitals and primary/community care, with more joint posts and less anxiety about protecting professional roles when responding to patient and community needs.
- Frontline practitioners have greater freedom to innovate and make decisions about

services and the care that they provide. This will need to be matched with greater accountability for individual professional judgement and the use of best available evidence to inform their practice.

- Effective leadership is evidenced if our services are to take on new roles, work differently and deliver the NHS plan improvements for patients, clients and communities. This will demand greater understanding of team development and the management capability to use human and financial resources creatively and to assess and manage risks accordingly within the parameters of 'safe practice'.

The workforce of the future will also prepare and deploy a range of competent assistant practitioners who will work in direct support of the professionally qualified primary care team. New roles are now emerging to support assistant practitioners to acquire a range of competencies that have been designed to enable them to respond to the needs of the local health/social care economy. Such roles interface with the development and implementation of new foundation degree programmes, informed by key health and social care imperatives including *Agenda for Change* (DH 2003a), and the *Knowledge and Skills Framework* (DH 2003b), and new emergent educational models supported and endorsed by the NHS.

As the scope of primary health care widens, opportunities for appropriately skilled and experienced primary care nurses to develop as advanced practitioners and nurse consultants will be provided. The challenge for the nurses themselves must be for them to articulate their skills, advance their practice (underpinned by evidence-based enquiry skills) and to market their contribution effectively to both their clients/patients and to commissioners of health/social care services.

New practice developments must therefore emerge to fulfil patient and provider agency expectations as increasingly complex care packages are transferred from the acute hospital sector to primary health care services and their associated provider services (DH 2008c). In order to ensure that nurses provide effective care to their clients, practitioners must ensure that they are effectively supervised in all areas of their practice and 'keep in touch' with the aims and objectives of their clients and senior managers. There are many ways to achieve this objective but perhaps the most successful has been the provision of clinical supervision and positive feedback from line managers. Clinical supervision has been recommended in various forms by the NMC for all of its nurses with the aim of providing staff with a framework within which to receive positive feedback on their performance and to share their own perceptions of how effective they consider their contribution to client care to be (NMC 2008).

The main professional challenges for primary care nurses may be summarised as the need to:

- Maintain and develop specialist/advanced diagnostic, clinical/therapeutic skills and competence
- Expand their knowledge and skills and to act on research-based best evidence to enhance their practice
- Recognise and accept personal accountability for nursing actions
- Pursue continuing professional education to enhance competence and patient safety
- Market skills to an increasingly diverse range of health and social care commissioners
- Promote public health/protection and assist in the development and maintenance of 'healthy communities'
- Engage in effective clinical supervision
- Exercise strategic leadership skills
- Constantly evaluate personal and collective performance

International influences on the health care agenda

The organisation of health care delivery and nursing activity in the UK is also influenced by a number of international agreements and agendas that are negotiated within the World Health Organization (WHO) and within the European Community (EC).

For example, the public health chapter of the EC Treaty of Economic Union (*European Parliament Committee Report on the Environment* [The Maastricht Treaty] 1993), requires all European countries to contribute to the promotion of health awareness and health protection by encouraging the design and implementation of local health initiatives and community health programmes. Such activities are directed towards action that prevents the incidence of major diseases, including drug dependence, by promoting research into their causes and means of transmission, as well as health information and education. Health has also been afforded enhanced status as a standing item on the European Parliament agenda in Brussels. Article 153 of the Treaty of Amsterdam 1999, commits the EU to achieving 'a high level of human health protection'.

European influences also regulate the movement of nurses between member states; systems and directives have also been agreed to enable European countries to ascribe mutual recognition to their pre-qualifying systems of nurse education. These systems have been designed to facilitate mutual harmonisation and recognition between countries in the EC and provide a shared framework for the preparation of nurse specialists throughout the region.

Within the wider context, the WHO also sets targets for health gain and health promotion. For example, in 1987, WHO published targets with the aim of improving the quality of health care delivery and surveillance for all world citizens. These targets have assisted in shaping the health care agenda in the UK and have facilitated the introduction of common standards for primary health services throughout the world. Other policy matters relate to the design of global health and nursing strategies based on the following principles:

- Equity – thus reducing the existence of inequalities between countries and within countries
- Health promotion – providing for the development of personal self-reliance and the acquisition of a positive sense of health

- Participation – requiring the active participation of world citizens in informing themselves (and others) about health matters
- Multi-sectoral cooperation – promoting international agreements on health targets, polices and strategies
- Primary health care – focusing attention on the importance of primary care delivery as the health care system closest to where clients live and work
- International cooperation – recognising that health problems cross international frontiers, e.g. pollution

Conclusion

This chapter has proposed that the 'reformed' health service requires a workforce that is both fit for practice and fit for purpose, equipped with competencies that will enable practitioners to function across a range of priority, interprofessional care pathways both within hospital and within primary care settings (including new polyclinics). In designing the new workforce we should be cognisant of the demand placed by service commissioners and providers to ensure flexibility within the workforce to accommodate to emergent needs in the population (DH 2008c,d).

The chapter has recognised that the demand for health care, influenced by changes in disease pattern and treatment response will evolve, based primarily on the co-delivery of health care in partnership between users, carers and clinicians. The NHS 'choice' agenda with emphasis being placed on home-based care in the community, has been a key driver for the government's vision of primary care services, which has been characterised with concepts relating to new sources of patient engagement, care packages for treatment and access arrangements to a multiplicity of care providers.

The reformed health agenda in England has been further influenced by the government's commissioned review of health care provision undertaken by Professor Lord Ara Darzi (DH 2008a,c,d). In his final report, *High Quality Care for All: NHS Next Stage Review*, a new vision for an empowered workforce, equipped with requisite skills and competencies is outlined. Key tenets for health care reform and new models of care delivery are expounded, impacting specifically within the community and its associated primary and social care services.

On the supply side we have noted the emergence of an increasingly diverse range of providers, including the role of the voluntary or 'third sector' and reliance on the commercial sector to provide substantial elements of diagnostic and treatment provision in the UK. Information technology has also made significant advances, which, in the next five years, will impact even further on patient care outcomes and service delivery. This will empower and inform patients and enable them to engage more effectively in judging health care performance and in assuming responsibility for personalised health care.

The importance of providing a competent workforce that is prepared to confront challenges relating to inequalities in health and social care treatment responses are also understood, as are the significant requirements for adherence to professional regulatory standards. Standards of proficiency, the enhancement of clinical skill competence and leadership, and the acquisition of clinical judgement skills in decision-making and care planning have also been identified as key drivers for change in care practice.

The key policy directives that have shaped our reformed health service in recent years have been derived from *The NHS Plan* of 2000, which has been updated significantly on an annual basis by our government health departments. For example, greater recognition has been given to supporting people with longer-term conditions, which was outlined in the DH health document (2005): *Supporting People with Long Term Conditions – Liberating the Talents for Nurses Who Care for People with Long Term Conditions*. Similarly this text has taken full account of emergent themes and trends from the DH's announcement (2006a) on modernising nursing careers (www.dh.gov.uk/cno).

More fundamental changes were envisaged by the DH in its 2006 publication *Our Health, Our Care, Our Say: A New Direction for Community Services*. These values have been analysed and embedded throughout the text.

More specifically, the Chief Nursing Officer's review of mental health nursing (2006c) and Ruth Northway's review of future directions for learning disability nursing (Northway *et al.* 2006) have been used to inform relevant chapters in this new edition. Nurses continue to be central to government plans as identified in DH's (2006a) *Modernising Nursing Careers*. For example, nurses play key roles in establishing new models of primary care and social enterprise and are integral to developing care pathways as part of the multi-disciplinary team. Following the successful implementation of national service frameworks, programmes of care policy have progressed to produce national competence standards identified by Skills for Health, which in turn inform educational curricula for primary care practitioners.

In summary the health service has engaged in a period of self-reflection and re-examination of personal and public values, thus reinforcing the need for clients to assume personal responsibility for their own social and health care needs. The reduction in dependency on inpatient care in our hospitals has assisted in the transfer of care to the community and to our naturally occurring neighbourhood support systems. Care in the community and investment in public health/primary care strategies will become an increasing feature of our health care philosophy and, in partnership with a rationalised (and smaller) acute sector, will provide the context for our health care system for the foreseeable future.

The significant role that the primary care trusts, strategic health authorities and social service departments play, further reinforces the government's commitment to primary care and the transformation of services. Lord Darzi in his vision for primary and community care, for example, advised that:

> 'Community services are in a central position to delivery the Next Stage Review of the NHS, and of critical importance in delivering our vision for the future of primary and community care... Increased influence for community staff in service transformation, through a commitment

to multi-professional engagement in practice based commissioning and the piloting of more integrated clinical collaborations.'

(DH 2008d, p. 1)

If this vision is to be achieved than the importance of leadership for primary care nursing must be acknowledged and responsive systems put in place to facilitate the emergence of innovative practice in local practice settings. Nurses must also continue to advocate for their clients, families and communities and engage in raising health-related issues for inclusion in local and government policy agendas. Above all they must demonstrate confidence and competence to assess risks and to practise safely in accordance with their professional code of practice (NMC 2008). Our primary care practitioners need to be prepared to respond to an increasingly well-informed public that is keen to have a bigger say in their care and treatment. The overall thrust of this new edition has been to re-focus and reform our understanding of primary care practice within the context of a rapidly evolving health service.

References

Department of Health (2000a) *The NHS Plan: A Plan for Investment, a Plan for Reform.* Department of Health, London.

Department of Health (2000b) *A Health Service of All the Talents: Developing the NHS Workforce.* Department of Health, London.

Department of Health (2002) *Liberating the Talents – Helping Primary Care Trusts and Nurses to Deliver the NHS Plan.* Department of Health, London.

Department of Health (2003a) *Agenda for Change – Modernising the NHS Pay System.* Department of Health, London.

Department of Health (2003b) *The Knowledge and Skills Framework.* Department of Health, London.

Department of Health (2005) *Supporting People with Long Term Conditions. Liberating the Talents of Nurses Who Care for People with Long Term Conditions.* Department of Health, London.

Department of Health (2006a) *Modernising Nursing Careers – Setting the Direction* Department of Health, London. Available at: www.dh.gov.uk/cno (accessed 20 Nov 2008).

Department of Health (2006b) *Our Health, Our Care, Our Say: A New Direction for Community Services.* Department of Health, London.

Department of Health (2006c) *From Values to Action: The Chief Nursing Officer's Review of Mental Health Nursing.* Gateway reference: 6140. Department of Health, London.

Department of Health (2007) *Our NHS Our Future: NHS Next Stage Review – Interim Report.* Lord Ara Darzi. Available at: www.dh.gov.uk/en/Publicationsandstatistics/Publications/PublicationsPolicyAndGuidance/dh_079077 (accessed 20 Nov 2008).

Department of Health (2008a) *High Quality Care For All: NHS Next Stage Review.* Final Report – Lord Ara Darzi, July, Cm7432. DH, London.

Department of Health (2008b) *The NHS in England: The Operating Framework for 2008/2009.* DH, London.

Department of Health (2008c) *NHS Next Stage Review: Our Vision for Primary and Community Care.* Gateway reference 10096. The Stationary Office, London.

Department of Health (2008d) *NHS Next Stage Review: Our Vision for Primary and Community Care: What it Means for Nurses, Midwives, Health Visitors and AHPs.* Gateway reference 10096. The Stationary Office, London.

Department of Health (2008e) *Direct Payments.* Gateway Reference: 9337. LAC (DH) 20081. Department of Health, London.

European Parliament Committee on the Environment, Public Health and Consumer Protection (1993) *Draft Report on Public Health Policy After Maastricht.* PE 205.804 Or, EN. European Parliament, Brussels.

European Parliament (1999) *Treaty of Amsterdam, Article 153,* Brussels.

Mathers, C. & Loncar, D. (2006) Projections of global mortality and burden of disease from 2002–2030. *PLoS Medicine,* **3**, 2011–2030.

NHS London (2007) *Healthcare for London: A Framework for Action.* Chair, Lord, Professor Ara Drazi, London.

Northway, R., Hutchinson, C. & Kingdon, A. (2006) *Shaping the Future: A Vision for Learning Disability Nursing.* UK Learning Disability Consultant Nurse Network, UK.

Nursing and Midwifery Council (2004) *Standards for Specialist Community Public Health Nursing,* (C/04/57). NMC, London.

Nursing and Midwifery Council (2007) *Advanced Nursing Practice,* update 19 June 2007. Available at: www.nmc-uk.org (accessed 20 Nov 2008).

Nursing and Midwifery Council (2008) *The Code – Standards of Conduct, Performance, and Ethics for Nurses and Midwives.* NMC, London.

Office for National Statistics (2007). Available at: www.statistics.gov.uk/cci/nugget.asp?id=1352 (accessed 20 Nov 2008).

The NHS and Community Care Act 1990. HMSO, London.

The Health Act 1999. HMSO, London.

Prime Minister's Office (2008) *Gordon Brown Sets Out Vision for The NHS*. Prime Minister's speech delivered on Monday, 7 January 2008 on the 60th Anniversary of the NHS at King's College, London.

Sang, B. (2005) *Fixing the Broken Triangle: Improving Patient and Public Involvement in Clinical Governance, Locally and Nationally*. In: Lugon, J. & Secker-Walker, P. (eds) *Clinical Governance in a Changing NHS*. RSM Press, London.

Standing Committee of Nurses of the EU (1994) *Public Health After Maastricht*. European Parliament, Brussels.

World Health Organization (1987) *Health for All. Declaration of WHO Conference on Primary Health Care*. Alma Ata, Geneva.

Chapter 2 **Social Policy**

Linda Burke, Jane Lopez and Elizabeth Treadwell

Introduction

The past 20 years have seen unprecedented change in health and social care policy, all of which has had an impact on community nurses. Not least of these changes has been the radical shift towards a primary care-led NHS. In the past, it appeared as if community nurses had been largely overlooked by policy makers (Walsh & Gough 2000), but with the election of the Labour Government in 1997, this all changed. It was emphatically stated by the Labour Government that nurses would be guaranteed a seat at the decision-making table. Successive policy documents (Department of Health [DH] 1997, 1998, 1999, 2000, 2004a, 2005b, 2006a,b, 2007a) have reinforced the message that nurses, midwives, health visitors and specialist community public health nurses have a crucial role in carrying out the government's plans for a new NHS.

Undoubtedly nurses can make a unique and valuable contribution to policy development because of their knowledge and experience of working so closely with patients. However, whether nurses will make the most of this opportunity remains to be seen. Historically, nurses have been absent from the policy-making arena (Maslin-Prothero & Masterson 1998) for reasons which may be related to the nursing profession's relatively low position of power in the hierarchy of health and social care organisations (Robinson J. 1992). Hennessy (2000) asserts that it is also partly because nurses themselves have not taken responsibility for having a role within policy-making, probably because they do not believe they have enough knowledge of the policy process.

It is essential that nurses learn about and develop understanding of social policy because the health of the patients and clients they interact with is affected by the many polices that are implemented in health and also in areas such as housing, employment, education, taxation, social security and the environment. Furthermore, it is only by having knowledge of policy that nurses will be able to influence and take on a more active role in policy-making and implementation.

The aim of this chapter is to provide community nurses with a broad understanding of the key developments in policy that have occurred within the health care sector. The chapter will concentrate on:

- The policy-making and implementation process
- Health care before 1948 and the evolution of the National Health Service (NHS)
- Health policy under the Conservative Government from 1979 to 1997
- Current and future health care policy under the Labour Government

This chapter focuses particularly on health policy because it has the most immediate relevance for community nursing. However, it is important to recognise that other areas of social policy also have a considerable impact on the health and well-being of clients.

The policy-making and implementation process

What is policy?

There are many different views about what constitutes a policy. Guba (1984) asserts that all policies fall into one or more of the following categories:

- Assertion of goals
- Standing decisions of a governing body
- Central guide to action
- Strategies to solve a problem
- Behaviours that have been sanctioned by a formal decision
- Norms of conduct
- Outputs of the policy-making system

There are two broad types of policy – universal and selective. Universal policies provide services or resources to everyone within a broad category, whereas selective policies focus on a clearly defined group (Gormley 1999). Universal policies can be seen to be more wasteful of resources but are more equitable, that is they attempt to provide an equal resource or service to everybody, whereas selective policies are based on the principle of equity, which means they target money at those perceived to be in the most need.

Social policies are generally considered as policies which provide a guide to organising the nation's resources for the perceived benefit of society. For example, Hennessy (2000) describes health policies as courses of action that are advantageous or expedient within the resources available to maintain or improve health. However, it is important to appreciate that just because something is labelled as social policy does not mean that it is necessarily beneficial for all of those on the receiving end. Policies are made within the prevailing ideological context of the government of the time which means they will reflect a particular view about what constitutes a good society and who is the most deserving of help (Titmus 1979).

Policies almost always suggest a course of action (Owen & Rogers 1999) but rarely prescribe what that action should be. Therefore, while policy includes the explicit decisions made by governments and their advisers, it also refers to the decisions and non-decisions made by managers and professionals, including nurses (Green & Thorogood 1998). This means that community nurses can play a significant part in shaping policy at all levels of health and social care organisations.

Who makes policy?

In order to set policy, groups manoeuvre to wield power, influence and control over each other. Such power is never equally shared and varies in each area of policy.

There are different theories of the distribution of power within society. They include pluralism, elitism, marxism and corporate theorism. Pluralists believe power is widely and equally distributed among different interest groups that organise themselves around an issue, with the state acting as a referee in the bargaining process. Elitists assert that power is disproportionately concentrated in the hands of a limited number of functional or occupational elite groups that acquire their power through control of economic resources. Marxists' fundamental beliefs are based on the perception that the state is an agent for domination by the capital-owning class over the working class. Finally, corporatist theory embraces the idea of the state working in conjunction with big business and other corporations, such as trade unions, to ensure private control of the means of production alongside public control.

While there is widespread agreement that, as in other fields of social welfare provision, the power of decision-making is not equally distributed in health care (Harrison & Ahmed 2000; Harrison *et al.* 1992), there is considerable debate about where the power of policy-making lies. Ham (1999) warns that it is important not to overemphasise the influence of political parties on policy-making, as ideology is often overruled by pragmatism. However, there is no doubt that the government does control the most important factor in making the policy a reality – the resources. This is done in a number of ways, by cash-limiting the NHS budget, ring-fencing money for specific causes, wage control and capital spending limits. Additionally, the question of how much power is devolved to a local level within the NHS is debated. In the UK, once a political policy is elected to power with a sufficient majority, it has almost entire control of policy. Furthermore, many commentators believe that the NHS is too politically sensitive an issue for the government to release its control over decision-making (Klein 2006).

Conversely, it can be argued that although ministers come and go, civil servants are here to stay. Their understanding of the system is far greater than that of the ministers they serve, and Ham (1999) argues it is they, not the government, who hold the real power. In addition to the civil service, the 1980s saw a growth in the number of quangos (quasi-autonomous non-governmental organisations). These are non-elected bodies made up of individuals usually appointed by the government. Mullard (1995) asserted that in 1993, quangos had responsibility for spending over 30% of the nation's income without any form of public accountability. There are also professional advisers, including representatives from nursing, allied health professionals and doctors. Medical influence within the NHS has long been recognised as the dominating power, as doctors not only influence policy at the centre but also at the periphery through clinical decision-making. It can be argued that the real power behind any health policy comes directly from the medical profession. However, since the introduction of general management into the NHS in 1984 (Department of Health and Social Security [DHSS] 1984) there has been an expansion in the power and influence of the manager and although the Labour Government has stated its commitment to the increasing the power of professionals in policy-making there is a view that this is more rhetoric than reality (Ferlie & Fitzgerald 2002).

Finally, business or organised interest groups (Dorey 2005) have widespread influence on policy-making. Their power is largely related to control over resources for investment and its ability to gain access to the centre of power. Such influence is still evident, for example, lobbying by supermarkets against a ban on advertising alcohol and the efforts of the food industry to continue to target advertising at children.

Consumer power is evident in pressure group activity, although there are concerns that such interest groups may exert influence on policy beyond their numbers. In addition, successive governments have given consumers a voice in local decision-making for health care, for example, through the Patient Advocacy and Liaison Service (DH 2000) and the recently introduced local involvement networks. Finally, the most powerful voice of the consumer could be said to be in the process of voting itself, although there are doubts about how representative the democratic process because of in-built inequalities within the state, such as wealth, education, the availability of information and the electoral and political system.

Policy-making therefore depends on the interplay of different voices and interests competing for priority. There is usually considerable interdependence of professional, political, managerial and public influences in decision-making. Nevertheless, it must be remembered that policy can be made with no consultation at all and often is.

How policy is made

In order to understand the complex process of policy development, theorists have used a number of different models: the rational comprehensive model, the incremental model and the bottom-up approach to policy development. Policy-making and implementation are sometimes viewed as separate processes but it can be argued that the distinction between construction and implementation of policy is unrealistic because often it is impossible to see where policy-making stops and implementation begins (Flynn 2007). Policy is often made and remade in the process of local implementation by the action of individuals and is the cumulative outcome of many decisions and responses by such individuals (Hogwood & Gunn 1984). Policy continues to evolve and change in the implementation phase (Ham & Hill 1993).

Rational model

The rational model owes much to the work of Pressman & Wildavsky (1973) who see the main value of this model in its potential as a radical model for implementing change and as a vehicle for strategic planning. Clear and achievable goals, a tendency towards centralised decision-making and the importance of achieving specified outcomes are the fundamental principles of this model. Policy, it is asserted, comes in at the top of the organisation and is successfully passed down to the operatives at the bottom who execute it in its pure form. Implementers are merely agents for those who have initiated the policy. This is associated with hierarchical concepts of organisation and has an emphasis on control, compliance and consent from the individuals within the organisation.

Criticisms of this model include the difficulty of agreeing values and goals and the fact that such goals will usually become distorted and modified once they are implemented. Furthermore, the reality that policy often comes from the bottom-up does not fit into this model. Finally, the lack of negotiation inherent in this structure is questionable.

Incremental model

The incremental model focuses on the principles of negotiation, interaction and agreement in decision-making, trial and error, pluralism and diffused authority and limited reliance on theory and ideology. Its main proponent is Charles Lindblom (Lindblom & Woodhouse 1993) who argues that policy is often made this way and that democracy is best achieved through this process. However, criticisms include its lack of analysis and long-term planning, the belief that all views are compromised and an over rosy view of the status quo.

Bottom-up model

The third model is the bottom-up model of policy implementation used by Barrett & Fudge (1981). The principle underpinning this model is that policy implementation is an interactive, iterative, evolutionary process. Policy implementation is a continuous process of action and interaction between a changing policy and implementing actors and agencies who are inherently difficult to control. Its central focus is on what is done – the activities and behaviour of groups and individuals, exploring the way action relates to policy rather than assuming it follows from policy. At any one time it may not be clear whether policy is influencing action or action influencing policy. To understand actions and responses there is a need to look at the actors involved, the agencies in which they operate and the factors which influence their behaviour (Barrett & Fudge 1981). The main critique of the bottom-up approach to policy implementation is that it overestimates the discretion of individuals to implement policy and pays too little attention to the legal, financial and structural constraints which set limits on their ability to act (Hogwood & Gunn 1984).

Policy-making can rarely be seen as fitting any theory completely. It is an untidy process of considerable complexity and rarely proceeds in an orderly, rational fashion. More often it consists of a web of decisions evolving over a period of time and throughout the implementation process. Policy implementation depends on a number of key factors: first, the policy itself and the political context and ideology of the time, and, second, the organisational culture, including the way the organisation is structured, how hierarchical it is and the style of the leader or manager, is important, as is the amount of discretion which individuals are allowed to interpret policy in the way they deem most appropriate and good communication channels within the organisation. The role of individuals is critical, as they may share the goals and values of the policy-makers and the organisation or have different priorities. Individuals or groups may have virtually autonomous power to shape the direction of policy, or at least to stand in the way of its effectiveness. This is particularly true of professional groups. Therefore, it is vital that the individual feels motivated and has the competence to implement the policy.

Another major issue to consider when implementing policy is the number of external constraints, for example, demographic change and new technology. Such factors may be out of the control of either policy-makers or implementers, but may have considerable impact on policy in practice. Clearly, policy implementation is a complex process in which factors as diverse as the individual, the resources, the organisation, the political context and, of course, the policy itself must be considered.

The evolution of the NHS

Pre-1948

By World War II a consensus was beginning to emerge that nationally coordinated health care provision was needed, because health care was not comprehensive or of good enough quality (Klein 2006). Before 1948, some national insurance and hospital, personal and domiciliary services had been introduced to address health and social care problems. However, the most significant change had been in public health services. The growth of industrialisation had led to overcrowding both in housing and in the workplace in factories. In such unsanitary conditions, diseases such as cholera and typhoid had been able to spread. In 1848, the government introduced the Public Health Act to ensure the adequate supply of water and sewerage systems and set up a Board of Health (Gormley 1999). Over the years legislation was introduced in housing and education, which also impacted on the general health of the population. This culminated in the work of William Beveridge, whose report in 1942 set out a plan to tackle the effects of what he described as the five giants: want, idleness, ignorance, squalor and disease.

Another aspect of health policy related to sickness insurance. In 1911, insurance coverage had been introduced to assist low-wage workers when they were sick and to pay for general practitioner (GP) services. Over the years this had been extended, but by 1939 there were still gaps in coverage, for example, the unemployed, self-employed and some women not in paid employment. Awareness was growing that provision needed to be available for all people.

Health care was provided in the home by GPs and district nurses. However, GPs charged fees to many and tended to be located in wealthier areas. District nurse services had been set up in the nineteenth century and health visitors were registered from 1907. They were organised by voluntary or charitable associations and, although the care was generally good, provision was far from uniform. The 1946 NHS Act had a big impact on district nursing as it obliged local authorities to provide a free home nursing service and enabled local authorities to set up health centres (Walsh & Gough 2000).

Hospital care was delivered by a mixture of voluntary and public, or municipal, institutions. Municipal hospitals began to be established in the 1860s and were available to those who could not afford to pay. However, some had developed from the old workhouses, which meant local people were often reluctant to use them. Voluntary hospitals were supported mainly by charitable donations and the contributions of wealthy people who were treated there. While they were respected institutions in the main, they had a number of problems. Those who could not afford to pay were expected to bring a letter of recommendation from a hospital subscriber and they provided very selective services, for example infectious disease and maternity care was often not available.

Two major problems of hospital provision were brought to a head by World War II. Distribution of hospital beds was haphazard. Often there were more beds in wealthy areas where need was less, and this led to competition between municipal and voluntary hospitals, particularly after 1930 when the running of workhouse hospitals had been taken over by local authorities. In addition, the voluntary hospitals were experiencing severe financial problems as the demand for hospital care outstripped the resources available.

The NHS

After World War II a Labour Government was elected under Clement Attlee, with an expectation that there would be considerable social reform. Plans for a national health service were underway before the war, but it was the arrival of Aneurin Bevan at the Ministry of Health that accelerated the process of reform. The NHS was established on 5 July 1948 and had a number of key aims (Fatchett 1999):

- The health of the whole population would be covered
- All services would be free at the point of delivery
- Provision would be comprehensive

- All services would be supplied and financed by the state
- The quality of the service would be improved to a good standard for all
- Services would be integrated, planned and distributed more effectively

The structure of the new health service was tripartite. GPs were self-employed, independent contractors and were funded directly from central government on a capitation and fee-for-service basis organised through family practitioner committees. Hospitals were run by hospital boards and organised by 14 new regional health boards reporting to the Department of Health. The third strand comprised the local authorities. Their power with respect to health care provision was reduced in that they no longer had responsibility for hospitals (Gormley 1999), but they now had a role in health promotion and prevention of ill-health which included health visiting, district nursing and environmental health. It is interesting that this role was seen as residual to the real business of health care, reflecting the ongoing view that health promotion was of secondary importance and effectively defining the NHS as an ill-health service. The tripartite structure was to cause problems for health care in the years to come, in that it separated health and social care and gave the government very little power over the gatekeepers to the NHS – the GPs.

Health care under the Conservative Government 1979–1997

In 1979 a Conservative Government was elected under Margaret Thatcher. Conservative social policy at that time reflected two strands of ideology – the neo-liberal and the neo-conservative. Neo-conservatives focused on the family as the centre of social life, the importance of traditional moral values and strong law and order. Neo-liberalism, or 'new right' thinking, was more concerned with rolling back the frontiers of the state, the necessity of competition and the market and the importance of introducing a business ethos into the public sector. New right thinking had its place within Conservative Party policy for some time (Friedman 1962,

Hayek 1982), but until the 1970s its effect was limited. From 1979, the influence of radical right think tanks, such as the Adam Smith Institute and the No Turning Back Group, was in the ascendency.

Policy towards the NHS from 1979 to 1989 did not reflect the principles of the new right as much as policy in other areas of welfare provision except in three areas. The first of these was an attempt to increase value for money in the NHS through general management, tighter monitoring and the pursuit of greater efficiency. Of these, the introduction in 1983 of general managers at regional, district and unit level, was the most controversial, as it was said to undermine clinical judgement and professional power (Harrison 1988). Alongside this came cost control initiatives such as the use of performance indicators and the introduction of clinical budgeting (Appleby 1992). These measures met with some success. There was a rise in day cases, average length of stay reduced from 9.4 days in 1978 to 7.3 in 1986 and the number of patients treated increased. Clinical staff became increasingly aware of the cost of treatment (Timmins 1996). Income generation was also encouraged, although the money earned in this way was relatively small adding less than 0.3% to NHS funds. The second policy thrust was stimulation of the private sector. Contracting out of ancillary services was compulsory from 1983, private nursing home sector use was encouraged and charges for prescriptions, dental and ophthalmic services increased. Alongside this, the percentage of people covered by some sort of private insurance increased from 3% of the population to 10% from 1979 to 1989 (Butler 1992).

Finally, the government attempted to control spending on the NHS, but with limited success. Although spending as a proportion of gross national product started to drop, it followed a trend which began in the mid-1970s under the Labour Government. Conversely, nurses experienced their best pay rises to date under the Conservatives and the Pay Review Body was introduced. Administrative reorganisation in 1979 and 1984 proved costly and the number of administrators rose threefold. Growth in the number of private nursing homes was matched by an increase in those qualifying for financial help, proving expensive to the Treasury, as did increases in prescription costs, where income raised was offset by the rising costs of those exempt from paying. Private contracting had to be made compulsory before it was widely adopted and even then fewer than 20% of contracts were awarded to outside contractors. Additionally, the social cost was high with many staff made redundant.

The internal market 1989–1997

In 1989, the Prime Minister, Margaret Thatcher, announced a cabinet-level review of the NHS, which resulted in the publication of the White Paper *Working for Patients* (DH 1989). The government was influenced by the ideas of an American, Alan Enthoven (1985), and the new right, which included more use of the private sector, greater management input, and the introduction of the internal market. A key area where neo-liberal ideas were ignored was regarding resources, as funding still primarily came from general taxation and there was no fundamental change to the basic principle of a free service at the point of delivery.

The most significant change was the introduction of the internal market to the NHS. This model still remains in England (although Scotland, Wales and Northern Ireland have changed this model as they now have their own departments with a mandate for health care organisation). A division was created between those agencies responsible for purchasing health care and those that were providers of services. Health authorities were main purchasers of health care, purchasing services on behalf of GPs plus all emergency treatment required by their population. They were supported by newly formed GP fundholders, who could purchase on their own behalf. Services could be purchased from any suppliers including the private sector and newly created NHS trust hospitals.

In theory, contracts were awarded on the basis of the best value for money, therefore knowledge of the price and quality of services was essential. To ensure this, managers were given much greater control over finances. Attention was given to performance indicators and the Family Health Services Authority gained a monitoring role over GPs. Additionally, incentives were introduced to the system, with money following the patient. Finally, to diversify supply and increase competition, the use of the private sector was developed through tax relief on private insurance for the over-65s.

It is highly debatable whether a truly 'free' market was actually created within the NHS, as the market was effectively managed in that trusts were told they must provide core services such as emergency departments, and education costs were removed from pricing decisions. Hospitals were not allowed free rein over their finances – borrowing and disposing of assets were only permissible within limits, and if deemed not against the public interest by the secretary of state (Robinson R. 1992). The question of whether the introduction of competition increased efficiency and saved money was curiously ignored, as were indications from the USA that competition actually increased costs (Robinson R. 1992). Therefore policies aimed at decreasing public spending and increasing the power of the market were potentially in conflict.

The Conservative Government claimed that power was devolved from the centre to the periphery as suppliers of health care could act independently of health authority control. However, it soon became apparent that the government was not prepared to decrease its control of such a politically sensitive institution as the NHS. Although policy-making and operational arms of health policy were separated by the creation of a policy board, which determined policy, and the National Health Service Management Executive (NHSME) dealing with implementation, the NHSME was directly accountable to the government and its control was increased by the replacement of the regional health authorities with regional offices of the NHSME staffed by civil servants. Consumer and professional representation was also decreased. Formal powers of the community health council were limited to consultation and lay representation on health authorities was reduced.

Professional representation was also cut as some professional groups, notably nurses, were no longer automatically represented on health authorities, and the role of doctors was substantially reduced. The chief medical officer and chief nursing officer were also excluded from membership of the NHSME (Butler 1992).

Problems of Conservative Party health care policy

There was some evidence that patients of GP fundholders received more choice of treatment. However, within a cash-limited budget, this treatment was provided at the expense of patients of non-fundholding GPs, resulting, it was claimed, in a two-tier system. These issues had to be weighed against the alleged improved efficiency of fundholders in reaching screening targets, receiving better information about hospital follow-up appointments and speeding up the process of receiving laboratory test results (Robinson & Scheuer 1992). The implementation of competition also proved expensive. Costs included:

- Employment of management consultants
- The expense of tax relief for older people
- The loss of economies of scale
- Administrative costs (which reached up to £300 million a year as the number of administrators trebled)
- Management costs

Furthermore, contracting had inherent inefficiencies in-built, in that it limited sharing of good practice and inhibited long-term planning and innovation. One year contracts proved an administrative nightmare because of the number of purchasers – over 100 health authorities and more than 3500 fundholders (DH 1997). One health authority reported issuing 60 000 invoices in one year! Lack of professional representation, the increase of secrecy clauses for staff and the invisibility of the patient in decision-making were also seen as major problems of the internal market (DH 1997). Therefore, in 1997, when the Labour Government was elected, they vowed to address these problems and create a 'new NHS'.

Labour Government health care policy

The New NHS: Modern, Dependable (DH 1997), describing the Labour Government's strategy for the NHS, was produced in November 1997. These intentions were further articulated in subsequent policies, for example, *The NHS Plan* (DH 2000), *The NHS Improvement Plan* (DH 2004a), *Our Health, Our Care, Our Say* (DH 2006a) and, most recently, *Our NHS Our Future* (DH 2007a). Within *The NHS Plan* the key principles of the NHS were outlined as:

- The NHS will provide a universal service for all based on clinical need, not ability to pay
- The NHS will provide a comprehensive range of services
- The NHS will shape its services around the needs and preferences of individual patients, their families and their carers
- The NHS will respond to needs of different populations
- The NHS will work continuously to improve quality services and to minimise errors
- The NHS will support and value its staff
- public funds for health care will be devoted solely to NHS patients
- The NHS will work together with others to ensure a seamless service for patients
- The NHS will help keep people healthy and work to reduce health inequalities
- The NHS will respect confidentiality of individual patients and provide open access to information about services, treatment and performance

Within the policies, community nurses are seen as central to the government's plans for developing this 'new NHS' and in transforming the rhetoric of the policy into the reality of practice.

Organisational change

The main thrust of Labour policy has been an espoused move towards decentralisation and ensuring that the structures within the NHS enable easier access to services for patients (DH 2001). To achieve this, organisational structures have been changed and new ones established.

First, the assemblies of Northern Ireland, Wales and Scotland now have their own departments with a mandate for health care. Within the English system the DH retains responsibility and accountability for health and social care. It has been reduced in size with an increasingly narrow core function of 'promoting effective stewardship of the nation's health' (DH 2004a). It has both legislative and regulatory powers and a remit for both standard and priority setting, while working to achieve its objectives of improving health status, improving care and achieving better value for all. The regional offices were closed down and ten strategic health authorities (SHAs) established, which no longer have responsibility for commissioning health care but have a managerial function on behalf of the secretary of state at a local level, linking with both the NHS and the DH. Their role is to lead the strategic development of local health services and monitor the performance of primary care trusts (PCTs) and NHS trusts, with the health authority chief executive answerable to the secretary of state. The original functions of the SHAs have been further modified to reflect the reform of the health care system. Strategically they have a role in leadership, organisational and workforce development, and have responsibility for managing, monitoring and improving local health care.

PCTs are seen as the lead organisation within the NHS and they bring together GPs, community nurses and other agencies involved in health and social care, in each geographical area to work together to improve the health of local people (DH 2001). Their main functions are to assess need, plan and secure all health services and improve the health of the local population and they have responsibility for the management, integration and development of all primary care services. They are also responsible for engaging local communities in decision-making and devolving power to frontline staff – notably community nurses. They are expected to work in partnership with other agencies to do this, in particular with other PCTs and with local authorities, and it is anticipated that they will form both care trusts to meet the needs of particular client groups, and joint PCT/local authority managed networks and/or teams to support people with long-term conditions. For children's services, joint commissioning should be carried out through children's trusts.

Since being established, PCTs have continued to evolve and there are now 152 PCTs in England, and these are responsible for spending a large percentage of the NHS budget. Part of their function is to use this budget to commission a range of comprehensive and equitable services that respond to local need and their role also requires them to directly provide services where this gives best value. Commissioning at a PCT level includes assessing population needs, identifying anticipated health outcomes and using public funds to procure, provide and manage services. It is a complex mechanism that now has become further devolved to involve GPs through practice-based commissioning (PBC), which continues the government's desire for better clinical engagement in the commissioning process. In 2007 the DH declared its intent to establish 'world-class commissioning' (DH 2007b) by laying out a range of competencies to be achieved by commissioning bodies. Under PBC, health care practices receive indicative budgets and will be able to see how much of their secondary care budget is going on hospital care. The intention is that it will give primary care professionals more control over resources and they can then free up money for local priorities. PBC will also include financial incentives for GPs to avoid patients staying in hospital. It is anticipated that the General Medical Services contract will assist PCTs in fulfilling this role as this national contract for GPs is outcomes based and gives PCTs the ability to shape services and increase primary care capacity to meet local needs (DH 2004b).

The main decision-making bodies within PCTs are professional executive committees or boards. These usually consist of an executive director and health professionals. Boards provide opportunities for community nurses to be proactive in policy decisions that shape and deliver services. Working with executive boards, community nurses have the potential to implement strategies that provide seamless care for patients with long-term health conditions, integrating new and innovative teams and services in response to changing need. Community nurses are well placed to facilitate and empower individuals and user groups within the population to be similarly involved in the commissioning. This role may change and increase in the near future as some services are separated from PCTs into arms length provider organisations.

There is some question as to whether PCTs are all able to take on this role effectively. Concerns have been raised whether members of PCTs work together effectively, and whether PCT members work for the organisation or represent professional interests (Burke & Harris 1999). The number of GP PCT members in relation to nurses is much higher, therefore nurses are worried that their views are ignored (McIntosh 1999). The need for consultation with each practice before decisions are made has implications for the speed with which the PCT agenda can move forward. In addition, the King's Fund has voiced concern about accountability in the commissioning process as PCTs spend approximately £58 billion with none of the accountability placed on local councils, which spend a similar amount of public money. In light of this, community nurses who engage in commissioning can help to monitor both the outputs and the outcomes of the commissioned service and also strengthen their contribution within decision-making processes.

Another issue of concern is the extent to which decentralisation is really taking place as SHAs have been reported as exerting undue pressure on PCTs under the guise of performance management. Although the government has talked about a supporting relationship and partnerships between SHAs and PCTs, there are some queries about the extent to which that will be possible if SHAs are accountable for PCT performance. Equally, Ferlie & Fitzgerald (2002) argue that central control is unlikely to diminish as monitoring, regulation and performance management continue to develop.

A further goal of the government is to improve access to GP services and this has been addressed in a number of ways including trying to make it easier to register with an open practice, same-day appointments and encouraging GPs to offer more flexible opening times. More controversially, the intention is to allow new providers such as social enterprises or commercial organisations to tender for service provision (DH 2006a).

NHS trusts are still responsible for the delivery of most health care but the aim is that trusts will increasingly become foundation trusts. Foundation trusts have a number of freedoms that NHS trusts do not have, for example, to borrow money and invest in new services, plus they are no longer performance managed by the DH but by an independent regulator. Their accountability is to local people, PCTs and the regulator. In order to help facilitate the target of an 18-week maximum waiting time the government intends that a further supplier of health care will be the independent sector through the development of independent sector treatment centres.

An additional change is the way in which payment will take place with the introduction of 'Payment by Results' (PbR). PbR emerged with the aims of increasing efficiency, choice for patients by creating diversity and competition among providers and transparency for the taxpayer about how their money is spent. National tariffs have been created for treatments and operations with the proviso that money follows patients. This was a significant change from the established pattern of locally negotiated block contracts and paved the way for offering patients a choice for secondary care referrals. Benefits and challenges of PbR have been identified at PCT level as it does encourage PCTs to work more closely with GP practices to avoid admissions. In addition, it continues the thrust towards setting up local specialised services, and it also encourages hospitals to treat as many people as possible as inpatients.

Patient involvement

From the start the Labour Government was determined to involve patients more in policy- and decision-making, and the development and monitoring of health services. The Health and

Social Care Act 2001 placed a duty on PCTs and NHS trusts to involve and consult with patients and the public and foundation trusts have also given the duty of engaging with local people. To facilitate this, a number of initiatives have taken place including the following.

- Setting up of the Commission for Patient and Public Involvement in Health in January 2003. This is an independent, non-departmental public body, sponsored by the DH, which aims to promote the involvement in health and health services of all sectors of the community
- Establishment of the Patient Advocacy and Liaison Services in every NHS trust and PCT to provide support and advice to patients and to respond to individual problems at both primary and secondary levels of health care delivery
- Strengthening of the Independent Complaints Advisory Service
- Patients' representatives sit on PCTs
- The competencies to be achieved by commissioning bodies (DH 2007b) include user involvement and PCTs have a fundamental duty to systematically and rigorously engage with the local population in the commissioning process to improve their health and well-being
- Trusts are obliged to collect regular feedback from patients
- Large-scale surveys of public views of the NHS
- Opening of trust and health authority meetings to the public

A further initiative, the Expert Patient Programme (EPP), emerged as strategy to promote self-care by patients with long-term health problems. Six-week programmes were designed to be user-led and structured to equip the patient with knowledge and skills for self-management. By 2004, the programme had been extended to include the parents of children with long-term health problems. Financial provision was not well thought out with funding of programmes becoming the responsibility of PCTs from 2004. Evaluation of the initiative (Lee *et al.* 2006)

indicates that patients who have attended the programme visit GP services fewer times, but, despite this, chronic health problems still dominate the nursing case load. However, within local settings, EPPs offer community nurses the potential to encourage patient participation in self-management and educational opportunities.

The setting up of the NHS Centre for Involvement in 2005, and the implementation of the Local Government and Public Involvement Act in 2007, has seen the replacement of Patients Forums with Local Involvement Networks(LINks). The power relationship between LINks and state-funded health and social care providers has been underpinned with government funding of £84 million, and purports to strengthen the voice of the people who use services. Vested with limited powers of entry to inspect care services, the network has a responsibility to investigate and act on areas of public concern, and to reflect the needs and views of local people in service development. Health and social care providers must respond accordingly in the provision of information and in response to LINks findings. It is important for community nurses working with patients in their own settings to note that this is very much about engaging with communities and individuals at local levels. Nurses engaged in the delivery of primary care are in an ideal position to identify, recruit and encourage users of services and individuals who will participate in initiatives.

A significant change which has been phased in since its introduction in *The NHS Plan* (DH 2000) is the principle of offering patients choice in their secondary health care provider. Following a referral from their GP for planned treatment, patients will be able to choose from any hospital or clinic from an NHS or foundation trust and from the independent sector. Patients can exercise this option as long as the provider reaches NHS standards and matches the NHS tariff. There is some scepticism about this partnership approach, which was exacerbated with the decision to disband community health councils. Recruitment across all groups, particularly clients with mental health problems and learning disabilities is challenging and funding to support this at trust and department levels remains difficult. There is also concern about how much particular individuals can be representative of the wider public and that there might be excessive influence of vocal groups over the direction in which the health service moves. Furthermore, it is still not known how much patients wish to be involved in making decisions about their care and whether they would rather leave these to the professionals. Nonetheless, the government is firmly committed to making this happen.

Increased focus on public health

From the early days of the Labour Government it was asserted that there needed to be a greater emphasis on public health (DH 1997). This may be because of the nature and size of the public health issues in the UK. Seventeen and a half million people in this country report a long-term condition, such as diabetes, asthma and arthritis (DH 2005a), and it has been estimated that the number of people over 65 years with a long-term condition doubles each decade. Smoking kills an estimated 86 500 people a year, and accounts for a third of all cancers. Up to 22 000 deaths and 150 000 hospital admissions each year are associated with alcohol misuse (DH 2006a), and 23%of people are obese (Longley *et al.* 2007). Poverty is a significant factor in determining life expectancy and inequalities are still considerable between social classes in England. Wanless (2004) has warned that failure to tackle public health could cost the NHS £50 billion.

The challenge for this government has been to find the balance between avoiding charges of intrusion into private lives, while ensuring the public good and mitigating the rising costs of avoidable ill-health. Eager to avoid the 'hector and lecture' approach (DH 2008b) or the nanny state label, the Labour Government has adopted a public health stance of stewardship or 'liberal paternalism' (Jochelson 2005), by introducing measures that set new social standards and help make changes for people who previously may have struggled to make them for themselves. Through differing measures of fiscal, regulatory and voluntary control, lifestyle issues such as smoking and alcohol have been addressed

with varying degrees of coercion. *Choosing Health* (DH 2004d) set targets to reduce smoking prevalence in the population and in July 2007 the government introduced a ban on smoking in enclosed public places and the workplace. The government is now considering legislation to control the packaging and display of cigarettes while reviewing access to vending machines.

Although obesity and alcohol consumption are high on the public health agenda, both industries have strong lobbies. However, closer partnerships with manufacturers have resulted in better labelling and prolonged discussion of the inclusion of salt and fat in foods. Politically, the need to continually balance NHS costs to the taxpayer is also problematic for the government, as public health demands funds; 'Healthy Weight, Healthy Lives', introduced in 2008 to tackle the rising trend in obesity, is underpinned by government funding of £372 million (DH 2008b).

To tackle long-term conditions, the government has introduced a 'long-term conditions model' (DH 2005a). The key features of this are stratification of care to meet identified patients' needs, using a case management approach to provide disease-specific care, joining up of health and social care, and supporting self-care. Community matrons have been appointed to lead case management, supported by multi-professional teams based in primary care with provision of specialist advice to manage care across all settings.

Concern over life expectancy at all stages of life, and the belief that inequalities in health are 'fundamentally unfair' (DH 2008b), ensured that strategies aimed at reducing avoidable mortality and morbidity have been the subject of successive reports and recommendations since the seminal work by Acheson in 1998. It is at this level that state intrusion is more widely seen as not just acceptable but necessary, with the current government using the authority of the state to identify expected outcomes and secure the necessary agreements between agencies and provision of services. The cumulative effects of low income and poor housing and life opportunities on morbidity and mortality are repeatedly researched and verified. To tackle these wider

determinants of health the government introduced initiatives, often in partnership with local
authorities (DH 2004a), aimed at improving
health, social care, housing, education services,
the environment and leisure resources. A range
of resources have been targeted at deprived
areas and groups and PCTs have frameworks
for assessing populations, identifying inequalities in health and planning services accordingly.
Health impact assessments provide a mechanism for monitoring progress and reviewing
the consequences of other service developments
and the Sure Start programme aimed to help the
development of services and improve health in
disadvantaged areas. However, although there
has been some progress in tackling child poverty, the gap in life expectancy between the bottom quintile and the population as a whole has
widened by 2% for males and 5% for females
(Longley *et al.* 2007).

An interesting development that may have an
impact in making sure that public health is an
the agenda of health care providers is that the
Healthcare Commission has a remit to review
the delivery of health improvement, reduction
of inequalities, public health delivery within
PCTs and progress made against smoking cessation and sexual health targets (Walker 2004).
Public health is also the seventh domain in the
DH's *Standards for Better Health* (DH 2004c),
against which the Healthcare Commission will
be making judgements about quality.

Community nurses will undoubtedly welcome
the wider perspective and political will given to
public health. Currently, they are engaged in a
wide range of educative and preventive activities, and their expertise is likely to be extended.
With the added dimensions of assessment and
partnerships with other agencies, nurses in
primary care settings now have the scope to
develop both individual and practice specific
health promotion activities and the lead role of
the community matron working with patients
with complex long-term conditions should add
to these opportunities. Public health is the area
in which community nurses are ideally placed
to become leaders within the field. They can
offer input not only in delivering public health

care but also in developing standards for public health. As the practitioners who work closest
to the patient, it can be argued that they are ideally placed to make a unique contribution at a
local and national level to public health policy
development that is sensitive and responsive
to patients' needs. The challenge will be to
develop a structured approach to measuring
the outcomes of their activities that balances the
ideological underpinnings of the government's
public health agenda with the political thrust of
its financial concerns.

Conclusion

There are indications that the changes and
the extra resources allocated by the Labour
Government to health care are beginning to have
an effect as maximum waiting times for operations has fallen from 18 months to nine months
and staff numbers have increased by more than
20% (DH 2004a). However, changes are likely
to continue within the NHS, particularly for
community nurses and, in order to fulfil their
roles effectively, community nurses will need to
be aware of the changes that are happening in
social policy and their potential impact on the
profession and, more importantly, on clients.

Lord Darzi (DH 2008a) has recently been asked
to review the NHS and develop a vision for the
next ten years around eight areas of care: maternity and newborn care; staying healthy; children's health; planned care; acute care; mental
health; long-term conditions; and end-of-life care.
Key messages that have come forward so far are:

- The need to deliver a wider range of more
  accessible and responsive services to meet
  local needs in community settings
- Allocation of resources to bring new GP
  practices (traditional or new private providers) to where they are most needed, starting with the 25% of PCTs with the poorest
  provision
- Greater flexibility in GP opening hours
  extending to evenings and weekends
- Investment in PCTs to develop 150 GP-led
  health centres, situated in accessible locations and offering a range of services to the

local population, including pre-bookable appointments, walk-in services and other services (DH 2007a)

Extending GP services and hours and providing more home-based care suggest workload implications for practice and community nurses, although the report's vision of networked polyclinics or enhanced GP services where patients can access a range of diagnostic and specialist services including mental health suggests a range of future career opportunities for all nurses. However, the British Medical Association (2007) was quick to note that the proposed changes will require different skills and capacities for nurses and these will need to be provided through training and, possibly, through the development of new and extended nursing roles.

In 2004 the Nursing and Midwifery Council opened a new part of the register for specialist community public health nurses and there is some debate that the standards of proficiency for these roles may be reviewed in the near future. In Scotland, an initiative is already underway in four pilot sites to test out a generic community nursing role, which integrates the skills of district nursing, public health nursing (health visiting and school nursing) and family health nursing within one discipline. *Modernising Nursing Careers* (DH 2006b) recognised that changes in services or the careers of other professional groups impact on how nurses 'take on new roles, work across boundaries and set up new services' (DH 2006b) particularly in the attempts to keep pace with current reforms. In the follow on from *Modernising Nursing Careers* the DH is currently engaged in consultation to consider moving nurses from all branches and locations along five pathways reflecting the main treatment categories for patients – and changes to pre-registration nursing education to reflect this are likely to follow.

The nursing profession must ensure that community nurses have the knowledge and skills to enable them to influence policy development and implementation and grasp the opportunities available for them within the NHS. This has implications for the education and continuing professional development of community nurses. It is therefore essential that community nurses engage in lifelong learning and develop further their own unique knowledge base so that they can continue to provide high-quality care to their clients and help shape the NHS of the future.

References

Acheson, Sir D. (1998) *Independent Inquiry into Inequalities in Health*. The Stationery Office and King's Fund, London.

Appleby, J. (1992) *Financing Health Care in the 1990s*. Open University Press, Buckingham.

Barrett, S. & Fudge, C. (1981) *Policy and Action: Essays on the Implementation of Public Policy*. Methuen, London.

British Medical Association (2007) Briefing Note. Professor Ara Darzi's Healthcare for London Review. Available at: www.bma.org.uk (accessed 7 March 2008).

Burke, L.M. & Harris, D. (1999) Education for Practice. In: *Specialists in Community Nursing: Current Issues in Community Nursing and Primary Health Care in Practice* (ed. J. Littlewood). Churchill Livingstone, Edinburgh, pp. 251–278.

Butler, J. (1992) *Policies and Politics: Before and After Working for Patients*. Open University Press, Buckingham.

Department of Health and Social Security (1984) *Implementation of the NHS Management Inquiry Report*. The Stationery Office, London.

Department of Health (1989) *Working for Patients*. The Stationery Office, London.

Department of Health (1997) *The New NHS, Modern, Dependable*. The Stationery Office, London.

Department of Health (1998) *A First Class Service: Quality in the New NHS*. HSC 1998/113. HMSO, London.

Department of Health (1999) *Making a Difference: Strengthening the Nursing, Midwifery and Health Visiting Contribution to Health and Healthcare*. The Stationery Office, London.

Department of Health (2000) *The NHS Plan: A Plan for Investment, A Plan for Reform*. The Stationery Office, London.

Department of Health (2001) *Shifting the Balance of Power Within the NHS*. The Stationery Office, London.

Department of Health (2004a) *The NHS Improvement Plan*. The Stationery Office, London.

Department of Health (2004b) *Delivering Investment in General Practice: Implementing the new GMS Contract.* The Stationery Office, London.

Department of Health (2004c) *Standards for Better Health: Health Care Standards for Services under the NHS.* The Stationery Office, London.

Department of Health (2004d) *Choosing Health: Making Healthier Choices Easier.* The Stationary Office, London.

Department of Health (2005a) *Supporting People with Long Term Conditions: An NHS and Social Care Model to Support Local Innovation and Integration.* The Stationary Office, London.

Department of Health (2005b) *Supporting People with Long Term Conditions: Liberating the Talents of Nurses who Care for People with Long Term Conditions.* The Stationary Office, London.

Department of Health (2006a) *Our Health, Our Care, Our Say: A New Direction for Community Services.* The Stationary Office, London.

Department of Health (2006b) *Modernising Nursing Careers.* The Stationery Office, London.

Department of Health (2007a) *Our NHS, Our Future: NHS Next Stage Review – Interim Report.* The Stationery Office, London.

Department of Health (2007b) *World Class Commissioning: Competencies.* The Stationery Office, London.

Department of Health (2008a) *High Quality Care for All: NHS Next Stage Review.* Final Report – Lord Ara Darzi. Cm7432. Department of Health, London.

Department of Health (2008b) *Healthy Weight, Healthy Lives. A Cross Government Strategy for England.* The Stationery Office, London.

Dorey, P. (2005) *Policy Making in Britain: An Introduction.* Sage Publications, London.

Enthoven, A. (1985) National Health Service market reform. *Health Affairs*, **10**, 60–70.

Fatchett, A. (1999) *Nursing in the New NHS, Modern, Dependable.* Baillière Tindall, London.

Ferlie, E. & Fitzgerald, L. (2002) The sustainability of the new public management in the UK. In: *New Public Management, Current Trends and Future Prospects* (eds K. Mclaughlin, K.S.P. Osborne & E. Ferlie). Routledge, London, pp. 341–353.

Flynn, N. (2007) *Public Sector Management*, 5th edn. Sage Publications, London.

Friedman, M. (1962) *Capitalism and Freedom.* University of Chicago Press, Chicago.

Gormley, K. (1999) The development of health and social care services. In: *Social Policy and Health Care* (ed. K. Gormley). Harcourt Brace, London, pp. 13–28.

Green, J. & Thorogood, N. (1998) *Analysing Health Policy.* Longman, London.

Guba, E.G. (1984) Cited in: Owen, J.M. & Rogers, J. (1999) *Program Evaluation: Forms and Approaches.* Sage Publications, London.

Ham, C. (1999) *Health Policy in Britain: The Politics and Organisation of the NHS*, 4th edn. Macmillan, Basingstoke.

Ham, C. & Hill, M. (1993) *The Policy Process in the Modern Capitalist State*, 2nd edn. Wheatsheaf Books, Sussex.

Harrison, S. (1988) *Managing the NHS, Shifting the Frontier.* Chapman and Hall, London.

Harrison, S., Hunter, D. & Pollit, C. (1992) *The Dynamics of British Health Policy.* Routledge, London.

Harrison, S. & Ahmed, W. (2000) Medical autonomy and the UK state 1975 to 2025. *Sociology*, **34**, 129–146.

Hayek, F.A. (1982) *The Constitution of Liberty.* Routledge and Kegan Paul, London.

Hennessy, D. (2000) The Emerging Themes. In: *Health Policy and Nursing: Influence, Development and Impact* (eds D. Hennessy & P. Spurgeon). Macmillan Press, Basingstoke, pp. 1–38.

Hogwood, B.W. & Gunn, L.A. (1984) *Policy Analysis for the Real World.* Oxford University Press, Oxford.

Jochelson, K. (2005) *Nanny or Steward? The Role of Government in Public Health.* King's Fund, London.

Klein, R. (2006) *The New Politics of the NHS: from Creation to Reinvention*, 5th edn. Radcliffe Publishing, Oxford.

Lee, V., Kennedy, A. & Rogers, A. (2006) Implementing and managing self management skills training within primary care organisations: a national survey of the Expert Patient Programme within its pilot phase. *Implementation Science*, **23**, 6.

Lindblom, C. & Woodhouse, E.J. (1993) *The Policy Making Process*, 3rd edn. Simon and Schuster Company, Englewood Cliffs, New Jersey.

Longley, M., Shaw, C. & Dolan, G. (2007) *Nursing: Towards 2015, Alternative Scenarios for Healthcare, Nursing and Nurse Education in the UK in 2015.* University of Glamorgan, Glamorgan.

Maslin-Prothero, S. & Masterson A. (1998) *Continuing care: developing a policy analysis for nursing. Journal of Advanced Nursing*, **28**, 548–53.

McIntosh, K. (1999) Only two PCG chairs to be held by nurses. *Health Service Journal*, **7**.

Mullard, M. (1995) Introduction. In: *Policy Making in Britain: An Introduction* (ed. M. Mullard). Routledge, London, pp. 1–9.

Owen, J.M. & Rogers, J. (1999) *Program Evaluation: Forms and Approaches*. Sage Publications, London.

Pressman, J. & Wildavsky, A. (1973) *Implementation*. University of California Press, Berkeley.

Robinson, J. (1992) *Introduction: Beginning The Study of Nursing Policy*. In: *Policy Issues in Nursing Education* (eds J. Robinson, A. Gray & R. Elkan). Open University Press, Milton Keynes, pp. 1–8.

Robinson, R. (1992) *Competition and Health Care: A Comparative Analysis of UK Planning and US Experience*. King's Fund, London.

Robinson, R. & Scheuer, M. (1992) A footnote for fund-holding. *Health Service Journal*, 19–20.

Timmins, N. (1996) *The Five Giants: A Biography of the Welfare State*. Fontana Press, London.

Titmus, R. (1979) *Commitment to Welfare*. Allen and Unwin, London.

Walker, A. (2004) Raise a glass to public health. *Health Service Journal*, 16–18.

Walsh, N. & Gough, P. (2000) In: *Health Policy and Nursing: Influence, Development and Impact* (eds D. Hennessy & P. Spurgeon). Macmillan Press, Basingstoke, pp. 1–38.

Wanless, D. (2004) *Securing Good Health for the Whole Population: A Final Report*. The Stationery Office, London.

Chapter 3 The Origins of Contemporary Primary Health Care

Professor Ann Taket

Introduction

This chapter traces the contemporary origins of primary health care and begins by exploring the concept of primary health care (PHC), linking this to relevant international and national policy documents, and introducing the concept of PHC developed by the World Health Organization (WHO). The chapter then focuses on the development of primary care in the UK. It explains how PHC is not just found within the National Health Service (NHS), reviews the different sectors involved in PHC, and then discusses the current structure of PHC in the NHS. Key concepts, including the primary health care team, primary care trusts (PCTs) and integrated heath and social care trusts, and the relevant current UK policy documents are introduced.

The chapter then moves on to discuss four important issues in the provision of primary health care in the community: health promotion; tackling health inequalities; health and regeneration; and tackling domestic violence. The author will explain why each of these issues is of particular significance and review briefly a number of studies/projects which illustrate what is happening/can be done; this will introduce a range of current research. The chapter concludes with a short review of challenges for the future, emphasising the important role that the nursing profession has to play in meeting these challenges. Readers are referred to Chapter 1 for a more detailed synopsis of recent UK primary care policy changes.

Primary health care – the concept

Providing a definition of PHC is not an easy matter. At its simplest, it is often understood as non-specialised health services, or alternatively as first-line health services. Thus, PHC is mainly provided outside hospitals to people who are living in the community. So far, so good. Matters become more complicated when the importance of the protection and promotion of health in communities as well as the provision of health care to those who are ill is acknowledged, and also when trying to itemise the type of services and activities that are included within PHC. This section introduces the concept of PHC that is central to the work of the WHO and to international health policies to which the UK government is a signatory; a brief chronology is provided in Box 3.1. This understanding of PHC is reflected in the *rhetoric* of current UK health policy, although there are some tensions between policy statements and the reality of policy implementation.

The basis for WHO's health policy is the objective enshrined in the WHO constitution: 'the attainment by all peoples of the highest possible level of health'. This provided the basis for a key resolution passed in 1977 by the World Health Assembly (the governing body of WHO), stating that the main social target of governments and WHO should be the attainment, 'by all the people of the world by the year 2000, of a level of health that will permit them to lead a socially and economically productive life'. The resolution become popularly known as 'health for all by the year 2000', (after the phrase 'health for all' originated by the then Director General of WHO, Halfdan Mahler), and later abbreviated as HFA2000 or HFA.

Although the concept of PHC had existed for some time, it was only around about the late 1960s and early 1970s that international health policy began to stress its particular importance.

Box 3.1	Health policy and PHC – a brief chronology until 1999
May 1977	World Health Assembly of the WHO first adopted the 'Health for All' policy goal (HFA or HFA2000): 'the main social target of governments and WHO in the following decades should be for all citizens of the world to attain by the year 2000 a level of health which will permit them to lead a socially and economically productive life'
1978	Alma Ata declaration on PHC (WHO/UNICEF 1978)
1979	Resolution in support of formulation of global, regional and national Health for All strategies adopted by World Health Assembly
1980	Adoption of regional strategies for Health for All
1981	Adoption of global Health for All strategy
1984	First set of European Health for All targets agreed (WHO/EURO 1985)
1986	Start of 'Healthy Cities' project Use of local level targets
1990–91	Revisions of European targets
1991	Adoption of second set of European targets – the common European health policy (WHO/EURO 1993)
1993	Adoption of EU Maastricht treaty, which contains a specific health component in terms of a new chapter on 'Public Health'
1997	EU Amsterdam treaty strengthens public health provisions, introducing a requirement for a high level of human health protection to be assured in *all* community policies and activities
1998	World Health Declaration adopted by World Health Assembly, Health for All policy for the twenty-first century, reaffirms commitment to PHC as defined in Alma Ata declaration; Health21 – the Health for All policy framework for the WHO European Region adopted by the European Regional Committee
1999	Health21 – the Health for All policy framework for the WHO European Region published (WHO/EURO 1999)

This arose out of concerns about the rising cost of health services and the lack of effectiveness of existing hospital-oriented health service systems in tackling priority health problems, together with the realisation that the services particularly needed in low-income countries were not specialised hospital-based care, but much more basic and less technically complex forms of care, with an emphasis on accessibility. Analysis of the failure of vertical disease control programmes (i.e. programmes focused on a single discrete disease and characterised by hierarchical organisation), such as WHO's global malaria campaign, contributed to the formulation of the PHC concept as the basic international strategy for health improvement (Gish 1992).

It was also argued that achieving 'health for all' would only be possible through a re-orientation of services towards the promotion and protection of health rather than an emphasis on the cure or care of those in ill-health. Thus a strengthening of community-based services, where protection and promotion can take place, began to be seen as essential. This increased emphasis on PHC applied equally to all countries (low or high income), and so, the predominant concern became the re-organisation of *all* health services with the aim of prioritising PHC. This represented a radical change from the earlier attitude which could be caricatured as: 'How can we continue to develop high technology medicine without spiralling costs and how can this be made available to poorer countries?'

A key event in the recognition of the importance of PHC was the 1978 conference held in Alma-Ata, in the former USSR. This was sponsored by WHO and Unicef (the United Nations Children's Fund), and attended by delegations from 134 governments and 67 UN organisations, specialised agencies and non-governmental organisations (NGOs) in official relations with WHO, including countries from all different stages of development. This conference reaffirmed health care as a fundamental right and reiterated that the inequalities that existed, both between and within countries, were unacceptable.

Alma-Ata was called at the time a 'historic collective expression of political will in the spirit of social equity' (WHO/UNICEF 1978). The conference was also important for its development of an improved understanding of the content of PHC, the key features of which are summarised in Box 3.2.

One tension within Europe has been between the role and influence of WHO and the European Union (EU) in health policy matters. The EU has dealt with health issues for four decades, initially with a very restricted health mandate, which was widened considerably by the Maastricht treaty (1993) and the Amsterdam treaty (1997). The Maastricht treaty gave the Community a new objective of making 'a contribution to the attainment of a high level of health protection' which is applicable to *all* Community policies. Article 129 of the treaty sets out a framework for Community public health activities in pursuit

---

Box 3.2   PHC – the Alma Ata concept

Eight essential elements in the PHC sector:

- Education about prevailing health problems and methods of prevention and control
- Promotion of food supply and proper nutrition
- Adequate supply of safe water and basic sanitation
- Maternal and child health services, including family planning
- Immunisation against major infectious diseases (diphtheria, tetanus, whooping cough, measles, polio, tuberculosis)
- Prevention and control of locally endemic diseases
- Appropriate treatment of common diseases and injuries
- Provision of essential drugs

Key features of PHC-based health services:

- Service provision in relation to needs of population, available and accessible to all in the community
- Should cover promotive, preventive, curative and rehabilitative services (with prominence given to promotion and prevention)
- Community participation, individually and collectively, in planning and implementation of health care
- Multi-sectoral approach, multi-factorial causation of ill-health and the importance of social and environmental factors should be recognised, coordinated action of health, education, agricultural, housing, sanitation, industry sectors is necessary
- Appropriate technology, (low cost, high quality essential drugs, self-reliance and affordability, in keeping with local culture, i.e. 'acceptable')
- Integration of different types of medical practitioner (non-allopathic and allopathic)
- Use of paramedics and community-based health workers

of this objective. The Article provides for the adoption of incentive measures, excluding any harmonisation of Member States' legislation, and recommendations. Finally, it stipulates that health protection requirements shall form a constituent part of other Community policies.

The legal basis of the Community's public health activities was further extended in the Amsterdam treaty, reflecting the evolving consensus on the importance of Community action in this field. With the continuing growth in membership of the EU, and the growth in concern with health matters through the Maastricht and Amsterdam treaties, an increased influence of the EU on health policy and health systems is clearly a real possibility. The mandate that the EU now possesses for health could be utilised to support the development of PHC. In practice it remains to be seen how this mandate will be used. Kokkonen & Kekomäki (1993) argue that there is considerable potential for legal and economic measures affecting health. Others conclude, however, that an expansion of the EU's role in health-related policies is likely to proceed only erratically. They argue that incrementalism, bargaining and compromises (Bomberg & Peterson 1993) dominate the process of policy formulation in the EU. Recent years have seen some closer links developing between the EU and WHO, but it remains to be seen how far this will. Some commentators (for example, Godlee 1995; Pannenborg 1991) have questioned the relevance of maintaining a WHO Regional Office in Europe with the increased health mandate of the EU.

Primary health care and the NHS

It should be obvious that, given the concept of PHC set out in the previous section, PHC is not just found within the NHS. This section begins with a review of different relevant actors in the UK context, and then move on to a discussion of the current structure of PHC in the NHS. This introduces primary health care teams, the 'primary care-led NHS', PCTs, integrated health and social care trusts, and local strategic partnerships.

Primary health care – multiple sectors and services

The Alma Ata conceptualisation of PHC was noticeable for its wide concern with factors supporting health, not limiting itself purely to health services. There is explicit mention of water supplies, basic sanitation, education and the food supply, as well as recognition of the multi-factorial causation of ill-health, including the importance of social and environmental factors. Achieving the promotion and protection of health, and successfully tackling health inequalities, requires action in *all* sectors of society.

The notion of health promotion is extremely important within the HFA policy framework and within PHC services along Alma Ata lines. This was an area where considerable policy development was needed, outcomes of which are reflected in the 1991 revisions to the European HFA targets (WHO/EURO 1993) and in the latest health policy framework for Europe, Health21 (WHO/EURO 1999); some of this work is considered later in this chapter. The 1999 public health White Paper included a recognition that 'major new Government policies should be assessed for their impact on health' (Secretary of State for Health [SoSfH] 1999, para 4.45). This use of health impact assessment represents an important step in encouraging all sectors to contribute to health promotion and protection.

Two particularly important elements in PHC delivery are settings-based approaches to health promotion, and the need for inter-sectoral or multi-sectoral collaboration with coordinated action of the health sector with other sectors in the economy, and the development of effective partnerships between the many different agencies involved. The use of settings-based approaches can be seen in the Healthy Schools and Healthy Workplaces initiatives, while initiatives such as New Deal, Sure Start, New Opportunities Funding, regeneration (Single Regeneration Budget [SRB]) funding and Neighbourhood Renewal are all designed to support partnership working.

The variety of different agencies and organisations that need to be brought together provides a major challenge. As Taket & White (2000) conclude in their review of different models for joint working or partnership, there is a 'complexity of factors that affect the outcomes of multiagency work'. While it is possible to identify barriers to, and facilitating factors for, successful outcomes (however defined), generally such facilitating factors are found to be neither necessary nor sufficient, and barriers, while preventing successful outcomes in some contexts, can also be found in other contexts where successful outcomes are obtained. Similar conclusions are supported by Henwood's (1999) review of the Community Care Development Programme. Hiscock & Pearson (1999), based on a study of joint working between health and social services carried out in 1994 and 1995, concluded that joint working can be jeopardised by staff's preoccupations with changes within their own organisations. In the current context of frequent organisational change in the NHS, this is particularly relevant. Examples of successful partnership working are discussed later in this chapter. *Partnership in Action* (Department of Health [DH] 1998) signalled the introduction of new flexibilities, available following the passing of Health Bill in January 1999, which helped remove the barriers to joint working between health and social services. A summary of the new possibilities is given in Box 3.3. The 1999 Health Act extended the existing duty of partnership between health authorities and local authorities to NHS trusts and PCTs, reflecting the need for partnership in service commissioning and delivery, as well as strategic planning (SoSfH 1999, para 10.14).

Primary health care within the NHS

The current organisation of PHC in the NHS was set up in the White Paper published in 1997 (SoSfH 1997). This promised: 'a system we have called "integrated care", based on partnership and driven by performance' (para 1.3), and set in motion a ten-year programme to 'renew and improve the NHS'. In the UK, PHC within the NHS is mainly, but not solely, provided outside hospitals to people who are living in the community. Sometimes services are provided to people in their homes, as when a family doctor makes a home call, or a community nurse visits a patient. PHC is often provided through local health centres or clinics, but is increasingly provided in the settings of everyday life – where people work, live, study and socialise (the settings-based approaches to health promotion mentioned above). Some PHC staff, particularly midwives, provide services across hospital and community settings.

PHC is also often the main gateway to care at the secondary and tertiary levels when people are ill. In health service systems such as the NHS, which include some kind of personal or family doctor (general practitioners [GPs] in the UK context), people who have a health problem and decide to seek help often approach this doctor first. PHC is especially relevant for promotion of public health and figures importantly in strategies of 'the new public health movement'. PHC is often (though not exclusively) based on relatively simple technologies and frequently requires an understanding of the social and environmental context for health as well as professional skill in techniques and procedures. For example, health promotion professionals working to reduce smoking will aim to encourage individuals to change their own behaviour and will also aim to promote change in public or private organisations, such as restrictions on smoking in public places or workplaces or on tobacco advertising. This work will require

---

Box 3.3 Removing the barriers to joint working, supporting partnership

- *Pooled budgets*: health (health authority or PCT) and social service (local authority) budgets
- *Lead commissioning*: one authority transfers funds and delegates functions to the other so that they can commission both health and social care
- *Integrated provision*: NHS trust or PCT provides social care services beyond the level possible previously or a social services in-house provider provides a limited range of community health services

communication and facilitation skills as much as medical knowledge.

Primary health care teams

The PHC team is a term used to describe the group of professionals most closely involved in providing PHC to an individual or family. Giving a precise definition is hard, since in different places the term will be understood in rather different senses reflecting the particular local configurations of services that exist. Figure 3.1 depicts what are usually always included (the 'core' NHS team) and other potential members. Notice that the concept is often limited to staff related to health and personal social services, although in line with earlier discussion, it would be more appropriate to include a much wider group: the receptionists and practice manager at a health centre; individuals, families, communities; workers in other sectors. Note also that with contracting and new funding flexibilities, some services provided by the voluntary or private sectors, or by local authorities, may be funded from NHS budgets.

NHS staff working in PHC may be employed by NHS hospital trusts, PCTs, integrated trusts, mental health trusts or general practices. Considerable variation exists across the country. PCTs, discussed below, which were introduced in the 1997 health White Paper, represent the core organising mechanism for the future.

Primary care trusts[1]

The structure of PHC in the NHS in England is now organised around PCTs, the first wave of which went live on 1 April 2000. PCTs

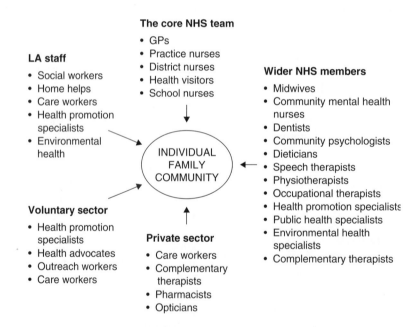

Note: The categories of staff listed under each heading are illustrative rather than exhaustive!

Figure 3.1 The primary care team – the National Health Service (NHS) core team and others potentially involved. Note: the categories of staff listed under each heading are illustrative rather than exhaustive! LA, local authority.

---

[1]The discussion here is in terms of England, structures are slightly different in other parts of the UK.

evolved out of the earlier primary care groups. PCTs were established as free-standing bodies accountable to the strategic health authority for commissioning care, and with added responsibility for the provision of community health services for their population. These services include district nursing, health visiting, physiotherapy, chiropody and speech therapy. Such trusts may include community health services transferred from NHS trusts. PCTs are able to run community hospitals and other community services. All or part of an existing community NHS trust may combine with a PCT in order to better integrate services and management support. Groups of PCTs sometimes also share services and management support.

PCTs covering all parts of England receive budgets directly from the DH. Since April 2002, PCTs have taken control of local health care whereas strategic health authorities monitor performance and standards. According to the DH (2002a) the main roles of PCTs are:

- Improving the health of the community
- Securing the provision of high-quality services
- Integrating health and social care locally

PCTs are required to have clear arrangements for public involvement including open meetings. PCTs are required to use a three-year planning cycle and to formulate local delivery plans (LDPs) that focus on the health and social care priorities set out in the DH's planning and priorities framework guidance (DH 2004). LDPs are then collated by strategic health authorities into a report for the whole strategic health authority area. There are currently 152 PCTs in England, and they control 80% of the NHS budget. The PCTs oversee 29 000 GPs and 18 000 NHS dentists. A nationally negotiated Quality and Outcomes Framework (QOF) is part of the contract PCTs have with GPs. It rewards best practice and improvement in quality. An example of more recent operational responsibilities may be found in the 2008/2009 NHS operating framework (DH 2008).

Current health policy places great emphasis on partnership and involvement, and the mechanisms of local strategic partnerships (LSPs) are designed to provide a focus for partnership working. An LSP is a single non-statutory, multi-agency body, which matches local authority boundaries, and aims to bring together at a local level the different parts of the public, private, community and voluntary sectors. LSPs are key to tackling deep-seated, multi-faceted problems, requiring a range of responses from different bodies. Local partners working through a LSP will be expected to take many of the major decisions about priorities and funding for their local area.

LSPs were central to the delivery of the New Commitment to Neighbourhood Renewal – National Strategy Action Plan (Standards and Effectiveness Unit [SEU] 2001). A five-year evaluation and action research programme of the LSPs was commissioned and results from this document showed the wide variety of different structures, membership and engagement achieved in the different LSPs, as well as the major challenges that LSPs face in terms of achieving transparency and involvement, and in shifting priorities in spending (Office of the Deputy Prime Minister [ODPM] 2004).

From the end of April 2004, the responsibilities of PCTs were increased to include being responsible authorities within local crime and disorder reduction partnerships (CDRPs). This places on PCTs the responsibility to work in partnership with other responsible authorities (police, fire and local authorities) to tackle crime, disorder and the misuse of drugs. The next section considers the work of these in relation to domestic violence.

Primary health care in the community – key issues and initiatives

As the previous section has indicated the organisation of PHC provision is changing, at what often seems, for those involved in it, a very rapid pace. This section picks up some of the important issues identified earlier, reviews briefly a number of studies/projects that illustrate current developments and introduces a range of current research. The issues to be addressed are: health promotion; tackling health inequalities; health and regeneration; and, contributing to CDRPs, the example of domestic violence.

Health promotion – everybody's business

As was mentioned earlier, the Alma-Ata concept of PHC stresses the importance of promoting and protecting health. A programme in health promotion was established in the WHO Regional Office for Europe in 1984, taking as its starting point the need to clarify some of the concepts and principles involved in the promotion of health. The definition of health promotion adopted was:

'the process of enabling people to increase control over, and to improve, their health. This perspective is derived from a conception of "health" as the extent to which an individual or group is able, on the one hand, to realise aspirations and satisfy needs, and, on the other hand, to change or cope with the environment. Health is, therefore, seen as a resource for everyday life, not the objective of living; it is a positive concept emphasising social and personal resources, as well as physical capacities.'

(WHO/EURO 1984, pp. 653–654)

Along with this comes a recognition that health promotion requires action not only within the health services, but within other sectors as well: 'health promotion… encompasses actions to protect or enhance health, including legal, fiscal, educational and social measures' (Whitehead 1989, p. 7). Elsewhere this type of model of health promotion has been referred to as the 'empowerment model' (Wallerstein 2006; Wallerstein & Bernstein 1988; Whitehead 1989), with the former linking it to Freire's pedagogy. The key features of the empowerment model are that it is positive, dynamic, enabling and participative. It aims to perform a delicate balancing act between recognising the constraints on healthy choices faced by people due to the environments (in the widest sense) in which they live and work, and strengthening people's

potential for taking action to improve their health (without slipping into victim-blaming). Health promotion programmes and initiatives therefore involve a wide spectrum of activities including advocacy, mediation, enabling, etc. This model of health promotion is the one underlying the various HFA policies (see chronology in Box 3.1). What is more debatable is how well this understanding has been taken up within UK health policy where there are still struggles over this model of health promotion (see for example: Kickbusch 1997; Naidoo 1986; Ziglio 1997).

Following on from work developing basic principles and concepts of health promotion, further work was initiated to explore mechanisms by which these might be put into practice. The first of these was a project aimed at exploring the concept of the 'healthy city' (Duhl 1986). This commenced in the European Region of the WHO in 1985, involving a small network of European cities (Tsouros 1990). By 1993, the project had grown rapidly, yielding 18 national networks and hundreds of towns and cities actively involved in Europe, North America, and, increasingly, low-income countries (Hancock 1993); it had also become known as the Healthy Cities movement, or Healthy Communities in some parts of the world. Besides the European Region, WHO has supported healthy city activities in the African Region, the Eastern Mediterranean Region and the Western Pacific Region (WHO 1994). The work has drawn explicitly on experience outside the health sector. The sources of this experience include community development workers, as well as broad social movements with origins in the community/voluntary sector, such as feminist, black and minority ethnic, civil rights and green organisations and groups. A valuable emphasis of much of the successful healthy cities work has been in stressing the importance of the local context for the selection of priorities for action and of the importance of achieving widespread involvement in, and commitment to, local action. This has particularly involved work around community participation and inter-sectoral collaboration, two of the themes of

HFA. The early work on healthy cities has since led on to the development of other approaches based in particular settings, such as health-promoting schools, workplaces and hospitals (WHO/EURO 1993).

Work in another area, 'healthy public policy', built on the earlier experience and responded to the danger of reducing health promotion to a variety of victim-blaming strategies by emphasising the importance of policy in all sectors in creating social, physical and economic environments where 'healthy choices become the easy choices':

'Healthy public policy is the policy challenge set by a new vision of public health. It refers to policy decisions in any sector or level of government that are characterised by an explicit concern for health and an accountability for health impact. It is expressed through horizontal strategies such as inter-sectoral cooperation and public participation.'

(Adelaide Conference on Healthy Public Policy 1988)

The notion of healthy public policy is argued to provide a foundation for promoting physical and social environments that support the adoption of healthy patterns of living (WHO/EURO 1993). Its aim is to ensure equitable access to the prerequisites for health, whether in the form of consumer goods, supportive living environments, or services that contribute to healthy living. It seeks to stimulate action and the development of specific mechanisms so that decision-makers at all levels and in all sectors are aware of the consequences for health of their decisions, and are willing to accept their share of responsibility for health in their communities. The commitment to health impact assessment for new policy (SoSfH 1999, para 4.45) reflects the UK government's intention to seek healthy public policy in the future.

Tackling health inequalities

Within the UK, major inequalities in health exist, by income, occupation, ethnicity, geography (the north–south divide). Many are persistent or even widening (Acheson *et al.* 1998). Of particular concern are the health inequalities experienced by groups whose needs are marginalised by mainstream service provision and/or those suffering social exclusion. Tackling health inequalities is one key challenge facing PHC, and requires the creation of effective partnerships, as well as effective inter-sectoral and multi-sectoral action.

A growing body of research demonstrates different ways in which the health of disadvantaged groups has been improved. Some studies have demonstrated the key role that voluntary sector organisations can play; one example is presented in Box 3.4, and others are reviewed by Taket (1999). Chapter 4 describes the important role that community development approaches can play in tackling health inequalities, also illustrated by the example in Box 3.4.

Health Action Zones (HAZs) have been one policy initiative aimed at stimulating innovation, and particularly at tackling health inequalities:

'New Health Action Zones will blaze the trail.… The accent will be on partnership and innovation, finding new ways to tackle health problems and reshape local services. Health Action Zones will be concentrated in areas of pronounced deprivation and poor health, reflecting the Government's commitment to tackle entrenched inequalities. An early task for each Health Action Zone will be to develop clear targets, agreed with the NHS Executive, for measurable improvements every year.'

(SoSfH 1997, para 10.6)

National and local evaluations of the achievements of HAZs (Barnes *et al.* 2005; Bauld & Judge 2002) have shown mixed success in identifying and implementing ways of reducing health inequalities, with the most successful innovations being integrated into mainstream service provision as the HAZ funding ended.

Health and regeneration

The next topic to be considered in this section relates to regeneration programmes. These provide an example of multi-sectoral initiatives

---

Box 3.4   Racial harassment as a health issue

Tower Hamlets Health Strategy Group (THHSG) is a voluntary organisation seeking to promote the health of the people of Tower Hamlets, East London.[2] A major part of the role of the group is undertaking action research projects to develop and evaluate appropriate innovatory forms of health-related service provision, which address previously unmet needs for underserved groups within the local communities. Its voluntary sector position has also facilitated the ability to challenge, where appropriate, professional views current in mainstream services. In estate-based health promotion work carried out in the late 1980s (under a community development philosophy, see Chapter 4) with Asian women living in local authority housing, a major issue raised by the women as affecting their lives was racial harassment. The women's strategy of avoidance by minimising time spent outside the home severely curtailed their activities and led to increasing feelings of isolation. The identification of racial harassment as a health issue was something that was initially resisted quite strongly by the health authority (demonstrating clearly the institutional racism affecting statutory services). After continued pressure from the THHSG, this was eventually accepted as a health issue that required a response on the part of the NHS, and was responded to through the provision of training to NHS workers about how to support individuals experiencing racial harassment.

The 1999 public health White Paper contains acknowledgement that tackling racial harassment still remains an issue – both outside and inside the NHS (SoSfH 1999, para 9.30).

---

that have considerable potential for addressing the health inequalities existing in particular localities. Funding to support regeneration programmes is available through the SRB scheme supported by the Department of Transport, Environment and the Regions.

Traditional regeneration programmes have concentrated on employment, on the physical environment, and on housing redevelopment. Obviously these have impacts, direct and indirect, on health. It is only comparatively recently however, that, during the 1990s, the design and implementation of regeneration programmes began to take health issues explicitly into account. A publication from a 1998 conference (Tower Hamlets Health Strategy Group/ Health Education Authority [THHSG/HEA] 1998) summarised much of the work in the field. This was then taken a step further, through the modification of the objectives allowed in programmes supported by SRB funding to include 'enhancing the quality of life, health and capacity to contribute to regeneration'. This expansion of the remit of SRB funding opened the door to a successful regeneration bid led by a health authority (now a strategic health authority) and

focused around the health sector. This example is described in Box 3.5. Other health authorities have since followed suit.

Contributing to Crime and Disorder Reduction Partnerships, the example of domestic violence

The last topic to be considered in this section is domestic violence as an example of the contribution that the heath service can make to CDRPs. Domestic violence is a major crime issue, accounting for almost a quarter (23%) of all reported violent crime (British Crime Survey [BCS] 2000), but it is also a generally unacknowledged public health issue. Intimate partner abuse, often termed domestic violence, is the abuse and control of a person by their current or former intimate partner. Partner abuse occurs in all types of relationships, both same sex and heterosexual. However, the highest prevalence is found for abuse against women, a review of population-based studies across the world, found that between 10% and 69% of women reported being physically assaulted by an intimate male partner at some time in their lives (Heise *et al.* 1999). Thus, for women, domestic

---

[2]Since 2000 the group has become Social Action for Health, see http://safh.org.uk/.

Box 3.5   Health and regeneration – the example of Redbridge and Waltham Forest

'The Health Ladder to Social Inclusion' was the first broad health-based SRB programme in the UK. It was led by City and East London Strategic Health Authority and was a seven-year programme, involving many different organisational partners, across public, voluntary and private sectors. The programme commenced in November 1999, and the major spending started in April 2000. Approximately £8 million SRB funding was involved, with at least an equivalent amount in matched funding from the various different partner agencies. The SRB involved projects in the following four main areas:

- Jobs and training
- Capacity building
- Access to PHC services
- Public health

The area covered by the SRB programme comprises 19 electoral wards, with a total population of approximately 215 000. This population has a higher proportion of black and minority ethnic residents than average for London (30% in Waltham Forest bid area and 34% in Redbridge bid area), and poorer health and greater mental health needs than other parts of these two local authority areas. The target groups for the SRB programme were:

- People experiencing social disadvantage in the SRB area (including homeless people and those living in temporary accommodation)
- Black and minority ethnic communities and refugee communities
- Young people
- Older people

The bid was the outcome of an extensive process of consultation and partnership working, involving statutory, voluntary, community and private sectors. It also built on the considerable experience of the Community Health Project in the South of Waltham Forest, which was recognised locally, nationally and internationally for its work with socially excluded communities, including refugees and black and minority ethnic communities. The SRB programme made use of the flexibilities introduced in 'Partnership in Action', (see Box 3.3).

---

violence has a higher lifetime prevalence than breast cancer.

Abuse is associated with both acute and chronic medical problems that are frequently treated in the health care system, with associated resource consequences. The cost for the NHS of physical injuries alone from domestic violence is estimated at around £1.2 billion a year (Walby 2004). Domestic violence affects women from all age groups, all ethnic and religious groups, at all income levels. It represents a health problem for those experiencing it, and health impacts are not limited to short-term injuries. Domestic violence can lead to acute and chronic physical injury, miscarriage, loss of hearing and vision, and physical disfigurement. It often leads to depression and alcoholism, and sometimes to suicide. Children are also affected – many women and children develop post-traumatic stress disorder, and experience years of distress. Despite the many opportunities for abused women to disclose in the health care setting, research has shown that approximately 3% to less than 10% of all abused women are identified by health care professionals (Yam 2000). These statistics show the unrealised opportunities for health care professionals to enable abused women to improve their lives.

Recently, there have been a number of projects within the health service, exploring how this important public health issue can be tackled, most particularly in primary care settings. There is an increasing body of research (see for example studies reviewed in Taket 2004; Taket *et al.* 2003, 2004) that demonstrates that health professionals can make an important difference to the health and well-being of women and children by providing information about the specialised services that exist, and enabling women to access specialised services.

A number of projects have investigated routine enquiry in health service settings, i.e. aiming to ask all women about experience, if any, of domestic violence, on her own in a private and confidential area, with a female interpreter if necessary. Routine enquiry can be carried out in many different ways: in well women clinics, in general practice by GPs or practice nurses, in the antenatal or maternity services setting to name just a few. The aim of routine enquiry is to facilitate, and not force, disclosure. It must remain the woman's choice as to if, when, and to whom, she discloses. Evaluations of projects have demonstrated that routine enquiry is feasible and sustainable, and acceptable to the vast majority of women (both those who have experienced abuse and those who have not). Many women report that, without being asked directly, they will not disclose their experience. Finding out about locally available specialised support services is important in helping women to consider their options, and receiving the clear message from trusted health professionals that domestic abuse is unacceptable, and *not* their fault, is extremely important. Although many health professionals, prior to training, are apprehensive about raising the topic, once trained and implementing routine enquiry, health professionals report that they find it useful.

Looking to the future

This short closing section offers a brief review of the challenges facing PHC for the future. Perhaps the single largest challenge facing PHC is that of reducing health inequalities, tackling particularly the multiply disadvantaged positions that black and minority ethnic groups often find themselves in. The importance of tackling inequalities has been fully recognised in health policy, and this chapter has earlier presented examples of some promising avenues of approach. Much work however remains to be done in evaluating the various initiatives underway and then acting on the knowledge

gained. This connects to the second challenge to be mentioned here, that of developing the evidence base for PHC practice, a task specifically for research as discussed in Chapter 6, which runs alongside the challenge of reshaping the delivery of PHC to utilise this evidence base in practice.

Another major challenge for all of those working within PHC is the pace of organisational change. Here a continuation of the tension between drive for seeking 'better' forms of organisation leading to a rapid succession of initiatives requiring changes, and letting one change settle in, before rolling out the next, can be expected. An enormous change agenda has already been set for the future following the prominent role that PCTs will now play in the reformed NHS, with the full implementation of the new GP contract, as well as initiatives such as the use of salaried GPs, the development of walk in centres, polyclinics and local diagnostic and treatment centres. Major changes can still be expected in the roles of different health professionals, and the development of the advanced practitioner in particular will open up new opportunities for nurses and others working in the community (DH 2007, 2008).

Another area remaining a challenge for the future is ensuring a truly multi-professional basis for the delivery of PHC. A continuation of changes in skill mix and role development within all professional groups can be expected as the NHS moves forward to reform future plans for service delivery. In talking of a 'primary care-led NHS', the WHO concept of PHC implies that it is important that this is led multi-professionally, and not reduced to a GP-led NHS. The dangers of a GP-led NHS are the perpetuation of a restricted understanding of PHC, and in particular, a lack of attention to protection and promotion of health (Box 3.6).

The WHO concept of PHC introduced in this chapter implies an extensive and important role for the nursing profession in PHC. The WHO Regional Office for Europe, the International Council of Nurses (ICN), and the International Council of Midwives (ICM), issued a joint call in February 2000, for a Europe-wide public

---

Box 3.6   Contradictions in policy?

'He [Tony Blair] promised that GPs were "central to the delivery of our vision for the health service", driving change and co-ordinating the different "levels of care" from basic community and social services through to the acute hospital sector and rehabilitation. The health secretary later amplified this, saying that GPs would be at the centre of a "single system shaped around the needs of the patient".'

(*Health Service Journal* HSJ 23/3/2000, p. 13, reporting the GP2000 conference).

'General practice is a fundamental part of health care. At its centre is the care provided to people who are ill or believe themselves to be ill, and at its heart a doctor-patient relationship based on mutual trust and personal attention focused on the individual.' John Chisholm, Chairman, General Practitioner Committee, British Medical Association, writing in the foreword to Mihill (2000), which forms a major part of the General Practitioner Committee's policy review process. It contains only four references to health promotion, only one of the many doctors quoted in the report explicitly mentions health promotion as a part of general practice.

Taken together these quotes illustrate the ambiguity surrounding the multi-professional nature of PHC and the importance of the promotion and protection of health within it. They seem explicitly to draw on a much more restricted notion of PHC than that envisaged within the WHO concept, and which is required to address health inequalities. As a further example of the potential difficulties, note the study of Barclay *et al.* (1999) into priorities for palliative care services, which found considerable differences between GPs and district nurses in terms of views on service adequacy and priorities for future development.

---

health campaign for nurses, health visitors and midwives. This is intended as an initiative to strengthen the impact that nurses, health visitors, and midwives have on improving health in the context of WHO's Health21 health for all policy framework. The campaign will emphasise the importance of developing effective teamwork skills and engaging in interdisciplinary teams to promote health, and provide care and treatment. It will also stress the overwhelming significance of developing 'family health nurses' as a force for health improvement throughout the European Region. In the UK, this is reflected in the recommendation that the health visitor develops a family-centred public health role (DH 2006, SoSfH 1999). In the words of Kirsten Stalknecht, President of ICN:

'It is clear that nurses and midwives are at the heart of most effective health care teams, especially the PHC team. Using their varied capacities and expertise, nurses and midwives working in many different capacities will make major contributions to Health21.

Nurse policy-makers, managers, educators and clinicians are already leading initiatives that improve the health of the population as a whole, and narrow the gap in health. The Health21 nurse and midwife movement will make all these contributions more visible and should inspire new initiatives.'

References

Acheson, D. *et al.* (1998) *Independent Inquiry into Inequalities in Health*. The Stationery Office, London.

Adelaide Conference on Healthy Public Policy (1988) *Report on Second International Conference on Health Promotion*. Adelaide, South Australia.

Barclay, S., Todd, C., McCabe, J. & Hunt, T. (1999) Primary care group commissioning of services: the differing priorities of general practitioners and district nurses for palliative care services. *British Journal of General Practice*, **49**, 181–186.

Barnes, M., Bauld, L., Benzeval, M., McKenzie, M. & Sullivan, H. (eds) (2005) *Health Action Zones: Partnerships for Health Equity*. Routledge, London.

Bauld, L. & Judge, K. (eds) (2002) *Learning from Health Action Zones*. Aeneas Press, Chichester.

British Crime Survey, 2000. Home Office, London.

Bomberg, E. & Peterson, J. (1993) Prevention from Above? The Role of the European Community. In: *Prevention, Health and British Politics* (ed. M. Mills). Avebury, Aldershot, pp. 140–160.

Department of Health (1998) *Partnership in Action: New Opportunities for Joint Working Between Health and Social Services.* Department of Health, London.

Department of Health (2002a) *Shifting the Balance of Power.* Department of Health, London.

Department of Health (2004) *National Standards, Local Action: Health and Social Care Standards and Planning Framework,* 2005/05–2007/08. Department of Health, London.

Department of Health (2006) *Our Health, Our Care, Our Say: A New Direction for Community Services.* Department of Health, London.

Department of Health (2007) *Our NHS Our Future: NHS Next Stage Review – Interim Report* – Lord Ara Darzi. Available at: www.dh.gov.uk/en/Publicati onsandstatistics/Publications/PublicationsPolicy AndGuidance/dh_079077 (accessed 20 November 2008).

Department of Health (2008) *The NHS in England: The Operating Framework for 2008/2009.* Department of Health, London.

Duhl, L.J. (1986) The healthy city: its function and its future. *Health Promotion,* **1**, 55–60.

Gish, O. (1992) Malaria eradication and the selective approach to health care: some lessons from Ethiopia. *International Journal of Health Services,* **22**, 179–192.

Godlee, F. (1995) The World Health Organization: WHO in Europe: does it have a role? *British Medical Journal,* **310**, 389–394.

Hancock, T. (1993) The evolution, impact and significance of the healthy cities/healthy communities movement. *Journal of Public Health Policy,* **14**, 5–18.

Heise, L., Ellsberg, M. & Gottemoeller, M. (1999) Ending violence against women. *Population Reports,* Series L, No 11. Johns Hopkins University School of Public Health, Population Information Program, Baltimore. Available at: www.jhuccp.org/pr/ l11edsum.shtml (accessed 12 February 2003).

Henwood, M. (1999) *The Community Care Development Programme: Building Partnerships for Success: An Evaluation Report to the Department Of Health.* Department of Health, London.

Hiscock, J. & Pearson, M. (1999) Looking inwards, looking outwards: Dismantling the 'Berlin Wall' between health and social services? *Social Policy and Administration,* **33**, 150–163.

Kickbusch, I. (1997) Think health: what makes the difference? *Health Promotion International,* **12**, 265–272.

Kokkonen, P.T. & Kekomäki, M. (1993) Legal and economic issues in European public health. In: *Europe Without Frontiers: The Implications for Health* (eds C.E.M. Normand & P. Vaughan). Wiley, London, pp. 35–43.

Mihill, C. (2000) *Shaping Tomorrow: Issues Facing General Practice in the New Millennium.* British Medical Association, London.

Naidoo, J. (1986) Limits to individualism. In: *The Politics of Health Education* (eds S. Rodmell & A. Watt). Routledge, London, pp. 17–37.

Office of the Deputy Prime Minister (2004) *LSP Evaluation and Action Research Programme, Case-Studies Interim Report: A Baseline of Practice.* Office of the Deputy Prime Minister, London.

Pannenborg, C.O. (1991) Shifting paradigms of international health. *Asia Pacific Journal of Public Health,* **5**, 176–184.

Regional Office for Europe. Reproduced in: *Measurement in Health Promotion and Protection* (1987) (eds T. Abelin *et al.*). World Health Organization, Copenhagen, pp. 653–658.

Standards and Effectiveness Unit (2001) *A New Commitment to Neighbourhood Renewal – National Strategy Action Plan.* Cabinet Office, London.

Secretary of State for Health (1997) *The New NHS: Modern, Dependable* (Cm 3807). The Stationery Office, London.

Secretary of State for Health (1999) *Saving Lives: Our Healthier Nation* (Cm 4386). The Stationery Office, London.

Taket, A.R. (1999) Tackling health inequalities in communities: the role of the voluntary sector. Paper Presented at Conference on 'Researching For Health: Challenges and Controversies'. Heriot-Watt University, Edinburgh.

Taket, A.R. (2004) *Tackling Domestic Violence: The Role of Health Professionals.* Home Office Development and Practice Report 32. Home Office, London. Available at www.homeoffice.gov.uk/rds/pdfs04/dpr32.pdf (accessed 20 November 2008).

Taket, A.R. & White, L.A. (2000) *Partnership and Participation: Decision-Making in the Multiagency Setting.* Wiley, Chichester.

Taket, A.R., Nurse, J., Smith, K., Watson, J., Shakespeare, J., Lavis, V., Cosgrove, K., Mulley, K. & Feder, G. (2003) Routinely asking women about domestic violence in health settings. *British Medical Journal,* **327**, 673–676.

Taket, A.R., Beringer, A., Irvine, A. & Garfield, S. (2004) *Tackling Domestic Violence: Exploring the Health Service Contribution. Evaluation of the Crime Reduction Programme Violence Against Women Initiative Health Projects.* Home Office Online Report 52/04. Available at www.homeoffice.gov.uk/rds/pdfs04/rdsolr5204.pdf (accessed 20 November 2008).

Tower Hamlets Health Strategy Group/Health Education Authority (1998) *Putting Health on the Regeneration Agenda: Proceedings of a Conference Held at London Guildhall University on 2nd April 1998.* Health Education Authority, London.

Tsouros, A.D. (1990) *World Health Organization Healthy Cities Project: A Project Becomes a Movement – Review of Progress 1987–1990.* SOGESS, Milan.

Walby, S. (2004) *The Cost of Domestic Violence.* University of Leeds, Leeds.

Wallerstein, N. (2006) What is the Evidence on Effectiveness of Empowerment to Improve Health? WHO Regional Office for Europe, Copenhagen. Health Evidence Network report. Available at www.euro.who.int/Document/E88086.pdf (accessed 5 June 2008).

Wallerstein, N. & Bernstein, E. (1988) Empowerment education: Freire's ideas adapted to health education. *Health Education Quarterly*, **15**, 379–394.

Whitehead, M. (1989) *Swimming Upstream: Trends and Prospects for Education in Health.* King's Fund, London.

World Health Organization (1994) *The Work of WHO 1992–1993 – Biennial Report of the Director General.* World Health Organization, Geneva.

WHO/EURO (1984) *Summary Report of the Working Group on Concepts and Principles of Health Promotion.* World Health Organization, Copenhagen.

WHO/EURO (1985) *Targets for health for all.* WHO Regional Office for Europe, Copenhagen.

WHO/EURO (1993) *Health for all Targets: The Health Policy for Europe.* Updated edition, September 1991. WHO Regional Office for Europe, Copenhagen.

WHO/EURO (1999) *Health 21 – The Health for all Policy Framework for the WHO European Region.* WHO Regional Office for Europe, Copenhagen.

WHO/UNICEF (1978) *Primary Health Care: Report of the International Conference on Primary Health Care, Alma-Ata.* World Health Organization, Geneva.

Yam, M. (2000) Seen but not heard: battered women's perceptions of the ED experience. *Journal of Emergency Nursing*, **26**, 464–470.

Ziglio, E. (1997) How to move towards evidence-based health promotion interventions. *Promotion and Education*, **4**, 29–33.

Chapter 4 Community Development in Public Health and Primary Care

Jane Wills

Introduction

Primary care organisations have been placed at the centre of health services development in the major changes that have taken place in the organisation of health services in recent years. In addition to their role in the treatment of ill health and the commissioning of secondary care services, they are also expected to take the lead in improving the health of their local populations. Public partnership and involvement is enshrined in health policy initiatives and the focus on a needs-led service has revived interest in community development approaches.

The NHS Plan (Department of Health [DH] 2000) set out the vision of a service where care is shaped around the convenience and concerns of patients, their carers and the public – where all will have more say over their own treatment and more influence over the way in which the organisation works. The rationale behind this draws on a growing understanding that:

- Patients' experience of care is intimately tied to the effectiveness of that care – patients' views can help to improve the impact of health care services
- The way care is provided affects more than satisfaction with care, but also patients' physiological, functional and psychological outcomes
- Health care services need to adapt to the changing needs and aspirations of better-informed and more assertive patients/public (Crawford *et al.* 2002; Florin & Dixon 2004; Harrison *et al.* 2002)

Participatory approaches to involvement can cover a broad spectrum of attitude and purpose. Taylor (2007) describes these as the consumerist approach in which people are asked for their views on specific issues or services, the representative approach where members of the public sit on advisory groups and committees to community development which involves active engagement with a defined group of people over an extended period of time in order to identify and tackle some of the issues that determine their health and quality of life. These moves to greater public involvement pose the twin challenges for the National Health Service (NHS) of transferring power and ensuring that decisions are representative of a public view. Many of the barriers to involvement are linked to the culture of health care professionals that fosters a belief in professional expertise and does not value lay understandings and priorities. Developing appropriate methods to effectively involve the public and their ability to recognise, evaluate and address health problems are further challenges.

This chapter commences with a short outline of the policy context for community development and approaches to health improvement and then explores the term 'community development' and the related concepts of social capital, capacity building and social inclusion. The second half of the chapter moves on to discuss some of the challenges and opportunities commonly associated with community development approaches including appropriate and compatible methods of evaluation. These will be illustrated by a brief case study of an innovative community health project.

The current context for community development practice

This section outlines the underlying themes of national policies and strategies and how they relate to communities and community development. The political philosophy of the Labour Government from 1997 embodied values of individual rights, duties and responsibilities as well as social justice and fairness. The concern to retreat from traditional welfare support led to a focus on greater choice, more devolved services and individual rights as consumers of services. These values have given rise to specific strategies and policy initiatives including:

- Devolved services allowing local flexibility and freedom, with additional 'earned autonomy' for best performing services
- Quality assurance and service accountability through clear standards and performance criteria
- Partnership working to erode professional barriers and enable the delivery of seamless services
- A positive focus on disadvantaged or excluded groups
- A community focus to build capacity and encourage communities to be active providers as well as users of services (Naidoo & Wills 2005)

Government policy has emphasised the importance of participation by users and the public in the modernisation agenda for health and social care. In 1998 the NHS Executive published a document on developing strategies for public participation in the NHS, which recommended using community development as a key part of health needs assessment and as a means of engaging communities in solving local health problems in partnership with statutory agencies (NHS Executive 1998). A significant lever was added through the Health and Social Care Act 2001 section 11 Strengthening Accountability (DH 2003), which was further enhanced by the Local Government and Public Involvement in Health Act 2007, by which each strategic health authority (SHA) and primary care trust (PCT) must proactively seek and build 'continuous and meaningful' engagement with patients to shape services (DH 2007). The Patient Advice and Liaison Service (PALS) offers a one stop advisory service in each hospital and PCT. This acts alongside an independent complaints advocacy service (ICAS). Local Involvement Networks (LINks) are the local bodies which gather the views of patients and users, ask for information from services and make recommendations on the commissioning of services. (Further information from www.nhs-centreforinvolvement.nhs.uk.) The commitment and recognition of the need for involvement as a key function of the modernisation agenda is summarised by the New Economics Foundation: 'Our institutions are starting to appreciate that a lack of accountability breeds a lack of legitimacy and trust. We are starting to understand that society is now so complex that no decision will stick unless it has involved everybody with a stake in it' (Lewis & Walker 1998).

Local government has also undergone a modernisation programme including a more responsive and community-oriented approach. A new duty has been imposed on local authorities under the Local Government Act 2000 to take the lead role in drawing up a community strategy alongside local neighbourhood strategies, to enhance local well-being through creating employment opportunities, reducing crime, improving housing and reducing the gap between the better off and disadvantaged areas. This process is overseen by a local strategic partnership that can enable 'local communities to articulate their needs and priorities' (Department of the Environment, Transport and Regions [DETR] 2000). The delivery plan for the community strategy is known as the Local Area Agreement.

Alongside this focus on involvement and participation there has been a renewed focus on 'the community' as the site where needs are both defined and met. The public health White Paper, *Choosing Health: Making Healthy Choices Easier* refers to how 'the environment we live in, our social networks, our sense of security, socio-economic circumstances, families and resources in our local neighbourhood can affect individual health' (DH 2004). Policy initiatives have attempted to address many of the characteristics of community. There has been a raft of regeneration initiatives intended to transform the country's most deprived and excluded areas. The sense that people have of community is also forged through everyday societal inter-actions and networks of friends, families and neighbours. Health inequalities are now clearly linked with the concept of social exclusion, the latter being defined as:

> 'What happens when individuals or areas suf-fer from a combination of linked problems such as unemployment, low incomes, poor housing, a high crime environment, poor health and family breakdown.'

> (www.socialexclusion.gov.uk)

This concept of social inclusion in which every-one, whatever their circumstances, is encour-aged to make use of opportunities to participate in society, has permeated policy. The govern-ment department of Communities and Local Government (www.communitiesgov.uk) is responsible, among other things, for build-ing sustainable communities, neighbourhood renewal and tackling anti-social behaviour. Working with and for communities through community development has now ceased to be seen as experimental and radical but much more mainstream in policy and service delivery and a vital public health function.

Defining the terms

This section discusses the key terms and concepts used when exploring the potential for promoting health in a participatory way: community, com-munity development and empowerment.

Defining community

The meaning of the word 'community' has also long been contested in sociological and policy terms. Jewkes & Murcott (1996) claim there are at least 55 different definitions in use. It is often conflated with neighbourhood yet many differ-ent kinds of communities exist. Geographically defined communities are convenient for agencies that want to work within boundaries, but living in the same place does not necessarily guaran-tee a common view. More recently, the emphasis has been on communities of interest with shared needs such as 'teenage mothers' or 'people with learning disabilities'. Marginalised communities

are those whose contributions are invisible. They may experience discrimination and may not make use of traditional or mainstream serv-ices. Examples of such groups are asylum seek-ers, gypsies and travellers, and homeless people. Other communities are those defined by: service use; shared interests or occupation; or by char-acteristics such as culture, religion and sexual orientation. Understanding who comprises the community and in what ways they share needs or concerns is vital to practice. Laverack (2004) identifies four characteristics of community:

- Spatial dimension, i.e. a place or location
- Interests, issues, identities that link other-wise heterogenous groups
- Shared needs and concerns that can be achieved through collective action
- Social interactions and relationships that bind people together

The question of who to involve in a 'commu-nity' is similarly complicated. Early attempts to increase participation focused on a strategy of involving those who were most accessible, who tended to be local leaders. For example, attempts to reach ethnic minority groups fre-quently employ strategies of contacting faith leaders or using existing groups that meet at religious buildings. Identifying 'activists' and those used to participating in groups – those in tenant groups or parents' associations – may also be seen as ways of increasing involvement and getting a 'lay voice'. Where there is no clear constituency these representatives tend to be drawn from voluntary sector agencies. 'These constraints result in the community representa-tives being drawn from one small part of the voluntary sector, the larger funded organisa-tions' (Jewkes & Murcott 1998).

Understanding the networks that exist within a community provides opportunities to iden-tify routes through which less visible mem-bers need to be engaged. Personal networks can both sustain communities and contribute to the effectiveness of community activity. It is not surprising then that there has been so much interest in the concept of social capital, the term used to describe networks and shared norms that facilitate coordination and cooperation for mutual benefit and create civic engagement. It is a relatively new concept that has aroused considerable debate about how it should be defined and measured. It originated with the work of Robert Putnam in Italy and the USA (Putnam 2000; Putnam *et al.* 1993). Putnam found that the very poor living in urban areas in the USA who have a few relatively intense family or neighbourhood ties are trapped in their poverty whereas those with a wider network of weaker contacts do better.

There is a body of evidence that suggests that low social capital and social exclusion arising from poverty or discrimination is linked to poor health. Wilkinson (1996, 2005) has argued that the level of inequality in a society is crucial in determining a range of factors, from the overall life expectancy of a population through to levels of violence and teenage birth rates. Low social status, poor friendship networks and difficult early childhood experience contribute to psychosocial insecurity, anxiety and people's sense of whether they are valued and appreciated. These are major sources of stress and may contribute to pathways which link a variety of social problems to relative deprivation and adverse health outcomes. It has also been demonstrated that where the levels of social capital are high, associated health benefits are evident. For example, reductions in infant mortality and increases in life expectancy (Putnam *et al.* 1993), lower levels of deaths from stroke, accidents and suicide and improved survival from heart disease (Kawachi & Kennedy 1997) and lower levels of common mental disorders (de Silva *et al.* 2005) have all been linked to social capital. For communities to be empowered and strengthened, there has to be a level of mutual trust and cooperation. In this way the concept of social capital is helpful as it provides a framework to examine the processes through which formal and informal social connections and networks can protect people against the worst effects of deprivation.

The related concept of 'community capacity' refers to the set of assets or strengths possessed by a community. 'Capacity building' is a systematic approach to build the confidence and ability of individuals, community and voluntary groups/organisations to influence decision-making and service delivery. This could include enabling communities to provide and manage services and programmes to meet community needs. So it may be used in a functional way to equip people for particular jobs through skills training or NVQ accreditation or it may involve personal or organisational development. The term 'releasing capacity' is therefore often preferred to reflect the view that local people are not 'empty vessels' and do have valuable experience, knowledge and skills.

Defining community development

This section discusses:

- Definitions of community development and community empowerment and how it differs from community-based health promotion
- Historical perspectives on community development
- Relationship between community development and patient and public involvement.

There is no one widely accepted definition of community development. The Standing Conference on Community Development published a definition of community development that clarifies it as a process:

> 'Community development is about building active and sustainable communities based on social justice and mutual respect. It is about changing power structures to remove the barriers that prevent people from participating in the issues that affect their lives. Community workers support individuals, groups and organizations in this process.'

> (Standing Conference on Community Development 2001 and at www.sccd.org.uk)

Some of the key principles underpinning 'community development' are summarised in Box 4.1.

The rise in popularity of community development approaches in the UK is relatively recent but it is a not a new concept. It can be traced back to late nineteenth century America

> **Box 4.1 Some key principles of community development**
>
> - A collective endeavour to identify and act on issues of concern to individuals and communities
> - Involves local leaders and local people to tackle the problems identified
> - Is emancipatory – empowering communities, building their confidence and capacity
> - Emphasises community participation in the promotion of more equitable and accessible services
> - Recognises the importance of social networks and social support
> - Provides support to challenge and influence the development and implementation of public policies
> - Requires organisations to respond to the identified needs of communities
> - Promotes social inclusion and emphasises tackling discrimination
> - Aims to reduce inequalities
> - Values 'joined up', inter-sectoral working

where its roots lie in colonialism and strategies for social control. At that time black self-help groups were organised by the Republican Party to improve agricultural productivity. This approach was extended to teach Native Americans better management of land, health and education with little emphasis on empowerment or autonomy (Community Practitioners and Health Visitors Association [CPHVA] 1999).

In the UK the rise of community development approaches can be traced to the Community Development Project launched by the Home Office in 1969. Twelve projects were funded to determine new ways of responding to the needs of those living in neighbourhoods with high social deprivation (Jones 1990). The underlying philosophy and principles were essentially radical, progressive and concerned with social equity, based on an analysis of the socioeconomic and political structures responsible for poverty. However, conflicts with government policy ensued and project workers began to question the government's intentions – control of the poor, defusion of the threat of racial and

urban unrest. Rather inauspiciously, funding for the projects was withdrawn (Tones & Tilford 2001). In the 1970s and early 1980s numerous community development health projects were set up, mostly funded and located outside the NHS. Inner city decline prompted projects to tackle neighbourhood renewal, sexual health, and youth and leisure provision. Key features of these projects reveal their radical dimensions:

- They are located outside the health professions
- They are concerned with inequalities in health and health care provision
- They promote a collective awareness of the social causes of ill-health
- They challenge the professional monopoly of information about health and ill-health
- Activities centre on work with small groups of local people (Rosenthal 1983).

An understanding of power and control in relation to, for example, the use and ownership of information, the role and agenda of professionals or the active discrimination against certain groups inform the theoretical basis of community development. Community development approaches have long been associated with the work of Paulo Freire, a Brazilian educationalist. Freire (1972) worked on literacy programmes with poor peasants in Peru and Brazil and saw education as the political and social means of changing power relationships. Women's health groups, the civil rights movement in the USA and many self-help groups were all examples of community participation and people coming together to campaign about issues within their community.

Community development as an approach thus needs to be distinguished from community-based health promotion. The latter has meant programmes or services reaching out to or located in communities as a means of breaking down the boundaries between organisations and users. These projects may be designed and delivered according to the needs of communities but tend to be set within government or health professionals' agendas (Gilchrist 2007). Community development prioritises issues identified by the community themselves and

Table 4.1 Characteristics of community-based versus community development models (after Labonte 1998)

Community-based	Community development
Problem, targets and action defined by sponsoring body	Problem, targets and action defined by community
Community seen as medium, venue or setting for intervention	Community itself the target of intervention in respect to capacity building and empowerment
Notion of 'community' relatively unproblematic	Community recognised as complex, changing, subject to power imbalances and conflict
Target largely individuals within either geographical area or specific subgroup in geographical area defined by sponsoring body	Target may be community structures or services and policies that impact on the health of the community
Activities largely health-oriented	Activities may be quite broad based, targeting wider factors with an impact on health, but with indirect health outcomes (empowerment, social capital)

seeks improvements in quality of life – material, environmental or social – that may indirectly lead to better health. They also help to address the problems that are collectively identified as being barriers to the concept of ownership of well-being. Table 4.1 illustrates some of the differences between community-based work and community development work.

The key process involved in community development is individual and community empowerment. 'Empowerment' is a notoriously slippery concept that is widely used but differently understood. In a broad sense it means 'individuals acting collectively to gain greater influence and control over the determinants of health and the quality of life in their community, and is an important goal in community action for health' (Nutbeam 1998). The process will aim to strengthen the range and quality of organisation in communities both at the level of networks and local activities but also increase participation and influence so that communities can begin to identify needs and lobby for change. If individuals are to become empowered, they need first of all to recognise their own powerlessness. Freire (1972) described this as 'conscientisation', a process of change in awareness and knowledge concerning a person's own position in the world in relation to others.

The rise in consciousness of their situation enables individuals to identify their own needs, rather than having them prescribed by others. At the organisational level the central tenets of empowerment are described as the exercise of power, information sharing and involvement in decision-making. This will, on the one hand, assist in empowering the individual within the organisation itself, and on the other enable the organisation to influence policies within the wider community (Israel *et al.* 1994).

Community development has radical roots, its intention is to bring about social and political change (Laverack 2007). On a critical note, the true nature of community development is beginning to be more widely contested. Is it driven by the democratic vision it espouses or is it a means of social engineering to promote 'competent and quiescent communities'? The mainstreaming of community development approaches far from resulting in government *by* communities may result in government *through* communities by which communities themselves get victimised and blamed for problems of neighbourhood decline or anti-social behaviour. Further, it has been argued that the decentralised decision-making that is such a feature of community development diverts attention away from the lack of control communities have over economic resources (Petersen 1994) and it becomes a means of 'gilding the ghetto' – having little impact on major health inequalities and merely focusing on the felt needs in one area or group.

The participatory and community development approach to promoting health uses a bottom-up grass roots perspective that enables and mobilises communities to take more control over their health whether this is the way in which services are delivered or tackling the causes of ill-health in a neighbourhood. The government's commitment to consultation and involvement is clear but this needs to be distinguished from empowerment where the objective is to strengthen communities. The ways in which communities are involved in decision-making and the design and delivery of programmes and services has been the subject of much debate. Several writers have developed typologies of participation (Arnstein 1969; Brager & Specht 1973; Wilcox 1994) that describe levels or stages of participation. These models make a hierarchical distinction between approaches to involvement according to the amount of power sharing involved and the degree of influence over decisions, attempting to distinguish between consultation, participation and empowerment. People can be involved in the services that affect or may affect them at a variety of levels and in a number of ways, ranging from very little to complex relationships:

- *Information* – ensuring that relevant information about service planning reaches the public, e.g. surveys, leaflets and focus groups
- *Consultation* – asking people's views and advice about plans, policies and services, e.g. Public meetings and consultation documents
- *Participation* – identifying a problem and asking the public to make a series of decisions within defined limits, e.g. the site of a health care facility
- *Partnership* – working together to set objectives, make plans and decide funding priorities, e.g. patients and carers in service planning groups
- *Delegated control* – giving authority and money to a community to plan services, choose providers and run the services

Box 4.2 illustrates the Ladder of Participation, applied to youth participation in a model developed by Hart (1992). It highlights the debate about levels of participation and their benefit for the individuals concerned and for decision-making. Somewhat controversially Hart suggests that shared decision-making by children with adults is the most desirable.

Box 4.2   Degrees of participation (extract from a UNICEF Innocenti Research Centre publication of Roger Hart's Ladder of Participation, sources: Earls & Carlson (2002, 76 citing Hart 1992) (Hart 1997)

8   **Youth-initiated, shared decisions with adults** is when projects or programs are initiated by youth and decision-making is shared among youth and adults. These projects empower youth while at the same time enabling them to access and learn from the life experience and expertise of adults

7   **Youth-initiated and directed** is when young people initiate and direct a project or program. Adults are involved only in a supportive role

6   **Adult-initiated,** shared decisions with youth is when projects or programs are initiated by adults but the decision-making is shared with the young people

5   **Consulted and informed** is when youth give advice on projects or programs designed and run by adults. The youth are informed about how their input will be used and the outcomes of the decisions made by adults

4   **Assigned but informed** is where youth are assigned a specific role and informed about how and why they are being involved

---

3   **Tokenism** is where young people appear to be given a voice, but in fact have little or no choice about what they do or how they participate

2   **Decoration** is where young people are used to help or "bolster" a cause in a relatively indirect way, although adults do not pretend that the cause is inspired by youth

1   **Manipulation** is where adults use youth to support causes and pretend that the causes are inspired by youth

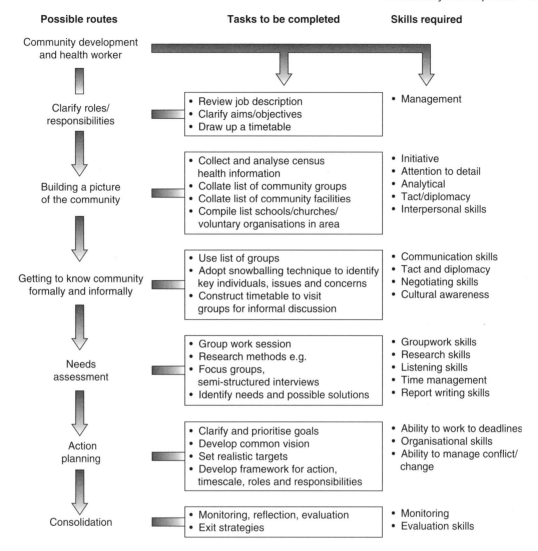

| Possible routes | Tasks to be completed | Skills required |

Figure 4.1   The route of community development work. From Jones, Siddell and Douglas, *The Challenge of Promoting Health*, second edition. 2002. With permission from Palgrave Macmillan.

Making it work – key issues in successful community development

Working within a community development framework can provide community practitioners with a number of opportunities and challenges. Some of these opportunities are about building partnerships and more responsive services. Some of the challenges relate to issues of professional autonomy, bureaucratic accountability, and fear of loss of professional power.

Figure 4.1 provides a useful framework illustrating the process of community development work. It identifies some of the tasks and skills involved in this process and the ways in which the practitioner enables the community to define and address issues. Forging alliances or partnerships with local people, other community workers, and voluntary and lay groups is fundamental to effective community development work. Practitioners need to build on their existing store of community knowledge to form partnerships and networks in order to identify health needs. In deprived communities, however, the motivation of local people to be involved or take any action may be low. This may be due to a perception that they cannot change anything, or that the agenda reflects PCT concerns, that they might be asked to step up 'the ladder of involvement' and do more than they want to or that they are outsiders to small cliques that are leading change in their community.

Successful community development also depends on an acknowledgement of the need to start with the priorities identified by the local community (see Chapter 22). Historically, a medical model of health that encourages a focus on pathology has dominated health and social care. This is at odds with a community development approach. A clear identification of community needs as a prerequisite is essential and must include issues wider than patterns of disease and illness and encompass a more social definition of health. The actual needs identified by a community may be radically different from the policy priorities and agendas of local authorities and primary care trusts.

The philosophy of community development holds that people should have a say and be involved in a meaningful way, and that their ideas and solutions to the problems facing them are listened to and action taken. For example, a needs assessment undertaken by the Leyton Community Health Project in East London identified that young people wanted:

- Direct access to information
- Support and guidance to promote mental health and physical well-being
- Young people having a say in service design and delivery
- Adults and professionals working alongside them to achieve these aims

As a result, a young peoples' pilot outreach project was set up and run by a nurse, a drugs outreach worker, a sexual health worker and a counsellor with a drop in session at a local school. The pilot project highlighted that action was needed on a number of fronts:

- Development of a less fragmented, more holistic approach to identifying and responding to young peoples' health needs

- Provision of health support in primary schools
- Independent access for young people (i.e. with no requirement for an adult to access the service on their behalf)
- Advocacy and brokerage into a range of other services
- Liaison with the Child and Adolescent Mental Health Service to bring their workers out into non-traditional settings in the community

Whilst young people had been involved in the setting up and advertising of the outreach project, a community health project manager drove it forward and developed it into a young peoples' independent access service named Face 2 Face. It had one central access point for young people in the community and six school based outreach 'drop in' clinics operating on a hub and spoke approach. This example raises questions about the role of the practitioner in community development and the extent to which they move beyond being a catalyst and facilitator.

The Leyton Community Health Project was nationally acclaimed as a best practice example and formed the basis of a further bid for regeneration funding. However it raises key questions about the sustainability of initiatives and their continued funding. Where new services have been developed as a result of community consultation their potential for exerting a powerful influence on mainstream service provision should be actively pursued as shown here in the development of the young people's service. However, once projects do become mainstream there is always the potential for them to become subject to organisational pressures and lose their drive and innovation.

Measuring the effects of community development initiatives on health is a complex undertaking. This is partly due to the need to measure changes in a broad range of social, economic and environmental factors encompassed within community development approaches, many of which may take years to be evident. More traditional research methodologies may also not be able to adequately reflect the need for outcome measures that are sympathetic to the differing agendas of the various interest groups involved. The extent to which evaluations of community development initiatives in the past have been well designed has been questioned as they do not necessarily address the community members' questions of 'Am I healthier?' or 'Is our community better than before?' (Dixon & Sindall 1994). Equally, evaluations that focus on outputs (often intangible) rather than process outcomes will fail to adequately reflect the successes and failures of community development work. There are frameworks for evaluating community development approaches to improving health and well-being. For example, the Achieving Better Community Development (ABCD) framework (Barr & Hashagen 2000) and the Learning Evaluation and Planning Model (LEAP; Box 4.3) (Hashagen 2003), both provide a structure within which community development work to promote health may be measured and evaluated.

Box 4.3   LEAP evaluation framework

The key outcomes are:
- Healthy people who have:
  — Awareness and knowledge
  — Confidence, choice and control
  — Independence and self-reliance
  — Connections to community
- Strong communities characterised by:
  — Community skills
  — Equalities
  — Community organisation
  — Community involvement
- Quality of life – likely to be context specific but include indicators in the following:
  — Community economy
  — Community services
  — Community health and safety
  — Community culture

The role of community health professionals

This section discusses:

- Why community nurses should be engaging in community development work
- How it relates to their scope of practice
- What are the competences and aptitudes required to carry out this kind of work

The past decade has seen an increase in community participation and collective action together with an expansion of community-based health projects. Initiatives arising from government strategies such as New Deal for Communities and Sure Start are attempting to address health inequalities and to assist in empowering local communities to establish elements of power and control over their own life circumstance.

The DH (2001b) health visitor and school nurse practice development initiative identified community development as an effective way to tackle the issues restricting people's health choices. It identified community health professionals, with their considerable knowledge and unique roles within the local communities they serve, as being in an ideal position to be at the forefront of these initiatives. They possess an abundance of knowledge about the health and social needs of their communities and about how those needs can be met. Their everyday experience of home visiting and their long-term knowledge of individuals, families and networks built up over time are valuable resources. As a result they are well placed to identify community leaders and build alliances with local groups. Community health practitioners also have a role to play in the recruitment and support of lay health workers from the local community who are key players in community health development programmes.

A fundamental shift is required, however, to enable practitioners to change their focus of practice in order to address not only the individual and the family but also the wider community. Community development necessitates a change in 'mind set' from a task- to a community-orientated form of practice recognising the individual as part of a collective group with specific needs. This may also pose an additional threat or challenge to practitioners who may find it difficult to relinquish their supposed superior knowledge and power (Jones & Wiggle 1987).

Practitioners wishing to be more proactive in their communities require skills, training and support to do so. In order for this to occur community development must become an integral part of the fundamental role of the community

Box 4.4 National Occupational Standards for Public Health: working with and for communities to improve health and well-being

- Facilitate the development of people and learning in communities
- Create opportunities for learning from practice
- Support communities to plan and take collective action
- Facilitate the development of community groups/networks
- Enable people to address issues related to health and well-being
- Enable people to improve others' health and well-being
- Work with individuals and others to minimise the effects of specific health conditions
- Involve communities as active partners in all aspects of improving health and well-being
- Empower communities to improve their own health and well-being
- Enable communities to develop their capacity to advocate for health and well-being

practitioner. One of the ten key areas in the National Occupational Standards for the Practice of Public Health is 'Working with and for Communities to Improve Health and Well-Being' (see www.skillsforhealth.org.uk) and the associated standards are listed in Box 4.4. The Federation for Community Development Learning have also developed a set of National Occupational Standards for Community Development Work designed for Community Development workers and activists, those adopting a community development approach within their work and those commissioning or managing community development work.

Not only does working in a community development approach necessitate new skills as illustrated in Box 4.5, but it can also pose organisational challenges. Employing authorities may view community development with some degree of scepticism (Naidoo & Wills 2009). This may contribute to the difficulty of obtaining an overall acceptability for community development within

Box 4.5 Skills required for community development	
Building relationships with key partners	Multi-agency, community and inter-professional joint planning and consultation
Appropriate organisational and leadership styles	Facilitative approach; conflict management; group work experience
Communication with people at different levels	Speaking the language of diverse groups and organisations
Humility	Accepting other people's ideas and knowledge; egalitarianism
Maintaining confidentiality	Awareness of potential dilemmas and conflicts of interest within and between groups
Flexibility	Working across boundaries; managing change
Negotiating skills	Dealing with resistance; setting realistic time-scales; not promising things you cannot deliver; securing organisational backing
Awareness of equal opportunities	Anti-discriminatory practice; sensitivity to issues of gender and race
Accountability	Clarity of roles and responsibilities
Advocacy/lobbying	Empowerment in everyday decision-making; providing choices about, and influence over, service provision
Evaluation skills	What have the benefits been to the community, short/long-term?
Research awareness	In-built, dynamic research approach; utilising evidence-based practice
Team working	Working and learning together
Interpersonal skills	Strengthening social relationships
Health promoter	Skilled in health needs assessment and building healthy public policies

the remit of professional practice. Although community involvement and civic engagement are an integral part of the policy framework, corporate agendas are not always compatible with the philosophy and aims of community development. Long-term involvement with communities is essential for strategies to develop and to be effective. However, this conflicts with the dominant political philosophy with its emphasis upon performance management, targets and the desire for immediate results. Crucially, this approach and the issues identified by communities may conflict with operational caseload demands or the traditional remit of the service. Much of community development work is resourced by short-term funded projects that do not recognise the time required to work successfully in this way. The funding for initiatives such as Sure Start and New Deal for Communities is longer term but there is vagueness about the sustainability of programmes once central funding is withdrawn.

Conclusion

Primary care organisations clearly recognise the importance of public involvement but historically have focused on individuals as patients and understand involvement from this perspective of consulting with patients as users of services. As well as being an unfamiliar field, public involvement may also be viewed as a threat to professional expertise and autonomy. The shift required is significant to move to a position where members of the public are valued as equal experts and public involvement is regarded as other than a 'time consuming indulgence'. Although there are detailed guidelines for involvement, for example *A Stronger Local Voice* (DH 2006), understanding how to engage local people is very dependent on individual practitioners. Yet reliance solely on the medical model of health and professional expertise ignores many fundamental socio-economic determinants of health and fosters an unhealthy dependency and passivity among patients. An understanding of the benefits of public involvement and skills in supporting public involvement and community development are vital aspects of the role of the community health practitioner today.

References

Arnstein, S. (1969) A ladder of citizen participation, *Journal of American Institute of Planners*, **35**, 216--224.

Barr, A. & Hashagen, S. (2000) *Achieving Better Community Development*, Community Development Foundation, London.

Brager, G. & Specht, H. (1973) *Community Organizing*. Columbia University Press, New York.

Community Practitioners and Health Visitors Association (1999) *Joined up Working: Community Development in Primary Care*. CPHVA, London.

Crawford, M.J., Manley, C., Weaver, T., Bhui, K., Fulop, N. & Tyrer, P. (2002) Systematic review of involving patients in the planning and development of health care. *British Medical Journal*, **325**, 1263–1265.

Department of the Environment, Transport and the Regions (2000) *Preparing Community Strategies: Guidance to Local Authorities*. DETR, London.

Department of Health (2000) *The NHS Plan: a Plan for Investment, a Plan for Reform*. Department of Health, London.

Department of Health (2001) *Health Visitor Practice Development Resource Pack*. Department of Health, London.

Department of Health (2003) *Strengthening Accountability: Involving Patients and the Public Practice Guidance*. Department of Health, London.

Department of Health (2004) *Choosing Health: Making Healthy Choices Easier*. Department of Health, London.

Department of Health (2006) *A Stronger Local Voice: A Framework for Creating a Stronger Local Voice in the Development of Health and Social Care Services*. Department of Health, London.

Department of Health (2007) *Local Government and Public Involvement in Health Act*. HMSO, London.

De Silva, M., MacKenzie, K., Harpham, T. & Huttly, S. (2005) Social capital and mental illness: a systematic review. *Journal of Epidemiology and Community Health*, **59**, 619–627

Dixon, J. & Sindall, C. (1994) Applying the logics of change to the evaluation of community development in health promotion. *Health Promotion International*, **9**, 297–309.

Florin, D. & Dixon, J. (2004) Public involvement in health care. *British Medical Journal*, **328**, 159–161.

Freire, P. (1972) *Pedagogy of the Oppressed*. Penguin, Harmondsworth.

Gilchrist, A. (2007) Community development and networking for health. In: *Public Health for the 21st Century: New Perspectives on Policy, Participation and Practice*, 2nd edition (eds J. Orme, J. Powell, P. Taylor & M. Grey). The Open University, Buckingham.

Harrison, S., Dowswell, G., & Milewa, T. (2002) Guest editorial: public and user involvement in the U.K. National Health Service. *Health and Social Care in the Community* **10**, 63–66.

Hart, R. (1992) *Children's Participation: From Tokenism to Citizenship*. UNICEF Innocenti Research Centre.

Hashagen, S. (2003) Frameworks for measuring community health and well being. In: *Public Health for the 21st Century: New Perspectives on Policy, Participation and Practice* (eds J. Orme, J. Powell, P. Taylor, T. Harrison & M. Grey). The Open University, Buckingham.

Israel, B., Checkoway, B., Schulz, A. & Zimmerman, M. (1994) Health education and community empowerment: conceptualising and measuring perceptions of individual, organisational, and community control. *Health Education Quarterly*, **21**, 149–170.

Jewkes, R. & Murcott, A. (1996) Meanings of community. *Social Science and Medicine*, **43**, 555–563.

Jewkes, R. & Murcott, A. (1998) Community representatives: representing the 'Community'. *Social Science and Medicine*, **46**, 843–858.

Jones, J. (1990) Community development and health education: concepts and philosophy. In: *Roots and Branches*, Papers from the OU/HEA Winter School on Community Development and Health. The Open University/Health Education Authority, Milton Keynes.

Jones, J. & Wiggle, I. (1987) The concept of politics of 'integrated community development'. *Community Development Journal*, **22**, 107–119.

Kawachi, I. & Kennedy, B. (1997) Socio-economic determinants of health: health and social cohesion: why care about income inequality? *British Medical Journal*, **314**, 1037.

Labonte, R. (1998)*A Community Development Approach to Health Promotion: A Background Paper on Practice Tensions, Strategic Models and Accountability Requirements for Health Authority Work in the Broad Determinants of Health*. Prepared for Health Education Board of Scotland, Research Unit on Health and Behaviour Change, University of Edinburgh.

Laverack, G. (2004) *Health Promotion Practice: Power and Empowerment*, Sage, London.

Laverack, G. (2007) *Health Promotion Practice: Building Empowered Communities*. Open University, Milton Keynes.

Lewis, J. & Walker, P. (1998) *Participation Works. 21 Techniques of Community Participation for the 21st Century*. New Economics Foundation, London.

Naidoo, J. & Wills, J. (2005) *Public Health and Health Promotion: Developing Practice*, 2nd edition. Ballière Tindall, London.

Naidoo, J. & Wills, J. (2009) *Health Promotion Foundations for Practice*, 3rd edition. Ballière Tindall, London.

NHS Executive (1998) *In the Public Interest: Developing a Strategy for Public Participation in the NHS*. Department of Health, Wetherby.

Nutbeam, D. (1998) Health Promotion Glossary. *Health Promotion International*, **13**, 349–364.

Petersen, A. (1994) Community Development in Health Promotion: Empowerment or Regulation? *Journal of Public Health*, **18**, 213–217.

Putnam, R. (2000) *Bowling Alone: The Collapse and Revival of American Community*. Simon Schuster, New York.

Putnam, R., Leonardi, R. & Nanetti, R.N. (1993) *Making Democracy Work: Civic Traditions in Modern Italy*. Princeton University Press, Princeton, New Jersey.

Rosenthal, H. (1983) Neighbourhood Health Projects: some new approaches to health and community work in parts of the UK. *Community Development Journal*, **13**, 122–131.

Standing Conference for Community Development (2001) *Strategic Framework for Community Development*. Standing Conference for Community Development, Sheffield.

Taylor, P. (2007) The lay contribution to public health. In: *Public Health for the 21st Century: New Perspectives on Policy, Participation and Practice*, 2nd edition (eds J. Orme, J. Powell, P. Taylor & M. Grey). The Open University, Buckingham.

Tones, K. & Tilford, S. (2001) *Health Promotion: Effectiveness, Efficiency and Equity*, 3rd edition. Chapman & Hall, London.

Wilcox, D. (1994) *A Guide to Effective Participation*. Pavilion, Brighton.

Wilkinson, R. (1996) *Unhealthy Societies*. Routledge, London.

Wilkinson, R. (2005) *The Impact of Inequality. How to make Sick Societies Healthier*. Routledge, London.

Chapter 5 **Health Needs Assessment and the Community Nurse**

Susie Sykes

Introduction

This chapter explores the concept of health needs assessments (HNA) as a tool for exploring, identifying and prioritising the health needs of communities and population groups and, in particular, the role that community nurses do and potentially could play in this process. In order to understand this, it is necessary to explore how HNAs fit into the current policy climate and to explore the range of approaches that dominate the thinking and practice that underpin HNAs.

Background and policy context

There have been increasing efforts over recent years to encourage the use of HNAs within the National Health Service (NHS). They have been encouraged as a tool to assess the health and social needs of local populations and as a means of obtaining accurate and appropriate information on which to base service development decisions and priorities. Driven by recognition of increased health and social care inequalities, limited resources within the NHS and increasing demands on health care (Macdowell *et al.* 2006) there is a need to ensure systems and processes are in place to inform health care-related decision-making and assess competing priorities.

Local health authorities have been required since the beginning of the 1990s to undertake systematic assessments of need to inform the commissioning process (Department of Health [DH] 1990), although since that time the role and expectations of these tools has increased. The government increasingly sees HNAs as a vital tool to apply to reduce health inequalities (Health Development Agency [HDA] 2005) and has placed renewed emphasis on local level cooperation and the use of evidence in policy and strategy making.

This focus, combined with public and user engagement, has driven the need to ensure that health care assessment is more fully imbedded in local decision-making (Jordan *et al.* 2002). Recent NHS reforms (DH 2007) have also taken this further with PCTs and local authorities, requiring them to work under a statutory obligation to produce a Joint Strategic Needs Assessment of the health and well-being of their local community with HNAs thus becoming an intrinsic part of the commissioning and strategic planning and priority-setting process across partners.

With the increased emphasis and interest in HNAs much work has been undertaken in recent years to develop systematic frameworks to support the rigorous and consistent use of this tool. This process has involved debate about the nature and approach that HNAs should take, and has resulted in some fundamental changes in the way in which HNAs are now conducted. While many different HNA approaches and professional frameworks exist, a common theme has emerged that is suggestive of a trend towards increased multi-agency and partnership approaches and increased community involvement and consultation. Furthermore HNAs can be seen to have evolved from their original role as a clinical tool for assessing health care needs, into a multi-faceted process that looks at both health and health care needs from what has been described as a 'multiple voices perspective'. (Horne & Costello 2003).

There is also increasing recognition that health and health care is everybody's business and more members of the inter-professional team have developed collaborative approaches to needs assessment (Horne & Costello 2003). HNAs may now include professionals from a wide range of different care sectors and professional levels

(Quigley *et al.* 2005). Health Needs Assessments are now regarded to be a core public health function and with the public health role of community nurses developing, their involvement in population-based HNA, as well as assessment of individual patient need, is likely to increase further in the future. In addition to an increased spectrum of professional involvement, the government's patient and public involvement agenda (DH 2000, 2006) has led local communities groups to become more actively engaged both as providers of data to inform the compilation of HNAs and as partners in the facilitation of the needs assessment process.

Defining health needs assessment

An HNA is frequently described as: 'a systematic review of the health issues facing a population leading to agreed priorities and resource allocation that will improve health and reduce inequalities' (Hooper & Longworth 2002). It seeks not only to describe the extent of disease and disability of local people, but to understand the patterns and inequalities that exist, the impact that these have on individuals and the community as a whole, and the perceptions and values that are placed on such issues by local people and the professionals who work with them (Rawaf & Marshall 1999). As such, it is not a one-off exercise but is a 'dynamic ongoing process' (Manitoba Health, p. 4) that involves a complex and pluralistic assessment of data on a continuous basis. It is a project that does not end on the completion of a report but which triggers planning and policy-making and which is reflected on continuously and amended over time (World Health Organization [WHO] 2001).

While the assessment of health care needs of individuals or families remains an important role for community nurses, the term HNA has become synonymous with assessments that look at whole populations. This might mean a geographical community but, equally, may mean assessing the needs of a community defined by social experience, setting, interest, characteristics or experience of a health condition (HDA

2005). The assessment of individual need may in turn contribute to the picture being built up of the whole community.

Despite attempts to provide consistent frameworks and guidelines for carrying out HNAs (Cavanagh & Chadwick 2005; Hooper & Longworth 2002) there exist a number of different approaches that inform the process and affect the types of data that might be gathered. In attempts to capture the distinction between various approaches, three are commonly cited: the epidemiological, comparative and corporate approaches (Naidoo & Wills 2009). In addition to these it is useful to consider asset-based (Macdowell *et al.* 2006) and empowerment-based approaches to needs assessment (Houston & Cowley 2002).

An epidemiological approach uses largely quantitative-type data in order to create an accurate description of the size and nature of a health-related problem and its distribution around a community. It is less concerned with community perspectives of the issue and often begins with a specific topic to be explored. Having identified the incidence and prevalence of a health problem, the epidemiological approach goes on to identify the effectiveness and cost-effectiveness of current interventions for the problem and identifies the current level of service provision. As such, its focus remains on health care needs rather than health needs. Reliance on this approach has been criticised for its narrow problem-based focus and for failing to identify any potential solutions to the issues identified (Robinson & Elkan 1996).

The comparative approach involves comparing the experience of poor health among one group with that of another, within or outwith the locality. If one group of people is not receiving a service or has poorer health outcomes than another group of people with similar demographic characteristics, the first can be said to have an explicit need (Robinson & Elkan 1996). A corporate approach may include the use of epidemiological and comparative data but goes on to explore the views of key stakeholders such as local health professionals, managers, commissioners and in some cases, users and local people.

Some argue that seeking the views of local people as part of an HNA, while important, does not go far enough and that in order for any interventions that follow to be successful, the community should be involved in identifying and prioritising their own needs as well as going on to identify appropriate actions to address those needs. As such, the empowerment approach seeks not to enable the community to identify the social context within which they experience health but also to explore their own health-creating potential and capacity (Houston & Cowley 2002).

A further approach that needs to be considered, and which can be seen to link into the empowerment framework, is that of the asset based model (Macdowell *et al.* 2006). The starting point of this approach is that assessment of need alone is not enough and that rather than taking a deficit approach which looks at what the community lacks, it should include an examination of the extent to which facilitators of health exist within the community itself. It therefore includes an assessment of the effectiveness of local community networks, the level of social capital, degrees of community cohesion and other resources upon which health can be built. It sees the community as a producer of health rather than being merely a consumer of services (Macdowell *et al.* 2006).

All of these approaches explore the needs of whole communities and current definitions of HNA emphasise this as a tool for population-based studies (Cavanagh & Chadwick 2005; Hooper & Longworth 2002). However, the place of applying an individual approach should not be ignored in any discussion of HNA (Jackson 2007; Naidoo & Wills 2009). The individual approach, while usually focused on a particular family or individual in order to determine need that will be responsive to health service intervention (Rowley 2005), can be an important element in building up a comprehensive picture of a community (Horne & Costello 2003).

Each approach is based on a different perspective and reflects different ways of conceptualising and thinking about both health and health needs as well as their relationship to health care, service provision and public health strategies.

Overlap exists between all of these approaches and in reality a HNA may incorporate elements of more than one method of enquiry. Some argue that what is needed is a balance of epidemiological data and appraisal of socio-economic information with that of the community's own 'lived experience' or perspective of health needs (Horne & Costello 2003). However, what is clear is that decisions about what approach to take will be informed by how both health and need are defined and perceived by those undertaking a HNA. These terms therefore need closer examination.

Perspectives of health and need

For many, health is viewed in biomedical terms as the absence of disease and disability and is determined primarily by physiological factors. A behavioural perspective, on the other hand, acknowledges the importance of this medical model but sees health as being influenced by the way in which people live their lives and therefore recognises behavioural as well as physiological determinants. An alternate perspective on health is a socio-economic approach that sees health as being primarily influenced by the social and economic environment within which people live and the constraints and opportunities such structural factors create.

Most professionals do not operate solely within the confines of just one of these perspectives but are likely to be influenced by one perspective more than another (Sykes 2007). However, the most dominant perspective held by any group leading an HNA will clearly influence the type of approach that is adopted. A position that incorporates a less biomedical model of health and acknowledges the socio-economic determinants of health will, for example, require the HNA team to adopt an approach that goes beyond the collection of epidemiological data and that explores both health and health care needs from multiple perspectives.

While the concept of need is acknowledged as an appropriate basis on which to make decisions (Hawtin & Percy-Smith 2007), as a concept, it is complex and contested. Bradshaw's (1972) taxonomy of need is often used to portray different types of need:

- Normative need – needs as they are defined by experts and professionals based on research and evidence. These may change over time or according to different professional groups
- Felt need – needs as they are defined by individuals and often associated with wants
- Expressed need – felt need that has become an action, seeking out some kind of resolution to the need
- Comparative need – determined by comparing the situation of one individual or group to that of another with similar characteristics. If one group is lacking in any area this becomes defined as a need

This taxonomy provides a useful way of considering the different perspectives that may emerge when exploring the needs related to a particular issue or population group from these different angles. Many thus argue that 'need' is a subjective concept that is both relative to both time and place (Robinson & Elkan 1996). This position creates dilemmas for the practitioner in reconciling the different conclusions that might be drawn form each perspective and may challenge emergent decisions.

There is not, however, a consensus on the notion of need as a subjective concept. Doyal & Gough (1991), for example, argue strongly that there are in fact objective and universal needs. They argue that the key goal for all people is to participate in society fully and that to do this they have two basic needs: the need for physical health and the need for autonomy, including mental health and cognitive skills. These, Doyal & Gough argue, are not driven by subjective values or positioning and do not alter with time or place but relate to everybody. They are, as such, both objective and universal. Doyal & Gough identify a number of intermediate needs that need to be fulfilled if the two ultimate needs are to be met, but again they argue that these are universal and objective. They acknowledge that the ways in which these needs can be met varies and can be met to different degrees or standards (Robinson & Elkan 1996).

A health economist perspective judges need against effectiveness, supply and demand (Billings 2002). Limited resources and the need to decide how to prioritise and allocate resources against competing demands is the key driver behind this position in a climate in which it is recognised that ever expanding health care needs cannot all be met in any health economy. Comparisons of the costs and benefits of different health interventions and the degree to which they can instigate change should, according to health economists, drive decision-making (Robinson & Elkan 1996). In such a model the ranking of need involves moral questions that cannot be dissociated from issues relating to economic drivers and value for money imperatives.

Tones & Green (2006) point out that given the debate about the concept of health and its determinants, and the lack of precise and agreed definitions of health needs, it should come as no surprise that there is not a consensus about the means by which health needs should be assessed. What is clear therefore is that in conducting a multi-agency partnership approach to HNA, discussion and clarification of these terms, which is not without contention, is needed before a process can be agreed on.

Reasons for and benefits of conducting health needs assessments

When deciding if a HNA is required it is important to understand the benefits and reasons for undertaking such an assessment. Traditionally HNAs have been seen as a tool used by decision-makers to justify the provision of existing services or to obtain additional funding (Jordan *et al.* 2002), but examination of their current use shows their benefits to be far more wide reaching.

As stated above, in many cases HNAs are a statutory requirement (DH 2007). However, notwithstanding this principle there is increasing recognition of the benefits that effective HNAs can bring to individuals, their carers and to service commissioners. Understanding the needs and issues facing a community is clearly essential if services, public health interventions and health protection programmes are to be effectively and appropriately planned, targeted and delivered. In a climate of limited resources and competing demands, there is a need to prioritise and to apply the principles of equity and social justice in decision-making and an HNA can provide the basis on which to do this (WHO 2001). The data also generate a baseline of information so that developments in services provision can be more rigorously evaluated and impacts and outcomes assessed.

HNAs can also provide an effective tool in challenging existing practice and in encouraging a broader view of how things can be done. Reviews of Health Visitors' experience of undertaking HNAs have shown, for example that they have not only resulted in a deeper knowledge of the community but have challenged the way existing services are delivered. Engagement with HNAs has also encouraged practitioners to engage in areas of practice that had not previously been regarded as their role. Others changed their perception of role importance as evidenced by the fact that issues not previously seen as a priority were identified as being important and things assumed to be a priority were shown not to be a major concern (Rowe & Carey 2004).

As well as being an important driver of the planning process, involvement in HNAs can enhance multi-agency working and facilitate an effective means of delivering coordinated and integrated responses to issues through the generation of improved communication and the development of a greater shared focus and understanding of priorities (Cavanagh & Chadwick 2005; Horne & Costello 2003). The links between services and the interdependence that might exist between them can be usefully mapped out and clarified through a partnership approach to HNA (Cowley & Houston 2003).

Approaches that incorporate community perspectives can effectively create a dialogue between service planners and the public and improve relations between the two. When managed appropriately, an opportunity to express needs can create a sense of involvement in decision-making and a stake in the services and projects that follow. This can also include an assessment of the community resources available to help address issues locally (Rawaf & Marshall 1999). If community participation is taken to the level of genuine involvement in decision-making, it can also create an understanding among the community about how decisions are made and how competing pressures have to be managed.

Finally, there are personal and professional benefits for those involved, particularly the opportunity to develop skills and to engage in personal and professional development. HNAs are a core public health skill, and involvement by community nurses can be an effective way of stepping out to reflect on their role (Rowe & Carey 2004) (Box 5.1) and develop a public health perspective of the population they serve, so enhancing their public health skills and function.

Box 5.1   Benefits of carrying out a health needs assessment

- Better understanding of the health and health care issues facing a community
- Better understanding of inequalities within a community
- Needs-led planning and development of interventions
- Needs-led prioritisation of issues
- Challenge existing practice and consider new ways of working
- More effective and equitable allocation of resources
- Contribute to effective partnership working
- Create shared understanding of need and priorities between partners
- Improved dialogue and understanding between community and decision-makers
- Identifies capacity within community to address issues
- Community involvement in decision-making
- Development of public health skills of professionals

Challenges associated with health needs assessments

The benefits identified above are dependent on the HNA being undertaken in a systematic and rigorous way; this process is not without diffi-culties and challenges. Frameworks for carrying out HNAs increasingly stress the importance of analysing multiple layers of data acquired through multi-agency working (Cavanagh & Chadwick 2005; DH 2007b; Hooper & Longworth 2002). The challenges of multi-agency work-ing are well documented (Atkinson *et al.* 2005; Delaney 1994) and, in particular, include the difficulty of achieving a shared language, com-munication difficulties, agreeing perspectives of health and need, limited resources and con-flict over staff time and availability, allocation of roles and responsibilities, competing priorities and organisational culture and commitment. Managing such challenges requires prior plan-ning and skilled management.

The effectiveness of HNA also rests in its abil-ity to influence strategic decisions. Yet there exists a danger that the target-driven culture of the health service with priorities already deter-mined centrally means that opportunities for findings to truly drive locally relevant decisions are perhaps limited. An HNA is a complex and time-consuming process, which requires care-ful planning and the allocation of its own set of resources. Commitment to provide these skills and resources may not always be forthcoming and timescales may not match management pri-orities and deadlines (Cavanagh & Chadwick 2005; Macdowell *et al.* 2006). The time required to undertaken such a project also impacts directly on those involved in conducting the HNA. Community nurses, for example, may find it difficult to prioritise this kind of work when still faced with their daily routine and direct care-related case load.

Assessing multiple layers and different types of data requires an acknowledgement that they may not all lead the assessor to a valid or reli-able conclusion. The competing perspectives of both need and the subjective experience of health means that, on some occasions compet-ing and sometimes conflicting conclusions may emerge (Raymond 2005). This may particularly be the case when using frameworks that seek to combine the epidemiological, corporate and community approaches to needs assessment.

The community perspective is increasingly accepted as an integral part of the HNA process but presents its own particular challenges. Care needs to be taken to avoid tokenism and there is a need to ensure that all sections of the commu-nity are represented. (A fuller discussion of the challenges of involving patients and public can be found in Chapter 24.)

The philosophy underpinning HNA requires reflection and expects professionals to critically evaluate existing services, practice and norms. For many this can in itself be a challenging process, particularly for those whose practice is well established. Resultant findings arising from the assessment that require a fundamental shift in approach to practice can, in some cases be difficult to implement and organisational cultures and norms can act as a constraint to change (Rowe & Carey 2004). A specific set of skills is required to both carrying out and being involved in HNA, particularly those that seek a community perspective. Some of these skills are listed in Box 5.2.

Box 5.2   Skills required to carry out a health needs assessment

- Partnership working skills
- Community involvement and liaison skills
- Project management skills
- Research skills including the ability to gather and analyse new and existing data
- Communication skills (at both community and strategic levels)
- Planning skills
- Reflective skills

The process of carrying out a health needs assessment

Robinson & Elkan (1996) advise that while it is important to acknowledge and explore the dif-ferent theoretical tensions that underpin any consideration of the assessment of health and need and the competing approaches to HNA that emerge from such deliberation, for practitioners, it is ultimately necessary to act and the practical elements that lie within a HNA need to be unpacked. The many frameworks that exist to support practitioners in undertaking rigorous and effective HNAs identify a variety of steps but from them some common stages emerge:

- Defining the population and the problem
- Planning the approach
- Review of existing data
- Collecting new data
- Analysing, assessing and prioritising
- Validation of findings
- Sharing findings
- Taking action
- Planning for ongoing monitoring and evaluation

Clarity is needed from the outset regarding the nature and characteristics of the community under scrutiny and its boundaries. Cavanagh & Chadwick (2005) identify the different types of populations that may be explored, including:

- Geographically defined populations
- Settings-based populations, such as schools, prisons and hospitals
- Shared social experience populations such as those based on homelessness, ethnicity, sexuality and so on
- Specific health experience populations, such as those based on particular diseases, mental health and disability

In addition, the public health issue to be explored needs to be made explicit. Larger-scale HNAs such as joint strategic needs assessments may begin with a blank canvass and have as their remit the examination of all issues affecting the health and well-being of a defined community (DH 2007b). Others may begin with a topic based focus such as sexual health needs or mental health needs. As with any good project planning, consensus on the aims and objectives from the outset is crucial to act as a point of reference to guide the project's work and to ensure there is a shared understanding among all stakeholders of the achievements being sought (Tones & Green 2006).

The planning stage of an HNA requires consideration of a number of issues. Key to this is identifying and gaining involvement and commitment of key stakeholders. The scale of the task involved in undertaking an HNA should not be underestimated and skills and resources need to be agreed from the outset, as well as agreement as to how findings will feed into local strategic decision-making processes. This planning stage should include agreement of the theoretical approach to be adopted and the appropriate needs assessment methods that will support this approach.

Before collecting new data, it is important to review existing data and ensure that there is no overlap with other local research being undertaken in the area (Health Canada 2000).The need for multiple layers of data required to understand and interpret diverse health needs has been frequently emphasised (Hawtin & Percy-Smith 2007; Horne & Costello 2003) and the processes for collecting data needs to be carefully mapped to both the approach chosen and the aims and objectives of the project. Table 5.1 shows how objectives can be broken down into research questions from which possible methods for collecting information can be identified and agreed on. Key to this decision needs to be consideration of who will undertake the assessment, including the skills, time and resources available. This process identifies the need to collect both quantitative and qualitative data if there is to be a commitment to understanding not only what the problems are, but why such problems exist and what possible solutions might be available to ameliorate or resolve them.

As stated above, one of the dilemmas of assessing need from different perspectives is that contradictory conclusions or competing priorities might emerge. Analysis of the findings is a fundamental stage that requires rigour and careful planning from the outset in order to avoid a normative perspective dominating the final conclusions. A number of criteria can be used for assessing priorities:

- How important is the issue in terms of numbers affected or potentially affected, the

Table 5.1   Mapping methods to objectives*

Objective	Research question	Possible methods
To gain a better understanding of the needs of the local community	What is the structure (age, gender, ethnicity) of the local population?	Analysis of census data
	What do we know about the employment status of the population?	Analysis of census data
	What local services do people currently use?	Survey, discussion group
	What do people think of local services?	Survey, discussion group
To identify what services are currently available in the local community	What services currently exist and where are they located?	Walkabout/observation
	Who provides them?	Council and other agencies directories of services
	Who makes use of local services? Are any groups excluded?	Interviews with service managers; discussion groups
To identify gaps in service provision	What additional services are needed by the local community?	Comparison of data on population with data from audit of services; survey; discussion groups

*From Hawlin & Percy-Smith, *Community Profiling a Practical Guide* © 2007. Reproduced with kind permission of Open University Press. All rights reserved.

degree to which people are affected, public concern about the issue and the financial cost?

- Are there services or interventions already in place to address the issue?
- Does the community have the requisite capacity and resources to help address the issue?
- How does it fit into local and national priorities?
- How far can the issue be addressed, i.e. is there an evidence base to show interventions could lead to health gain and what is the potential for this?

In order to ensure validity and acceptability of the conclusions, a process of reflecting findings back to the community and gaining a further tier of feedback and input can be valuable (Cowley & Houston 2003).

The fundamental purpose of an HNA should be to inform strategic decision-making and therefore the process cannot end with the drawing of conclusions. Findings need to be disseminated, linked firmly into the planning cycle

and used as baseline data to evaluate actions and interventions that follow. Risk assessments also need to be undertaken to ensure that the planned policies or interventions do in fact address the issues raised without causing additional health hazards and to explore the relative risks of different options (De Rosa & Hansen 2003). As such the HNA is an ongoing process to be built on and integrated into practice. It should not be seen as a comfortable linear process but one that has a number of steps which inform each other and which require refinement and adaptation as the work progresses (Rawaf & Marshall 1999).

While each HNA will take on a different format and approach there are features that have been shown to be characteristic of effective HNA processes. Research by Jordan *et al.* (2002) categorises these in two overarching themes of quality and context. Quality incorporates those features that ensure that robust data collection and analysis processes are in place that stand up to scrutiny and enable the conclusions to make a solid case for change. Such features include clarity of aims and objectives, reliable data that are linked to objectives, decisive leadership and academic support where relevant. The theme of context refers to those features and circumstances that set the scene for the project. In particular, this relates to support for the topic chosen, collaboration, inclusivity, ownership and commitment by the stakeholders, the linkage of the HNA to local level priorities and essentially that the HNA is tied to resources and potential service improvement.

Participatory approaches

As discussed in Chapter 26, participation and involvement of patients and the public is not only enshrined within public health and health promotion frameworks (WHO 1986, 1997) but is now embraced within government policy, and all NHS bodies are required to involve and consult with patients and the public in the design, development and delivery of services (DH 2007). Participation can be seen not only as the right of individuals and communities to input into a process that affects their health and well-being but also as a tool to ensure relevancy, understanding and acceptability of subsequent interventions and strategies (Watson 2002).

Participation in HNAs by the public can range from simply being a source of information, to provide answers to questions about their perceptions of need as posed by professionals leading an HNA process to a less tokenistic and more influential role in deciding what local 'experienced' needs are and how they should be prioritised (Tones & Green 2006). One tool that encourages such community ownership is that of rapid appraisal. Rapid appraisal techniques are based on principles of equity, participation and multi-agency collaboration, and acknowledge the need for local knowledge. The model uses a qualitative approach and aims to move away from professional dominance and gain an insight into a community's perspective of its own need in a short space of time (Bowling 2000), potentially within about ten days. This speed is not achieved through compromising standards or limiting scope, but rather through drawing on a wide range of skills and resources

to both carry out and inform the assessment process, triangulating different research methods to draw rigorous conclusions.

While the term rapid appraisal has become an umbrella term for a number of different processes that vary in the degree to which they are participatory, there are some common key stages. Rapid appraisal regards communities as systems that can be deconstructed for exploration and uses iterative processes based on discussion and repetition. Ong & Humphris (1994) have identified the key stages involved in rapid appraisal that demonstrate this iterative workshop-based process and the degree to which analysis takes place in the field:

(1) Identify a rapid appraisal team that includes a broad range of skills and perspectives
(2) Workshop 1 – team members agree target agree, key informants to be interviewed and questions to be asked
(3) Fieldwork – interviews with informants including professionals working with the community, community leaders such as faith leaders, community groups leaders and so on, and people with an insight into local informal networks, e.g. local trades people, lollypop person
(4) Data analysis
(5) Workshop 2 – preliminary needs list agreed
(6) Fieldwork – needs are taken back to the community, validity checked and informants asked to prioritise
(7) Analysis using triangulation
(8) Workshop 3 – results are discussed and proposals made
(9) Open meeting – action plans formulated

While the exact process may vary, the underpinning values of rapid appraisal remain: that individuals need to be understood within their social context; that public involvement is inextricably linked to the rapid appraisal process; that wider perspective than that provided by the health service is needed including local workers outside the health service and key informants; and that assessment of need should be about the promotion of equality (Murray 1999)

The role of the community nurse

Raymond (2005) identifies three constraints to the contribution community nurses can make to the HNA process:

- Their perception of their position as agents of both social control and social change
- The extent to which their potential contribution is recognised and sought by commissioners
- The ability of community nurses to articulate their knowledge in language familiar to such commissioners

Studies suggest that such barriers do indeed exist and that for many community nurses their involvement is restricted to epidemiological or health care-related individual needs assessments, rather than participating in broader community-based needs assessments that look beyond health care needs to needs relating to health and well-being (Cowley *et al.* 2004; Rowe & Carey 2004). However, there is much evidence to support the view that the contribution of the community nurse in HNAs is both key to the process and entirely appropriate and relevant for their 'reformed' role and as such is a key function that should become increasingly integral to their work.

Rowe & Carey (2004) argue that the challenge is not for community nurses, and in particular health visitors, to embrace HNA as a new role and skill but rather to 'rediscover and apply their HNA capabilities' (p. 185). HNA and its application to practice has long been taught as part of health visitors' education, and all community nurses are accustomed to undertaking caseload profiles of individual families or individuals (Billings 1996). With the move to a more public health approach to primary care and the requirement for community nurses to take a more collective view of health, their increased involvement in HNAs, which take a more holistic view of health and explore the needs of populations rather than just individuals, is perhaps inevitable.

Many argue that community nurses are well placed to contribute to, and in many cases lead, the HNA process and that they are holders of valuable information. Information gathered as part of a nurse's case load provides both qualitative and quantitative data that are current and can be used to paint a detailed picture of sections of a community. Community nurses participate as part of the community (Robinson & Elkan 1996) and through their work are in touch with many families and individuals and also organisations within a community. Not only are their contacts potentially large in numerical terms but these relationships can also be rich in depth and understanding. Community nurses are in a position to observe the informal systems and structures that operate within a community, thus enabling them to observe issues that might go unnoticed through a formal checklist-based approach to needs assessment. The relationship between the nurse and a family is such that not only do they have an understanding of what health issues affect the families they are working with, but they are also in a position to begin to understand the causes of the presenting problems and the challenges to the delivery of effective care (Percy-Smith & Sanderson 1992). In particular, they may contribute valuable insight into the health and social care inequalities that impact on different people and care groups.

Community nurses are also uniquely positioned at the interface between a community and strategic decision-makers. They are therefore able to transmit information about the community in an upwards direction and can also observe the impact of policies and interventions on the community (Robinson & Elkan 1996). This understanding of how policy is received and reacted is key if an HNA is to identify acceptable solutions related to proposed service improvements, as well as needs. Nurses are particularly well placed to observe and assess any potential risks that may be associated with the implementation of particular policies or planned responses (Hesman 2007; Raymond 2005).

As the assets-based approach identifies, solutions require resources and many of these resources may already exist within a community. While some resources, such as those provided by local support groups and facilities are tangible and fairly easy to identify, others are less formal and more fluid. Social capital and local networks have also been shown to be important local resources used within community development work to address issues from within a community (Ledwith 2005). Community nurses may be well placed to understand the nature of such networks, or at least to indicate where closer observation and intelligence gathering are required.

The experience of community nurses and their involvement in the settings within which people live their lives provides for a sophisticated understanding of the link between health needs and the socio-economic environment within which they occur. Not only are community nurses able to observe the wider determinants of health but, as Cowley *et al.* (2004) showed, they can also elicit and describe the complexity of such needs on the basis of wholeness or holism. This broad view of both health and need reflects the movement that HNAs have taken away from an over-reliance on epidemiological data to the incorporation of wider community perspectives that incorporates consideration of both wider health and social well-being needs.

Not only then are community nurses well placed to provide data to inform the construction of HNAs, but they potentially have a level of insight and understanding that can enable HNAs to move beyond the compilation of a profile of issues to the provision of a holistic assessment that can facilitate change. While the above suggests a role for community nurses as a provider of information to the HNA process, the potential also exists for this role to extend to enable them to assume the role of HNA facilitators leading multi-agency assessment and planning processes.

Conclusions

This chapter has demonstrated the growing importance of HNAs as a tool for assessing the wider health and social needs of a population, which goes beyond their traditional role of identifying the health care needs of individuals. The new statutory requirements for local authorities and primary care trusts to produce joint strategic needs assessments is evidence of this. While acknowledging the many different frameworks and approaches to HNA, based partly on different perceptions of health and need, this chapter has identified key stages that are common across frameworks and which can be used as a basis for good practice.

An examination of the process of HNA identifies many challenges, particularly when working in partnership. The fundamental challenge is ensuring findings do actually go on to influence decision-making and planning. However, strategies that are based on rigorous, multi-faceted HNAs are more likely to be targeted, relevant and acceptable to the local community.

Any discussion of HNA needs to include consideration of the roles played by different organisations and professionals. While the role of the community nurse has traditionally often been limited to assessing the health care needs of individuals, there is potential for their role to be far more influential. Not only are they the holder of key formal and informal data that should be fed into a local HNA, but they are skilled and well positioned in roles that increasingly incorporate public health functions, to lead multidisciplinary HNA projects that lead directly into strategic decision-making.

References

Atkinson, M., Doherty, P. & Kinder, K. (2005) Multi agency working; models, challenges and key factors for success. *Journal of Early Childhood Research*, **3**, 7–17.

Billings, J. (1996) *Profiling for Health; The Process and Practice*. Health Visitors Association, London.

Billings, J. (2002) Profiling health needs. In: *Public Health in Policy and Practice; a sourcebook for Health Visitors and Community Nurses* (ed. S. Cowley). Ballière Tindall, London.

Bowling, A. (2000) *Research Methods in Health*. Open University Press, Buckingham.

Bradshaw, J. (1972) The concept of social need. *New Society*, **496**, 640–643.

Cavanagh, S. & Chadwick, K. (2005) *Health Needs Assessment*. Health Development Agency, London.

Cowley, S. & Houston, A. (2003) A structured health needs assessment tool: acceptability and effectiveness for health visitors. *Journal of Advanced Nursing*, **43**, 82–92.

Cowley, S., Mitcheson, J. & Houston, A. (2004) Structuring health needs assessment: the medicalisation of health visiting. *Sociology of Health and Illness*, **26**, 503–526.

Delaney, F. (1994) Making connections: research into intersectoral collaboration. *Health Education Journal*, **53**, 474–485.

Department of Health (1990) *The NHS and Community Care Act*. The Stationery Office, London.

Department of Health (2000) *Shifting the Balance of Power*. The Stationery Office, London.

Department of Health (2006) *A Stronger Local Voice: A Framework for Creating a Stronger Local Voice in the Development of Health and Social Care Services*. Department of Health, London.

Department of Health (2007) The Local Government and Health Act 2007. The Stationery Office, London.

Department of Health (2007b) *Guidance on Joint Strategic Needs Assessment*. Department of Health, London.

De Rosa, C. & Hansen, T. (2003) The impact of 20 years of risk assessment on public health. *Human and Ecological Risk Assessment*, **9**, 1219–1228.

Doyal, L. & Gough, I. (1991) *A Theory of Human Need*. MacMillan, London.

Hawtin, M. & Percy-Smith, J. (2007) *Community Profiling: A Practical Guide*. Open University Press, Berkshire.

Health Canada (2000) *Community Health Needs Assessment: A Guide for First Nations and Inuit Health Authorities*. Health Canada, Canada.

Health Development Agency (2005) *Clarifying Approaches to Health Needs Assessment, Health Impact Assessment, Integrated Impact Assessment, Health Equity Audit and Race Equality Impact Assessment*. Health Development Agency, London.

Hesman, A. (2007) Protecting the health of the population. In: *Vital Notes for Nurses, Promoting Health* (ed. J. Wills) (2007). Blackwell Publishing, Oxford.

Hooper, J. & Longworth, P. (2002) *Health Needs Assessment Workbook*. Health Development Agency, London.

Horne, M. & Costello, J. (2003) A public health approach to health needs assessment at the interface of primary care and community development: findings from an action research study. *Primary Health Care Research and Development*, **4**, 340–352.

Houston, A. & Cowley, S. (2002) An empowerment model to needs assessment in health visiting practice. *Journal of Clinical Nursing*, **11**, 640–650.

Jackson, L. (2007) Promoting health for communities. In: *Vital Notes for Nurses; Promoting Health* (ed. J. Wills) (2007). Blackwell Publishing, Oxford.

Jordan, J., Wright, J., Ayres, P., Hawkings, M., Thomson, R., Wilkinson, J. & Williams, R. (2002) Health needs assessment and needs-led health service change: a survey of projects involving public health doctors. *Journal of Health Service Research Policy*, **7**, 71–80.

Ledwith, M. (2005) *Community Development, a Critical Approach*. The Policy Press, Bristol.

Macdowell, W., Bonell, C. & Davies, M. (2006) *Health Promotion Practice*. Open University Press, Berkshire.

Manitoba Health (no publishing date given) *Community Health Needs Assessment Guidelines*. Manitoba Health, Manitoba. Available at: www.gov.mb.ca/health/rha/chnag.pdf (accessed March 2007).

Murray, S. (1999) Experiences with 'rapid appraisal' in primary care; involving the public in health needs, orientating staff and educating medical students. *British Medical Journal*, **318**, 440–444.

Naidoo, J. & Wills, J. (2009) *Health Promotion; Foundations for Practice*, 2nd edition. Ballière Tindall, London.

Ong, B.N. & Humphris, G. (1994) Prioritising needs within communities: rapid appraisal methodologies in health. In: *Researching the People's Health* (eds J. Popay & G. Williams) (1994). Routledge, London.

Percy-Smith, J. & Sanderson, I. (1992) *Understanding Local Needs*. Institute for Public Policy Research, London.

Quigley, R., Cavanagh, S., Harrison, D., Taylor, L. & Pottle, M. (2005) *Clarifying Approaches to Health Needs Assessment, Health Impact Assessment, Integrated Impact Assessment, Health Equity Audit and Race Equality Impact Assessment*. Health Development Agency, London.

Rawaf, S. & Marshall, F. (1999) Drug misuse: the ten steps for needs assessment. *Public Health Medicine*, **1**, 21–26.

Raymond, E. (2005) Health needs assessment, risk assessment and public health. In: *Community Health Care Nursing* (eds D. Sines, F. Appleby & M. Frost). Blackwell Publishing, Oxford.

Robinson, J. & Elkan, R. (1996) *Health Needs Assessment; Theory and Practice*. Chuchill-Livingstone, London.

Rowe, A. & Carey, L. (2004) The effect of population-based needs assessment on health visitor practice. *Primary Health Care Research and Development*, **5**, 179–186.

Rowley, C. (2005) Health needs assessment. *Journal of Community Nursing*, **19: 6**, 11–14.

Sykes, S. (2007) Approaches to promoting health. In: *Vital Notes for Nurses; Promoting Health* (ed. J. Wills) (2007). Blackwell Publishing, Oxford.

Tones, K. & Green, J. (2006) *Health Promotion; Planning and Strategies*. Sage, London.

Watson (2002) Normative needs assessment: is this an appropriate way in which to meet the new public health agenda?. *International Journal of Health Promotion and Education*, **40**, 4–8.

World Health Organization (1986) *Ottawa Charter for Health Promotion*. World Health Organization, Copenhagen.

World Health Organization (1997) *The Jakarta Convention on Leading Health Promotion into the 21st Century*. World Health Organization, Geneva.

World Health Organization (2001) *Community Health Needs Assessment; An Introductory Guide for the Health Nurse in Europe*. World Health Organization, Copenhagen.

Chapter 6 Research Perspectives Applied to Primary Health Care

Dr Vasso Vydelingum, Professor Pam Smith and Pat Colliety

Introduction

This chapter will help the reader to make links between research, policy and practice as described elsewhere in this book. The chapter can also be read as a 'stand-alone' text that provides the community health care practitioner with the necessary information to consider research methodologies, methods and findings as they apply in everyday practice.

The chapter considers:

- Priorities for nursing and primary health care research.
- The knowledge base for primary health care practitioners.
- Reflective practice and research mindedness.
- The research process with selected research examples that demonstrate the application of the research process and use of research in community nursing practice.
- General research issues.

Priorities for nursing and health care research

Over the past decade, government policy and strategy in the UK have put primary care and public health high on the agenda of health and social care delivery (Department of Health [DH] 2004a–d, 2006a). This agenda is supported by the emphasis on the utilisation of existing staff in new ways and the evolution of new roles in order to align nursing careers with the National Health Service (NHS) careers framework and ensure that nursing careers reflect the pathways followed by service users and patients (DH 2006b, 2007a).

There are also changes to funding primary care through the General Medical Services (GMS) contract which shifts the focus from doctors to take account of practice workloads and patients' needs (DH 2004b, 2006a–d, 2007c). The review of the role of health visitors (DH 2007b) again reinforced the importance of public health within the government's policy agenda, while the government document *Choosing Health: Making Healthy Choices Easier* (DH 2004c) has emphasised the need for public health work with children and young people. This agenda has been supported by a research and development strategy to set priorities and promote a research culture to move the base of clinical practice from ritualistic to evidence-based practice and improve the quality of care for patients, clients and communities (DH 2005a, 2006e–g, 2008a,b).

Well-established features of the evidence-based health care landscape include the Cochrane Collaboration, which originated in Oxford in the 1990s and undertakes systematic reviews of trial findings and disseminates them among clinicians and purchasers, and the NHS Centre for Reviews and Dissemination at the University of York. The aim of the York centre is 'to promote the application of research-based knowledge in health care'. This knowledge not only relates to evidence on the effectiveness of treatments but also service delivery and organisation. The National Institute for Health and Clinical Excellence (NICE) is another key feature of the government's drive to raise the profile of evidence-based health care and to ensure that only those interventions with a proven track record of effectiveness are adopted. There are also internet-based discussion groups to support this agenda, such as the public health group (public-health@jiscmail.ac.uk) and the evidence-based health group (evidence-based-health@jiscmail.ac.uk).

Smith *et al.* (2004) are cautious of the messianic flavour of the evidence-based health movement and invite other approaches to capture evidence, through narratives and participatory action research to both complement and offer alternatives to the 'gold standard' of systematic reviews, meta-analysis and randomised controlled trials (RCTs). Narrative and participatory action research, as we shall see later, have much to offer the community nurse practitioner.

Readers will be familiar with the changing discourse of health promotion and public health. This discourse dates back at least to the 1976 policy document *Prevention and Health: Everybody's Business* when responsibility for maintaining health and well-being was explicitly shifted from a collective responsibility at the level of government and firmly placed on individual shoulders. A subsequent document, the *Health of the Nation* (DH 1992), was criticised for its narrow focus on five prescribed areas: coronary heart disease and stroke; cancers; mental illness; human immunodeficiency virus (HIV)/acquired immune deficiency syndrome (AIDS); and accidents. Research and development programmes were set up for each of these areas in order to document and reduce their incidence and investigate treatment outcomes. The responsibility for these programmes was devolved to the regional health authorities, which, in 1996, were incorporated into the Department of Health.

Harris (1993) believed that changes during the early 1990s within the NHS offered opportunities to redress the balance between hospital-dominated research programmes of the past and population-based primary care and by inference, public health research of the future. Historically, there has certainly been a dearth of research in the field of community nursing in favour of topics associated with the care of hospitalised adults. The White Paper *Saving Lives: Our Healthier Nation* recognised that social and economic issues play a major role in the nation's health (DH 1999a). Public health initiatives have been a key feature under the auspices of the health development agency and the continued interest in the development of strategies and toolkits to move the agenda forward.

As Wanless (2004) has so clearly highlighted, the emphasis for public health practice has to shift from a focus on individual needs to that of the whole population in order to recognise, understand and tackle inequality. *Choosing Health* (DH 2004c) reflects this changing ideology of public health and identifies ways in which individuals and communities can be helped to optimise their health, and the importance of public health approaches is also reflected in policy documents such as *Every Child Matters* (DH 2004a) and national service frameworks. Resources such as the public health electronic library (www.library. nhs.uk/publichealth/), the NHS electronic libraries (www.library.nhs.uk) and the primary care electronic library (www.nelhpc.sghms. ac.uk) ensure that information about these and other initiatives is widely disseminated.

A growing recognition of the impact of the increasing number of people with long-term conditions (LTCs) is another area that has been reflected in government policy and research, for example the DH document *Supporting People with Long Term Conditions* (DH 2005c). This document offers examples from social care, the NHS and international initiatives with the aim of helping local health communities improve services for people with long-term conditions. Complementing this is *Raising the Profile of Long Term Conditions Care: A Compendium of Information* which focused on the outcomes that people with LTCs said they want from services and describes how more effective management of LTCs in a number of areas is delivering high-quality, personalised care (DH 2005b).

As part of implementing the government's framework to put patients and frontline staff 'at the heart of the NHS', the government published *The NHS Improvement Plan: Putting People At The Heart Of Public Services* (DH 2004d) which set the priorities for 2004–8. Key points were the identification of primary care trusts (PCTs) as taking a lead role in the changes because of their 'unique position across community, hospital and primary care' and at the interface of the NHS and local authority. The need to develop both existing staff and new roles to support innovative services such as Hospital at Home and Hospital at Night while taking account of the reduction in junior doctors' hours were also identified. Within the NHS there is a move away from working with traditional roles towards looking at what needs to be done and who is the most appropriate person to do it, all of which must be underpinned by a sound evidence base. Subsequent policy documents such as *Our Health, Our Care, Our Say* and *Care Outside Hospital* reflect this approach too (DH 2006a,c).

Our Health, Our Care, Our Say: A New Direction for Community Services (DH 2006a) has recommended a substantial transfer of NHS functions to the community, proposing that upto 15 million outpatient attendances should be delivered in community settings. While PCTs develop the necessary infrastructures to shift specialist care, it is suggested that most of the control of local health resources be granted to general practices via practice-based commissioning, to avoid fragmentation of services. PCTs will be given the incentives for managing the change through the mechanism of payment by results and such plans require considerable investment in infrastructure and training and would result in fundamental changes in working practices for many health care professionals. The recent announcement (BBC News 1 April 2008) about health screening for the over 40s, may be part of the new initiatives for a greater focus on primary care prevention. Everyone aged 40–74 in England will be offered health checks for heart disease, stroke, diabetes and kidney disease under new government plans, with a full roll out in 2009.

Partnerships with communities and individuals working together with health authorities, local authorities and the voluntary sector are seen as key to improving health and promoting equity. Schools, workplaces and neighbourhoods are identified as the key settings for action. Professionals from different agencies are expected to work together to achieve this. The imperative for partnership working has been given further impetus in the wake of such tragedies as Victoria Climbié, whose cruel treatment and subsequent death at the hands

of her great-aunt went undetected because of a lack of integrated working between the police, health and social services. Although at the time of writing (December 2008) the official inquiry into the death of Baby P in the same borough has not yet taken place, newspaper reports suggest that similar failings in communication and integrated working occurred. A report (*Guardian* 2 December 2008) commissioned at the conclusion of the Old Bailey trial of the toddler's death highlighted the following failings:

- Failure to identify children and young people at immediate risk of harm and to act on the evidence
- Agencies working in isolation from another and without effective coordination
- Poor gathering, recording and sharing of information
- Inconsistent quality of frontline procedures and insufficient evidence of supervision by senior management
- Insufficient challenge by the local safeguarding children's board to council members and frontline staff
- Poor child protection plans
- Failures to ensure all requirements of the inquiry into Victoria Climbié's murder were met

Readers would be well advised to read the report of the official inquiry into the death of Baby P when it is published and consider what the similarities are to Victoria Climbié's case and what recommendations follow.

Joint assessments between community nurses and social care staff to ensure that patients' health and social needs are considered and the creation of children's trusts to promote effective communication and coordination between all those working with children as highlighted by the Laming report (DH 2003) are examples of how working partnerships can be developed. The emergence of new roles for NHS staff and the new mechanism for funding primary care discussed above, further enhance the partnership process. The development of children's trusts, encompassing health, education and social services as well as the voluntary sector, has also been supported by policy (DH 2004a), as have the development of Sure Start and Extended Schools initiatives.

The NHS Reform and Health Care Professions Act 2002, as well as defining the distribution of functions between strategic health authorities and PCTs, also extended the role of the Commission for Health Improvement, and reformed the structures for patient and public involvement in the NHS. Additionally, it provided for joint working between NHS bodies and the prison service and reformed the regulation of the health care professions, including the establishment and functions of the Council for the Regulation of Health Care Professionals; further evidence of the government's agenda for patient and public involvement and partnership working.

Sir Liam Donaldson (2006) argued that partnerships between health care providers and recipients were key to developing effective health care as:

'patients, and the citizens from whom they are drawn, are the paymasters and commissioners of all that we collectively do. As the thrust of governmental policy seeks to devolve decision-making back to communities and individuals, the centrality of the patient becomes ever clearer. I am encouraged by what I see as a paradigm shift in the world around us: the old-fashioned professionalism, often critiqued as paternalistic and distant – a closed shop, has genuinely given way to a new, inclusive and patient-centred concept of professionalism'.

A further factor to consider in relation to the changing milieu of health care provision is the emergence of Social Enterprise organisations, which are not-for-profit organisations which supply services to the NHS through the commissioning process (Social Enterprise Coalition 2008). The drive towards a plurality of providers is reflected in a number of government policies, for example *Our Health, Our Care, Our Say* (DH 2006a), which specifically discusses encouraging innovation and allowing different providers to supply services.

Since its election in 1997 and its continued office until the current time the New Labour

Government has introduced a number of cornerstone documents that continue to confirm the prominence of evidence-based practice, research, quality and audit as components of clinical governance (DH 2008b). These are regularly updated and can be accessed via the Department of Health website (www.dh.gov.uk/en/Publichealth/Patientsafety/Clinicalgovernance).

In 1997 *The NHS Modern, Dependable* stated:

'The NHS Research and Development strategy aims to create a knowledge-based health service in which clinical, managerial and policy decisions are underpinned by sound information about research findings and scientific developments.'

(DH 1997)

The NHS Research and Development strategy has subsequently shifted its emphasis to support these initiatives (DH 2006e,f, 2008a,b). Active research programmes are encouraged, based on locally defined priorities and alliances in order to develop specialist research which 'reflect consultation with NHS users and staff'. The need for a capacity building strategy to take the proposed research forward is also acknowledged.

The increased prominence of public health policy, the development of new roles and new funding models all lead to a renewed emphasis on a broad sweep research agenda to incorporate the associated fields of primary care, health promotion and public health to ensure the rhetoric matches the reality.

The importance of research skills to community nurses and public health practitioners is highlighted by a study undertaken by the three authors of this chapter (Vydelingum *et al.* 2004). They were commissioned by the local strategic health authority to create a vision for public health and undertake an audit of public health skills among the local community nursing staff. This included school nurses, practice nurses, health visitors and district nurses who all identified a range of research, epidemiological and change management skills as being essential for taking the new public health agenda forward.

Changes to local working arrangements such as meeting targets for first contact, public health and chronic disease management, as outlined in the report *Liberating the Talents* (DH 2002), and subsequent documents such as *The NHS Improvement Plan* (DH 2004d), *Liberating the Talents for Nurses Who Care for People with Long Term Conditions* (DH 2005d) also highlight the need for new skills as part of the development of new community nursing roles.

For example, the impact of the new roles on nursing practice and perception are captured in the following quotation featured in a paper by Franks and Smith (2002). A nurse consultant working in the care of older people describes the scope of her new role that allows her to work collaboratively with other professions thus:

'central to this job is trying to forge links between health and social care. I work with entire ward teams of nurses, domestic staff as well as strategically with the PCT (Primary Care Trust). I have told people about my role – the community team, other professionals, trust boards, voluntary organisations… and I'm still doing it two years later.'

From a reading of government policy therefore, there is clearly a need to identify an appropriate knowledge base and flexible and innovative research methodologies and methods for investigating a range of issues associated with health service reform in general and public health and primary care in particular. The next section examines the knowledge, methodologies and methods required to fulfil the research requirements of the current primary health care and public health agendas.

The knowledge base for public health and primary health care practitioners

Primary health care practitioners constantly have to respond to complexities of clinical situations, political changes, societal demands and economic challenges such as increased migration, refugees and asylum seekers. Consequently they need to draw on knowledge from a range of disciplines including medicine, epidemiology, psychology, sociology and anthropology. The field is complex and as such needs a multidisciplinary approach to its practice, education and research.

Epidemiology, often described as the cornerstone science of public health (Mulhall 1996) is concerned with the occurrence, distribution and determinants of states of health and disease in human groups and populations (Abramson & Abramson 1999). Scientific knowledge, which predominates in medicine and epidemiology, is associated with facts and theories. On closer scrutiny these are not necessarily set in tablets of stone, as the risk factor literature illustrates. For example, stress, which prevailed as a risk factor in the development of peptic ulcers for decades, was overturned during the 1990s in favour of a bacterial model of disease causation. Researchers demonstrated that there was a strong association between the organism *Helicobacter pylori* and the occurrence of the condition (Moore 1995). The discovery of this new information was not welcomed by the drug companies at first and indeed financial reasons may have played a part in delaying the uptake of the bacterial rather than the stress theory of causation.

Practitioners need to 'accept that the information and research we talk about today is based on yesterday's understanding'. It is also necessary 'to understand the limitations of our present knowledge' and acquire 'skills to evaluate new information and research findings and to apply this to tomorrow's situations' (Rees 1992). As clients and patients are becoming well informed through the media and the internet, primary health care practitioners are no longer the only holders of evidence or information about diseases and treatments. They need to become more familiar therefore with critical appraisal of the literature, research methodologies, methods and findings and evaluate them in the light of practice. Rogers (2005) suggests that nurses have been sharing knowledge and experience with others through 'on the job' learning and this form of knowledge has been critical in the development of nursing. Ways of doing this are through reflective practice and increasing research mindedness. The practitioner who combines reflection and research mindedness is in a good position to apply research to practice and undertake research to generate knowledge to advance practice.

Reflective practice and research mindedness

Reflective practice described by Benner (1984) and Schön (1987) assists practitioners to work in a reflective and analytic way to recognise their field knowledge, evaluate research findings and guide future practice. Researchers work in similar ways, moving between the field, the literature and their data to make interpretations to generate findings and guide future research.

Research mindedness is defined by the Royal College of Nursing's research group as 'a critical and questioning approach to one's work, the desire and ability to find out about the latest research in the area and apply it as appropriate' (Royal College of Nursing [RCN] 1982). Such a view is also shared by Parahoo (2006), suggesting that research mindedness involves an attitude and an ability to ask questions of one's practice but not necessarily all having to carry out research. Practitioners need to be involved in practice-based inquiry; however, Freshwater & Bishop (2003) contend that practitioners may be involved at different levels. This may range from knowing what good evidence is and using such evidence to guide practice, how and where to find it and how to evaluate it, to undertaking research to produce evidence that will inform practice. To achieve this, practitioners require a good understanding on the most suitable research methodology and methods.

For the primary health care practitioner who shares many similar work experiences to social workers the elements of research mindedness identified in a textbook for social work practitioners seem particularly relevant (see Box 6.1). Although Everitt and colleagues published their textbook in 1992 their original insights on reflective practice and critical thinking are still as pertinent today. This definition of research mindedness reflects an integrated approach to research-based practice. The emphasis for the

authors is clearly not simply on doing research but on using its theoretical perspectives and methods to think analytically about and inform practice. Research mindedness also allows practitioners to identify their own knowledge and expertise that would otherwise go unrecognised and undetected. Being research minded therefore encourages reflective practice and critical thinking, challenges the status quo and constructs arguments to defend resources and assist decision-making (Smith 1997).

Box 6.1   The characteristics of the research-minded practitioner (Everitt et al. 1992)

- Constantly defining and making explicit their objectives and hypotheses
- Treat their explanations of the social world as hypotheses – that is, as tentative and open to be tested against evidence
- Aware of their expertise and knowledge and that of others
- Bring to the fore theories that help make sense of social need, resources and assist in decision-making with regard to strategies
- Thoughtful, reflecting on data and theory and contributing to their development and refinement
- Scrutinise and analyse available data and information
- Mindful of the pervasiveness of ideology and values in the way we see and understand the world

Everitt *et al. Applied Research for Better Practice*, 1992, Macmillan. Reproduced with permission of Palgrave Macmillan.

Evidence-based approaches to primary health care practice have been formalised in the rise in nurse prescribing powers through the introduction of extended nurse and supplementary prescribing to provide patients with quicker and more efficient access to medication (DH 2003). The contribution community nurses make to the monitoring and evaluation of health care has long been demonstrated, as evidenced in a series of papers compiled by the Health

Visitors' Association (HVA 1994). Local practitioner knowledge, described as qualitative (p. 47) and anecdotal (p. 49) was identified as being particularly valuable. A later document (HVA 1995) cited by Kendall (1997) aimed to accumulate evidence to demonstrate the effectiveness of health visiting to decision-makers. However, the authors of the report were seriously challenged in their endeavours. Kendall attributes this to the difficulty of demonstrating the person or family-centred activity of health visiting, practice nursing or district nursing, which does not fit with the type of evidence associated with the 'gold standard' of systematic reviews. Decision-makers are more familiar with this form of evidence and need to be convinced, as Popay and colleagues (1998) suggest, of the importance of 'subjective meaning, description of social context, and attention to lay knowledge' which qualitative research can offer. How then can reflective, research-minded practitioners go one step further to systematise and consolidate their local knowledge into research questions, projects and evidence? The research process provides a helpful framework that can be used for this purpose.

The research process

The practitioner can begin the research process by keeping a reflective diary to accumulate qualitative and anecdotal evidence for the purposes of informing decision-makers, evaluating and assuring quality of care. Reflection and research mindedness are part of the process by which an evidence-based approach to practice is assured. An evidence-based approach to practice means having information from research that will assist in this process. Indeed one could argue that the application of research findings to practice, evidence-based practice, is the key to high-quality, safe health care.

Macleod-Clark & Hockey's (1989) definition of research described it as 'an attempt to increase the body of knowledge, i.e. what is currently known about nursing by the discovery of new facts and relationships through a process of systematic scientific enquiry'. For Macleod-Clark and Hockey 'the essential characteristic of research is its scientific nature'.

Czuber-Dochan and colleagues also chose the DH (1993) definition of research as the acquisition of knowledge that includes 'gaining information, clarification and illumination as well as translating it (research) directly into policy or practice'. This last point suggests the important role practitioners play in critically assessing the relevance of research for practice.

Drawing on these and other texts, Czuber-Dochan and colleagues characterise research as:

- A process
- Scientific
- Objective
- Systematic
- Problem solving
- Advancement of knowledge
- Exploration of facts and relationships
- An enquiring attitude

Czuber-Dochan and colleagues (1997) concluded: 'As the list above indicates, we adopted a broad concept of research because we saw it as being representative of the "real world" of nursing. We believed that conceptualising research in this way would provide opportunities to embrace both the art and the science of nursing knowledge. It would also support the notion that nursing, like research was a diverse activity that takes place in a variety of settings'. Upton (1999) suggests that the process of achieving evidence-based practice is through practitioner's knowledge and skills upon critical reading and analysis of literature in an effort to provide effective care. However, before the research can be applied, information and knowledge needs to be generated. The research process refers to the different stages involved in undertaking a research project. Like any process however, although the project is represented as being divided into distinct stages, which follow on from each other, often they are not mutually exclusive and there may be some overlap between them.

The stages of the research process can be grouped in the following way:

- Identifying the research problem and formulating a research question
- Selecting an appropriate research approach or methodology

- Designing the study
- Developing data collecting methods and techniques
- Collecting data
- Data management, analysis and interpretation
- Writing, research presentation and dissemination

In a text written by an interdisciplinary group of authors from education, sociology, science policy and political science, the shift from the conventional, scientific mode of knowledge (referred to as mode 1) to a new mode of knowledge (referred to as mode 2) is described (Gibbons *et al.* 1994). Mode 1 refers to the hypothetico-deductive linear approaches to knowledge production that are common in academic research. Hypotheses are devised and tested in order to verify theories, make predictions and discover a body of independent objective knowledge. The new mode of knowledge production is described as 'non-linear' in that it does not depend on hypothesis and theory testing. Rather, the production of mode 2 type knowledge requires reflexivity, interdisciplinarity and values difference. It can take place in a variety of settings such as factories, hospitals and health centres, and draws on a range of sources and processes (including information technology) to support a research agenda that is committed to exploring and legitimating different knowledge forms.

Similarly, it is important to recognise that the usual convention of describing the stages of research as a linear process is also limited and needs to be sufficiently flexible to manage the production of mode 2 knowledge. As Smith (2004, p. 114) notes 'Multiple stakeholders with their competing values, agendas and expectations are involved in the new production of knowledge', and there is an increasing recognition that research designs and approaches need to be sufficiently flexible and responsive to carry out investigations across organisations, disciplines and professions. Similarly, it is important to recognise that the usual convention of describing the stages of research as a linear process is also limited, and needs to be sufficiently flexible to manage the production of mode 2 knowledge.

Within the UK, the National Institute for Health Research (www.nihr.ac.uk/) is the government body that commissions and funds NHS and social care research that underpins the delivery of public health and personal social services. Its stated role is to:

> 'to develop the research evidence to support decision-making by patients, professionals and policy makers, make this evidence available, and encourage its uptake and use. Our key objective is to improve the quality, relevance, and focus of research in the NHS and social care by distributing funds in a transparent way after open competition and peer review'

> (NIHR 2008)

The NIHR makes explicit reference to its links to the NHS Purchasing and Supplies Agency (Centre for Evidence Based Purchasing), NICE, the National Institute for Innovation and Improvement, PCTs and other health care providers. It also states that it supports initiatives that increase the potential for the dissemination of research, all of which emphasise the importance of evidence-based practice rather than research per se.

Kitson (2008) investigated what influenced the way nurses implemented research into practice in New Zealand and Australia and found that the key issues were strategic policy influences, activities within leading academic units and responses in practice areas. She also found that the health policy-makers were influenced by the trend towards explicit consideration of clinical effectiveness and evidence-based practice. She argues that more work needs to be done in relation to the implementation of research in practice and that issues such as ownership, culture, practice, championing as well as the organisation itself are key to this. In the next section, the stages of the research process and a range of research methodologies and methods associated with different types of knowledge are considered.

Taking the research process forward

The research process is a conventional but convenient framework in which to consider research paradigms, approaches and methods when reading about and/or planning a project. The process involves identifying a topic, specifying underlying theories, formulating questions, selecting a suitable approach, specifying methods and devising a plan to take the study forward. This will depend to some extent on whether a qualitative or quantitative research approach is adopted. Ultimately, however, the choice of methodologies and methods depends on the researcher's preference and also on the purpose of the research, the topic under study, the subject discipline, the funding body and the resources available. Careful consideration of time and financial budgeting, secretarial support and obtaining ethical clearance are required when planning the research and will repay itself with interest over the remainder of the study. Within this chapter there are examples of research studies demonstrating the application of different aspects of the research process to primary health care practice.

Identifying the research problem: where do research questions come from?

Holloway & Wheeler (2002) suggest that certain criteria should be considered when identifying a research problem. They argue that the topic must be relevant, be of interest to the researcher and the question must be researchable. Brink & Wood (1994, p. 2) define a researchable question as 'an explicit query about a problem or issue that can be challenged, examined and analysed and that will yield useful new information'. Potential topics for research stem from the thoughts, observations and practice experiences of the community nurse. For example, the authors of this chapter undertook a study to explore the education needs of public health practitioners (Vydelingum *et al.* 2004). The study was funded by the public health directorate of the local strategic health authority and the aims were to identify a vision for public health for PCTs, audit the public health skills of the local workforce and implement the vision through proposed practitioner development programmes. The findings were then fed back to both the public health practitioners and the trust managers, and an action plan developed.

Another study (Scholes *et al.* 2008) evaluated an education initiative, the development of modules to support nurses developing skills in physical assessment that had been jointly developed by local trusts and education institutions and supported by the strategic health authority. The trusts had asked for the modules to be developed to support specific needs, such as the development of Hospital at Night services, the development of the community matron's role and planning to meet the changing demands generated by the changes to junior hospital doctor hours.

The role of the literature review

Polit & Beck (2008) note that researchers rarely conduct research in an intellectual vacuum, therefore it is important to establish what knowledge base exists in a particular subject area. Thus, a literature review is undertaken to familiarise oneself with the literature by locating the evidence, appraising it and drawing conclusions about the current evidence. In both the examples cited above, the literature review helped the authors to refine the research question, and previous work provided ideas and approaches to the research as well as examples of data analysis tools and analysis that had been used successfully. For example Vydelingum *et al.* (2004) found that the key issues from the literature review were:

- Government policies have located health promotion and public health at the centre of the debate
- The need to implement the NHS plan and the standards of the national service frameworks requires practitioners with public health roles, skills and functions
- Involvement of public health practitioners in local initiatives has revealed knowledge and skills deficits
- Some community nursing services, such as district nursing and midwifery, provide holistic care based mostly on a reactive and referral-led service
- Health visitors, school nurses and practice nurses have greater involvement in public health

Vydelingum *et al.* also drew on the work of Dunkley & Baird (2000) and Meyrick *et al.* (2001) to develop an audit tool and validate their findings. Scholes *et al.* (2008) explored the government's policy agenda to support the development of new roles, for example community matrons and debated the concepts of advanced and specialist roles. The issues of out-of-hours and unscheduled care were also considered. Scholes *et al.* used a responsive evaluation model which seeks to capture the views of a range of stakeholders about the impact of an evaluation.

Conducting a literature review is a systematic process which includes starting with a research question and a plan or a search strategy. Key words are used to search from databases and refined to make the search more focused. Inclusion and exclusion criteria need to be identified. Grey literature or non-empirical evidence is also sought and can be found in opinion articles, case report, clinical case notes and local health authority or NHS trusts reports. However, the bulk of the search of the literature nowadays is done through electronic searching, through databases.

The world wide web and revolution in computer technology have influenced the ways in which information is accessed and disseminated. Surfing the net is a quick way of gathering information on research, nursing, and just about anything else imaginable at the touch of a button. Many comprehensive computerised databases are available, including a number of research journals. Some tried and tested databases are: CINAHL, MEDLINE, BIDS and EMBASE. These databases are available as CD-ROMs and also online. Online search engines allow search terms or keywords to be typed in and produce lists of results. The National electronic Library for Health, which had opened up an exciting gateway not only to research but also to policy, practice and education literature, now operates as the National Library for Health (www.library.nhs.uk/). The Public Health Library is part of that electronic gateway. An associated part of the electronic age is the growth of the network culture and the possibility to work with colleagues at a distance through the internet. Further discussion on the world wide web and a range of useful databases are presented at the end of this chapter.

Selecting an appropriate research methodology and approach

Silverman (2005) defines methodology as a general approach to studying research topics which is concerned with the philosophy and theory that drives the research rather than the nuts and bolts of data collection and analysis, e.g. specific techniques such as observation, interviewing and audio recording (i.e. the methods).

Paradigm, a term used by the physicist turned philosopher of science, Kuhn (1970), is defined in two basic ways: first, as the range of beliefs, assumptions, values and techniques shared by a scientific community; and second, as the procedures used to solve specific problems and take theories to their logical conclusion. In short, paradigm pertains to the worldview and practical endeavours that drive research. Simply, paradigm can be described as a way of looking at natural phenomena that encompasses a set of philosophical assumptions which guide a researcher's approach to inquiry, (Polit & Beck 2008). Guba & Lincoln (1994) state: 'Paradigm issues are crucial; no inquirer, we maintain, ought to go about the business of inquiry without being clear about just what paradigm informs and guides his or her approach' (p. 116).

For behavioural psychologists, epidemiologists studying the distribution of diseases in populations and clinicians conducting clinical trials, the methodology of choice is likely to involve experimentation, careful observation, measurement and control of the phenomena under study. Because this type of methodology is associated with numbers and counting, it is described as 'quantitative'. It is also associated with scientific enquiry underpinned by positivist philosophy and hypothetico-deductionism. That this is an over-simplification of the nature of scientific enquiry is made evident in the writings of Medawar, an eminent and influential medical scientist, who encourages researchers to think creatively and take risks. He writes:

'The word "science" itself is used as a general name for, on the one hand, the procedures of science – adventures of thought and stratagems of inquiry that go into the advancement of learning – and on the other hand, the substantive body of knowledge that is the outcome of this complex endeavour.'

(Medawar 1984, p. 3)

Similarly, methodologies used in epidemiological studies may include descriptive and explanatory surveys as well as experiments which serve three main purposes: for community diagnosis; aetiology; evaluation of health care. The preferred methodologies of social scientists such as anthropologists and sociologists are more likely to be interactive or 'qualitative'. Such methodologies include ethnography, grounded theory and phenomenology, which involve participant observation and in-depth interviewing to describe and explain qualities of phenomena. Critical social theory, feminisms, symbolic interactionism and interpretive hermeneutics underpin these methodologies. For further explanations see, for example: Bryman (2008), Gilbert (2001), Greenfield (2002), Holloway & Wheeler (2002), Neuman (2006).

Issues about paradigms are not without controversy. While it is argued that positivist (quantitative) and naturalistic (qualitative) paradigms should not be mixed, Atkinson (1995) had earlier argued that such simplistic polarisation is unhelpful. Some commentators suggest that nursing requires its own methodologies and methods to generate knowledge that is uniquely nursing whilst others suggest this limits the nature and scope of inquiry (Cotter & Smith 1998). Similar issues have been debated within the field of health services research (HSR). Popay *et al.* (1998) argue convincingly for the need for interdisciplinary working in order to embrace a pluralistic approach to the study of health across a range of different approaches and methods. In particular, they note the increasing recognition given to qualitative research and the contribution it can make to the field (Black 1994). There is also a growing literature supporting the use of both paradigms within studies in order to capture the full richness of the data (Bryman 2007; Fielding & Schreier 2001; Kelle 2001). This shift towards a less rigid approach to methodological paradigms is good news for primary care practitioners who need to understand not only

the 'what?' and 'how many?' which may be determined by quantitative methodologies, but also the 'why?' and 'how' which may be determined by qualitative approaches.

Evidence

Before designing a study, it is essential to consider the existing body of knowledge on the topic area for research. It is important to review the literature, as discussed earlier, and critically appraise the evidence, synthesise the results and draw conclusions. Such an exercise would identify gaps in either knowledge on the topic area, methodology or theoretical understanding. If there is no or very little published literature on the topic, then a literature search on areas or topics closely related to the research topic should be conducted. For example, a health visitor wishing to study parents' experiences of using cranial osteopathy on their children may find very little published material on the topic owing the recent introduction of such services. However, he or she may find that a literature search on parents' experiences of using alternative therapies for their children quite informative. It is worth noting at this stage the hierarchy of evidence (Box 6.2). The hierarchy is usually based on the scientific rigour of the studies and the ability of the results to be generalised to the wider population.

Box 6.2   Hierarchy of evidence

(1) Randomised controlled trials (RCT) with double blinding (clinical trials)
(2) Well-designed RCTs with pseudo-randomisation
(3) Well-designed RCTs with no randomisation
(4) Cohort studies – prospective and retrospective studies with controls
(5) Qualitative studies
(6) Case studies
(7) Expert opinions
(8) Anecdotes

Examples of these different types of evidence are presented by Smith *et al.* (2004) in their book, *Shaping the Facts: Evidence-based Nursing and Health Care*. James *et al.* (2004) refer to Archie Cochrane's monograph *Effectiveness*

Table 6.1   Levels of evidence according to the National Institute for Health and Clinical Excellence (Marks 2002)

Level	Criteria
1a	Systematic review and meta-analysis of randomised controlled trials
1b	At least one randomised controlled trial
2a	At least one well-designed controlled study without randomisation
2b	At least one other type of well-designed quasi-experimental study
3	Well-designed non-experimental descriptive studies, such as comparative studies, correlation studies or case studies
4	Expert committee reports or opinions and/or clinical experience of respected authorities

and Efficiency, which so strongly influenced the evidence-based practice movement and after whom the Cochrane collaboration was named. They point out that it is often forgotten that Cochrane wrote about the importance of so called 'softer skills' in ensuring quality health care as the following quotation demonstrates:

> 'In "cure" outcome plays an important part in determining quality, but it is certainly not the whole story. The really important factors are kindliness and the ability to communicate.'

> (Cochrane 1972, p. 28)

The hierarchies of evidence described in Box 6.2 as qualitative studies, expert opinions and anecdotes can often best capture the 'softer skills' of kindliness and communication identified by Cochrane. Investigating such concepts usually falls outside the remit of RCTs and cohort studies. But even here Pope *et al.* (2004) show there to be exceptions to the rule. They describe the innovative RCT undertaken by feminist scholar Ann Oakley in which she demonstrated the connection between social relations and the health and well-being of women and their babies (Oakley 1992). Baum (1995) points out that public health as a focus of study is complex and requires the integration of qualitative and quantitative methods not only to describe, but also to understand, communities.

Hierarchies of evidence are not uncomplicated, as various organisations may have their own standards and it would seem that it is a bit like horses for courses. NICE (2002), in its attempt to use existing evidence to produce guidelines for practice, has set up different criteria for evaluating evidence (Table 6.1).

Designing the study

When designing a research study it is important that an appropriate research design is selected to take account of the type of research question being considered and the type of evidence required. Examples of research designs frequently used in primary health care research include: experiments and clinical trials; descriptive and explanatory surveys; case studies; participatory approaches. Many of these designs are concerned with evaluation, which is a key interest of primary care research. As Daly and colleagues (1992) observe: 'We would argue that when a given problem is studied, different approaches to research will ask different data and use different frames of analysis.'

Experiments, RCTs and quasi-experiments

The experimental approach, referred to as the 'randomised controlled trial', has been widely applied to the study of interventions on human subjects, and a double-blind RCT is seen as a gold standard in the hierarchy of evidence. However, Oakley notes: 'The RCT has been increasingly promoted over the last twenty years as the major evaluative tool within medicine' (p. 27). In order to decide on the specific design for the trial, researchers need to be clear from the outset of their aims and should have one or two clearly stated objectives (Crichton 1990). Study design incorporates every stage of the study including decisions about sampling, size, the techniques by which the subjects will be allocated to a treatment (or non-treatment group), how the intervention will be introduced, statistical applications required and the methods by which the outcome of the study will be evaluated.

The phenomena under study (smoking and lung cancer; occupational groups and attitudes to child care) are broken down or reduced to smaller components known as 'variables'. Smoking, for example, may be broken down into variables such as type and number of cigarettes smoked and over how many years; lung cancer may be examined in relation to variables such as the victim's age and class status. The variables are chosen because they are assumed to have explanatory value that will contribute to theory testing, prediction and new knowledge. Smoking would be the independent or explanatory variable and cancer the dependent variable.

Subjects recruited to take part in studies need to be representative of the population from which they are drawn and bear sufficient similarity to the type of individuals likely to benefit from the intervention. Clear inclusion criteria therefore should be identified for this purpose. It is important that variables related to class, age, gender and ethnicity are taken into consideration. Normally, a randomised sample is utilised in an experimental study.

It has been shown that studies have been undertaken with a bias towards white middle class males with a risk that the needs of women, ethnic minority groups and older people will be overlooked. The famous Framingham Heart Study undertaken in the USA, for example, provided detailed knowledge of the risk factors associated with cardiovascular disease in white middle class men but did not take sufficient account of the specific risks for women and people of different ethnic backgrounds (www. framinghamheartstudy.org/).

An RCT of people with strokes who had not been admitted to hospital assessed the impact of offering them a package of occupational therapy for up to five months, compared with a control group who received 'routine practice' (Walker *et al.* 1999). The results were very encouraging

in that the measures used to assess activities of daily living and 'carer strain' suggested that the intervention had more favourable results compared with the people in the control group. The main differences between an experimental and a quasi-experimental design are that both approaches involve an intervention, however, a quasi-experimental study does not include randomisation in its sampling frame and such studies are referred to as controlled trials without randomisation; quasi-experiments also do not have control groups in their design.

A 'placebo' group may be added to the experimental and control groups. The placebo group receives a modified version of the treatment or intervention. The reason to introduce a placebo group into the study design is two-fold. First, it helps to discount bias on the part of researcher or patient in their judgement (whether favourable or otherwise) towards the experimental intervention. Second, it provides a control for the frequency of spontaneous changes that may occur in the patient, independent of the intervention under study. Placebos are often used in experimental studies for testing the effectiveness of drugs or other interventions.

Oakley (quoted in Watts 1999) argues for RCTs to evaluate health promotion interventions rather than the qualitative approaches that have traditionally been favoured in this field. To prove her point she cites evidence that suggests health promotion can actually be harmful (e.g. health visitors' rigorous attempts to prevent old people falling down and breaking bones actually seemed to increase the fracture rate). Her conclusion therefore is that 'the case for evaluation in health promotion is even stronger than elsewhere in medicine because the people you are dealing with are not ill in the first place' (p. 30). Oakley has since spearheaded web-based databases comprising systematic reviews, which demonstrate the effectiveness of promoting health, and a trials register of interventions (http://eppi.ioe. ac.uk). The databases are regularly updated and submitted to the Cochrane Collaboration for Health Promotion and Public Health.

Health impact assessment (HIA) is an evaluation strategy designed to measure the effects of public policies on individual and community health. It has been described as 'great for addressing inequalities'. HIA is recommended in *Saving Lives: Our Healthier Nation* (DH 1999a) and is of two types: prospective (the impact of a new policy on health is evaluated ahead of its introduction to maximise the potential benefits) and retrospective (the impact of a policy is monitored following its introduction). HIA can also be used to inform better decisions for future policy and practice at a local, national and international level (Taylor & Blair-Stevens 2002). Because HIA is such an important part of government commitment to implementing an effective public health agenda, primary care practitioners need to be aware of the methodologies currently being developed. These methodologies can be applied to a variety of projects, policies and programmes and are represented diagrammatically in Box 6.3 (DH 1999b).

Box 6.3   Evaluative tools (with permission from the DH)

The choice of evaluative technique in any appraisal of policy will depend partly on the question to be addressed and partly on availability of data. These approaches to evaluation are summarised here:

- *Cost effectiveness analysis* (CEA): If alternative (non-health care) policies yield the same type of effect, but at different volumes, then CEA is the appropriate evaluative technique, and the output of the analysis will be expressed in terms of cost effectiveness (CEA) ratios, i.e. 'cost per unit of effect'
- *Cost utility analysis* (CUA): This is a special case of cost effectiveness analysis where the effects are measured in some generic way such as quality adjusted life years (QALYS)
- *Cost benefit analysis* (CBA): This type of analysis enables an assessment to be made of the worth of implementing a policy or not (rather than implementing policy A vs. policy B). CBA converts all costs and benefits to monetary terms: if the value of the costs exceeds the value of the benefits then this suggests that it is not worthwhile to implement the policy

---

The Health Development Agency has taken on the leadership of the health impact assessment initiative. There is now an entire website (www.hiagateway.org.uk) dedicated to its dissemination and implementation. The website contains case studies written by practitioners and policy-makers with personal experience of using HIA. The case studies present examples of how using HIA has provided opportunities to increase community participation as well as a mechanism to evaluate the impact of a range of cross-sectoral initiatives including transport, air quality, nutrition and sports facilities (www.hiagateway.org.uk/contacts/personal_experiences). The case studies illustrate the broad remit of public health and the need for the community practitioner to be aware of local initiatives that may impact on and go beyond, their own roles.

Surveys

Most people are familiar with surveys either as investigators or respondents. There are two types: the descriptive survey used to collect biographical, demographic and attitudinal information and the explanatory survey set up to find out 'why?' The Office for National Statistics regularly conducts a whole range of routine and special surveys. The national census is the prime example of a survey that describes the total population. More usually a representative sample has to be drawn. Controversially, in the 1991 census a whole generation of young men was lost from the census data because they 'disappeared' from the electoral register rather than pay the unpopular and expensive poll tax. Valuable resources were then lost from the inner cities because the level of deprivation was underestimated (Hanlon 1994). The 2001 Census (www.statistics.gov.uk/census2001) revealed very useful information which could be invaluable for community health care practitioners, in terms of ideas for further research, such as:

- Almost 30% of households in England and Wales contained dependent children and one in nine had children under 5
- Almost one-quarter of households in England and Wales consisted of pensioners

only and the region with the highest proportion was the south-west (27%)

- More than five million people provided unpaid care for a relative, friend or neighbour with one-fifth of them giving more than 50 hours a week
- Over one-fifth of family households in London had no adult in work. In the boroughs of Tower Hamlets, Islington, Hackney, Newham and Haringey, there were fewer than one in three adults in these households in work
- Women remain 'clustered' in low-paid occupations and are more likely to work part-time, while men tend to work long hours in jobs that pay more

However, the census also contained errors or less useful information such as the fact that around 390,000 people gave their religion as Jedi – amounting to 0.7% of people in England and Wales. Star Wars' fans thought Jedi would be recognised as an official religion but this has not happened.

Sapsford & Abbott (1998) describe the Dingwall & Fox study (1996), as a quasi-experiment or type of explanatory survey. This was because the study design manipulated variables to compare health visitor and social worker perceptions of child protection. Twenty participants from each profession were asked to rate what they thought was going on in 20 vignettes. The vignettes, used as proxies for child protection cases, described a set of circumstances or incidents related to child neglect and violence. The findings suggested there were many areas of overlap in views of, and approaches to, dealing with child protection issues, between social workers and health visitors, and that organisational rather than training differences might account for their reported difficulties in working together (Dingwall & Fox 1986) – a finding supported by the Laming Report (2003).

Clinical trials and surveys more often have large samples so they can claim generalisability but Dingwall and Fox make no such claim. Rather they 'hope to establish the value of the approach and to show that the results are sufficiently interesting to justify further investigations'. Gomm

et al. (2000) suggest that experimental methods are the only ones capable of investigating causality, as it is impossible to decide whether such and such health and social care interventions are effective if it is unclear what causes and what effects were. It is important for practitioners to realise that small-scale studies, are valuable for giving insights on local situations while identifying areas for further enquiry.

Case study

Case studies allow the researcher to gain in-depth perspectives on a situation or an incident (Bell 2005; Parahoo 2006). The case study can be combined with a range of qualitative methodologies. Ethnography for example involves participant observation and interviewing during extended periods of fieldwork.

Scholes *et al.* (2008) used a case study approach in their evaluation study whereby the focus of the case study was the organisation rather than the individual, thus allowing a picture of the cumulative experiences to be built up. Data were collected by participant observation and interviews with a range of stakeholders and analysed within the prism of the organisations involved.

Different methodologies and methods give new insights

Knutsson *et al.* (2008) undertook a study which looked at children's experiences and needs when visiting relatives on an intensive care unit. The study found that the children did not appear to be frightened by the visit, instead 'it generated feelings of release and relief' (p. 155). This hermeneutic study allowed the author's insight into the thoughts and feelings of the child respondents, thus establishing what the children thought rather than what adults thought the children thought!

In relation to LTCs, epidemiological data provide information about how many people have a particular condition, how old they and where they live. Studies such as that by Clark *et al.* (2008) complement that data. Clark *et al.* looked at the complexities of informal care giving for people with chronic heart failure using semi-structured interviews with informal carers. Clark *et al.*

concluded that the management of heart failure was a shared and ongoing responsibility between the patient and the carer and although the carer had limited clinical knowledge, their expertise was in the effect of the condition on the patient.

Participatory approaches for community research

A number of research approaches are available to primary health care researchers that involve local participants and contribute to empowering and improving their lives and communities. Community participation is also a key health promotion concept (Pearson 2008; Strachin *et al.* 2007). Readers will be familiar with action research, a popular methodology with health care researchers (Bell 2005; Parahoo 2006). Action research is usually associated with participatory and collective forms of research although at its most extreme it can be set up as an experiment in which an 'intervention' is tested and its outcomes monitored (Coghlan & Brannick 2005).

The central tenet of action research is the cyclical process of intervention, evaluation and feedback with researchers and participants working closely together. Action and other participatory forms of research balance generalisable knowledge and benefit to the community by collaborating as experts and as equals in the research process (Macaulay *et al.* 1999). The public health agenda described above with its emphasis on partnership working and the major NHS reorganisations that are currently underway, particularly within the PCTs, suggests the appropriateness to the community practitioner of understanding the principles of action research to gain insights into the process of developing complex relationships and managing change.

Participatory appraisal

Participatory appraisal, a community research approach, encapsulates the current government commitment to eliminate social exclusion and reduce poverty. It involves multi-agency and partnership working to assess need and involve local communities in order to effect and evaluate change. It also demonstrates the range of methods available to primary health care practitioners.

Pain & Francis (2003) describe participatory appraisal (PA) as: 'participatory approaches (methodologies and epistemologies) that aim to effect change for and with research participants'. Investigators involved in participatory methods are concerned with issues of empowerment and the relationship between research and action. The aim of PA is to enable those from marginalised groups to make their needs known while at the same time encourage debate within communities and agencies involved in developmental work with them.

Feurstein's model of participatory evaluation has been adapted by Smithies & Adams (1993) to systematise an approach that is subject to competing agendas and unpredictable outcomes while maintaining a commitment to community development. The model is presented as a cyclical process and emphasises the importance of capacity building to equip local people to develop local initiatives. The model offers a framework that evaluates and builds on any initiatives forthcoming from the PA.

Data collection methods

Methods are the techniques of doing research: asking questions, observing people and groups, analysing case records, sifting through historical documents and local newspapers (Bell 2005; Field & Morse 1994; Parahoo 2006; Pope & Mays 2000). A variety of research methods can be used within a study, irrespective of the underlying paradigm and approach. The multi-method research approach is described as 'triangulation', by which more than one method is used and/or groups of people studied within the same project (Foss & Ellefsen 2002). This has the advantage of validating the findings as data are collected from a variety of sources, paradigms and subjects, thus affording a more comprehensive understanding of the phenomenon being studied.

Data management, analysis and interpretation

How data are analysed in a study will depend on the research questions being asked and the methodologies and methods being used. Data analysis is often the most time consuming part of the research. For example, if it takes two months to collect data, it is likely to take four months to analyse and interpret them. In order for researchers to retrieve their data easily and accurately for analysis and interpretation, it is important that, during data collection, they develop systems to ensure this. In quantitative studies, it is likely that the data are coded, collected and recorded on standardised forms, for example self-administered questionnaires and structured interview schedules.

In qualitative studies, the researcher develops ways of recording fieldwork notes during participant observation, such as by keeping index cards to record observations as events take place, for example mealtimes in a day nursery. Interviews are (with the participants' permission) most often tape-recorded and then transcribed to facilitate analysis of the interview contents.

In large-sample surveys, data are likely to be stored in a computer. This will potentially ease and speed up data analysis. If the sample is small, it may be quicker to analyse the data by hand. Data, it should be remembered, are only as good as the operator who enters them into the computer and the logic that inspires decisions about statistical tests. Preparing data for analysis may also be very time-consuming. Data analysis produces summary statistics (e.g. frequencies and average – mean, median and modes) and appropriate statistical significance tests (Greenhalgh 2006).

Statistical analysis can be undertaken using such programs as SPSS (Statistical Package for the Social Sciences) and Minitab, and textual analysis, can be undertaken with, for example, the Nvivo and MaxQda programs, which are constantly being revised. Statistical tests are based on probability theory, and a statistician is usually consulted to advise on the appropriate test given the sample size, type of data and questions being asked. In short, the data are manipulated statistically in order to ensure the results have not occurred by chance. The importance of logic in interpreting results cannot be underestimated. A 'significant' result does not mean that 'cause' and 'effect' are automatically established. First the researcher must ensure that a number of conditions are met if causality between variables

is to be demonstrated. Sometimes an accidental link may bind independent and dependent variables together in a 'spurious' relationship, or confounding of results or muddling the picture (Greenhalgh 2006).

The hallmark of the qualitative research process is that coding and analysis take place alongside data collection. The researcher then decides what future data should be collected, and from where and whom they should be obtained. During the process, in-depth descriptions, interpretations and theoretical perspectives are generated. Phenomena are then described through narratives and accounts as a way of understanding, explaining and making inferences. Latent and content analysis can be used to analyse transcripts and develop themes and categories (Field & Morse 1994; Holloway & Wheeler 2002).

Melia (1982) in her now classic study used grounded theory, further developed by Strauss & Corbin (1994), and in-depth interviews to study student nurse socialisation. Analysis yielded six conceptual categories, which were then used as a framework for presenting substantive issues raised by the students. The categories were: 'learning and working', 'getting the work done', 'learning the rules', 'nursing in the dark', 'just passing through', 'doing nursing' and 'being professional'. From 'nursing in the dark', for example, she derived further categories, which she labeled 'coping with the dark', 'fobbing off the patient' and 'awareness contexts'.

In PA, analysis is collaborative and collective and, as described in the example below, permits a variety of needs and concerns to be expressed. Processed data are referred to as 'findings' or 'results'. Methods of data analysis vary according to the underlying research approach. Qualitative research is presented through words and narratives, quantitative research through numbers and statistical manipulations and also in tables and graphs (Greenhalgh 2006; Holloway & Wheeler 2002).

A multi-method evaluation of a clinical educational innovation

A multi-method evaluation was undertaken by Scholes *et al.* (2008) to evaluate the impact on practice of an education innovation, the development of physical assessment skills modules for nurses. The approach was a 360 degree evaluation and as many stakeholders as possible were involved in the evaluation. Interviews, both face to face and telephone, were undertaken with the alumnae of the course, the general practitioners or other medical staff they worked with and, where appropriate patients and carers. The nurses' managers were also interviewed in order to determine if their expectations of the nurses post-course had been met. Observations of the interactions between the nurses and the patients they were examining were also undertaken. The sample was purposive and recruitment relied on local contacts. The multi-method approach allowed the researchers to build up a picture of the impact of the nurses' development of physical assessment skills on a range of stakeholders. Comparisons were made between the findings and the literature.

Different perspectives were elicited by the different methods. Interviews allowed the researchers and participants to explore issues related to the topic in more depth; the telephone interviews were more focused and used a more predetermined format. However, the telephone interviews, by saving on travel time, allowed the researchers to widen their sample using the semi-structured schedule that had been employed during face-to-face interviews.

Example of PA

Pain & Francis (2003) undertook a project with homeless young people, young people who had been excluded from school and people who were working with these young people. The aim of the project was to explore the experiences of homeless and excluded young people in order to understand the experiences of victimisation and concerns about crime and disorder. The authors employed a range of data collection methods such as interviews and observations. However, they also used participatory diagramming, whereby the young people used tools such as post-its and coloured pens to identify, discuss and prioritise issues. Where solutions were identified, the participants were encouraged to act on them if they wanted to. The data from the project were verified with the participants.

General research issues

Validity, reliability and generalisability

Regardless of methodological considerations, all researchers must consider issues of validity and reliability. In quantitative research, reliability refers to the extent to which methods and settings are consistent over time, across groups and between researchers. Validity refers to the accuracy and truth of the data being produced in terms of the concepts being investigated, the people and objects being studied and the methods of data collection and analysis being used. For qualitative researchers the social context in which data are collected is important to consider. During field observations for example, as researchers become increasingly familiar with the research setting, they are able to check the accuracy and recurrence of data in a number of different situations and from a variety of participant perspectives.

Validity and reliability are important concepts in large-scale studies, such as clinical trials and surveys, if the studies are to be generalisable. This is a particular concern in undertaking systematic reviews to ensure the robustness of the findings. Meta-analyses take account of these issues by reviewing the populations, methodologies and findings of a number of studies on a given topic. Statistical analysis is then applied to assess the significance of the combined results.

Results from qualitative research are not usually generalisable to the wider population due to the small sample sizes and contextualised nature of the findings. However, such findings have theoretical generalisability in terms of their ability to relate the results to raise awareness about experiences of others and the implications for practice. One of the authors conducted a phenomenological study (Vydelingum 2000) and despite the small purposive sample, the findings of this study have nonetheless given important insights into the experiences of South Asian patients in hospital. The isolation and loneliness encountered by patients due to communication difficulties should make nurses more aware of such experiences and hopefully discuss these issues with relatives. Nurses would be able to pay more attention to the information given to South Asian patients and relatives about their conditions and aftercare, and ensure that supportive domiciliary services are mobilised.

In qualitative research, concepts of validity and reliability are not easily transferable. There is a lot of debate and controversy about the best ways to evaluate qualitative research (Koch 1994; Sandelowski 1993). However, Guba & Lincoln (1989) proposed four main methods for establishing rigour in qualitative studies: dependability, credibility, transferability and confirmability.

- *Dependability* (reliability): findings of the study need to be consistent and correct to be dependable, so that anyone reading the study will be able to evaluate the sufficiency of the analysis and results from the research process
- *Credibility* (internal validity): the extent to which readers and participants can recognise the meaning that they give to the situations or contexts or the 'truth value' of the results
- *Transferability* (generalisability): how the results in one context could be 'transferred' to comparable situations or participants. In some cases, due the small-scale samples utilised, theoretical transferability could be achieved
- *Confirmability* (objectivity): this method requires an audit or decision trail for readers who can judge the study for the intellectual honesty, researchers' bias and openness to sensitivity to the methods

Presentation and dissemination

Presentation and research dissemination are essential so that findings are made available to be used and applied by others. Researchers may change their style of presentation according to their audience. One of the authors wrote her research for two journals: the *Journal of Advanced Nursing* (Smith 1987, 1991) and *Nursing Times* (Smith 1989). To the non-researcher, the article in the first journal may appear 'jargonistic', using language that is difficult to understand. In the *Nursing Times* article, the language is more accessible and easier to understand by the field-level practitioner. The issue of whether researchers should write in the first or third person is discussed by Webb (1992). The convention in quantitative research is to maintain objectivity and authority by writing in the third person. Qualitative, and particularly feminist, researchers prefer to write in the first person. In this way, they write themselves into their research accounts and make their methods and findings more transparent to the reader.

The notion of networks is an important part of the modernised health service and has been set up for the purposes of practitioners sharing expertise and knowledge across NHS trusts. The public health networks have been set up primarily to allow public health specialists and practitioners across PCTs 'to share good practice, manage public health knowledge and very importantly act as a source of learning and professional development' (DH 2004e, p. 39). These networks also offer contacts with universities to support research, education and development and joint-cross boundary collaborations across PCTs.

The internet or world wide web

The internet is useful for gathering and sharing information on web pages, by email, in forum discussions and newsgroups. It also influences the way research is conducted and disseminated. Although there has been massive investment in information technology, some practitioners still do not have access to the internet and inequalities still exist between different parts of the country and different professional groups. This situation is improving as the NHS commits itself to ensuring that its employees have access to email and a vast range of electronically accessible databases. It is essential that access and training are provided to practitioners because of the many uses of information technology and the net. Because information develops at such a fast rate, information published in more traditional media, such as books and journals, is in danger of being out of date before it is published.

Professional, ethical and information sharing issues are associated with research on the net. At present, it is extremely difficult to regulate the internet or hold individuals or companies responsible for unethical research practices. Copyright on the net is ambiguous, meaning not only is most information free and transcends boundaries, but also individuals and companies are not accountable for bad press of individuals, libellous remarks or improper research and unethical practices. Web-service providers say they are unable to regulate what goes on their notice boards or is discussed in forums. The main message to be taken from this by potential researchers is to be extremely cautious about the information received and transmitted via the internet. Currently, large amounts of information are available and positive and negative uses of the Internet must be considered.

Research proposals

Monkley-Poole (1997) suggests:

'There can be many reasons for writing a proposal apart from "pure" research. For example, similar principles can be applied to writing proposals to obtain resources to introduce change into clinical practice or undertake an audit of services. Proposals can also be submitted to request funding to support study leave or attendance at a conference. In the health service, the move to the market with its emphasis on evidence based health care suggests the need for practitioners to attract monies to fund research and to clearly identify and document research activities being undertaken in the clinical areas.'

A proposal puts forward the argument for why a piece of research is worth doing, how it will add to the body of knowledge and the plans and procedures necessary to successfully complete it. The applicant also includes short curriculum vitae to demonstrate that he or she has the necessary experience for the job. When writing any proposal it is important to consider the membership of the panel or committee who will be taking decisions based on its content since each member will have different backgrounds and biases. It is important to be clear and explicit when putting together the proposal especially if the people making decisions about it are likely to be unfamiliar with its approach. Another source of guidance for preparing and submitting a research proposal is provided by Punch (2000).

Funding

Researchers with an interest in particular topics will apply for funding when tenders are advertised. These are found in a variety of places,

such as nursing journals including the *Nursing Times* and *Nursing Standard*. Newspapers such as the *Guardian* or *The Times Higher Education Supplement* are also good sources of information about funding.

In addition, several websites can assist in identifying funding sources and their purposes such as the Charities Aid Foundation (www.cafonline. org) and www.trustfunding.org.uk which had replaced the *Directory of Grant Making Trusts*. The *Association of Medical Research Charities Handbook* (AMRC 2004) has also been replaced electronically. All the information previously contained in the handbook is now available on the organisation's website (www.amrc.org.uk). Guidelines supplied by funding organisations will contain the relevant information to inform the applicant. These guidelines may also indicate the preferred philosophical and methodological approach to be employed.

Individual funding bodies invite submissions at different times of the year and may offer varying degrees of financial support. It is important, therefore, for the applicant to be realistic when estimating the budget and to request resources that will satisfy anticipated need as 'top-up' funds after the event may not be forthcoming. One source of funding that had been open to nurses especially for the study of education and practice-based research was the English National Board for Nursing, Midwifery and Health Visiting, now incorporated into DH funding initiatives and, to a lesser extent, the United Kingdom Central Council for Nursing, Midwifery and Health Visiting, now superseded by the Nursing and Midwifery Council.

An important source of funding is the NHS Service Delivery and Organisation (SDO) research and development programme administered by the London School of Hygiene and Tropical Medicine (LSHTM). Useful advice is provided on its website (www.sdo.lshtm.ac.uk).

The association of the LSHTM with the SDO R&D programme is an example of how funding for research programmes is administered through higher education establishments. Universities may also have research committees that allocate monies to local staff in response to competitive bids. The CHAIN (communication, help, advice, information network), now administered through the NHS University, is an excellent news source on research contacts, bids and specialist practice that it is well worth subscribing to (chain@nhsu .org.uk).

Charities such as the Florence Nightingale Foundation are specifically committed to funding research, travel, training and projects (www.flor-ence-nightingale-foundation.org.uk) while the Foundation of Nursing Studies is committed to supporting practice development, small scale research projects, dissemination and implementation (FoNS 1996, www.fons.org).

Ethical issues

Irrespective of paradigm, approach or method, research proposals should always be scrutinised for their ethical implications and submitted to an ethics committee for approval prior to commencement of the study. It is perhaps worth noting that people involved in research are called different things depending on the research design, for example, they are called *subjects* in experimental studies, *respondents* in surveys and *participants* in qualitative research such as ethnography or phenomenology, and by virtue of what they are called can give you an indication of the type of activities involved. Research subjects should also be fully informed of the study's implications before giving their written consent and be able to withdraw without prejudice at any time. Participant observation should not be covert and researchers using this method should be clear about their role.

All research activity must comply with the Research Governance Framework for Health and Social Care (DH 2001), as in general terms, health authorities and PCTs owe a direct and non-delegable duty of care to NHS patients. The framework clarifies responsibilities and accountabilities that define the setting in which negligence might occur and refers to the responsibility of researchers' employers.

Health authorities are required to set up multi-centre research ethics committees (MRECs) and local research ethics committees (LRECs) to protect both subjects and researchers. The multi-centre committees cover a cluster of health

authorities and the researcher applies to one of these committees when the research is being undertaken in more than one site. When the research is being undertaken in one site only the researcher applies to the appropriate local trust based committee. She or he must also apply to the local research and development committee for permission to commence fieldwork and to request an honorary contract. Ethics committees are also found in universities and students carrying out research as part of an academic award are expected to apply to their respective university ethics committees. Professional bodies, such as the Royal College of Physicians and the Royal College of Nursing, produce guidelines to assist researchers in considering the ethical dimensions of their research proposals (RCN 1993). Similar guidelines are available from the British Psychological Society and the British Sociological Association for researchers. ARVAC (Association for Research in the Voluntary and Community Sector) has a set of ethical guidelines sensitive to the complex needs of the sector and which focus on the research subjects' rights. Researchers are urged to take account of equal opportunities, in terms of race, gender, disability and sexual orientation and the principles, values, objectives and agendas of the participants. The development of 'mutually beneficial relationships' between researchers and researched, set within the wider 'social, political and economic setting', are seen as key (ARVAC 2000, www.arvac.org.uk).

Unexpected ethical consequences can result from 'neutral', seemingly theoretical science; for example, the application of theoretical physics to the development of the atom bomb did untold harm and formed no part of Einstein's original intentions. Similarly, Darwin's theory of evolution was used by many Victorian biologists to advance pejorative racial stereotypes. This was especially true in Australia during the nineteenth century. Social Darwinism, as it was known, put forward racist stereotypes of aboriginal inferiority that tried to establish European cultural dominance. This approach continues to this day.

Unlike obviously intrusive clinical trials, and research practices such as giving placebos rather than treatment or testing drugs with unknown side effects, qualitative research not involving patients or clients is often seen as exempt from the need to be scrutinised by an ethics committee. However, ethical implications of covert research, i.e. research undertaken without the subjects' knowledge, are apparent when findings are reported without subjects ever having known they were being observed.

Consider, too, the ethical implications of interviews about feelings and emotions and the need to consider the participant's view with respect to research on women involving cervical screening (Howson 1999) or young women's experiences of abortion (Harden & Ogden 1999). Such interviews need to be carefully managed so as not to distress the interviewee.

Ethics committees

Ethics committees are set up to regulate good ethical practice in the conduct of health care research. In the UK the National Research Ethics Service (NRES) collaborates with colleagues to maintain a UK-wide system of ethical review that protects the safety, dignity and well-being of research participants, while facilitating and promoting ethical research within the NHS. Through the granting of ethical approval, ethics committees are ensuring that health care research adheres to the basic principles of the Helsinki Declaration and the EU convention on Human Rights.

The Human Rights Act 1998, active since 2000, contains numerous articles that are relevant to health care research. Protection of right to life (Article 2), prohibition of torture or degrading treatment or punishment (Article 30), the right to liberty and security (Article 5), the right to respect for private and family life (Article 8) and freedom of thought, conscience and religion (Article 9) should be included for consideration in study proposals to protect the interests and well-being of research participants. Further information on the requirements for ethics committees is available on local PCT websites and the DH and NRES websites (www.nres.npsa.nhs.uk/).

Ethics committees require researchers to prepare written proposals to demonstrate the proposed study's adherence to ethical principles, such as autonomy, consent, justice, beneficence and non-malevolence. Practically, this may involve the signing of a consent form, following a full explanation of events, before the research commences. Informed consent signifies that the potential participants have had the opportunity to get satisfactory information or explanation about the research, their roles and expectations clarified. It is also important for researchers to allow the participants sufficient time to consider the information before making a decision and they should also be offered guarantees that a refusal to participate in the research will not jeopardise the care or service they receive. Any nurse is within his or her rights to ask to see the consent form before allowing researchers access to patients.

Research on people with mental health problems, with a learning disability or with children is problematic. This is because these groups are vulnerable to improper research practices. There is the issue of whether children, the learning disabled and mental health service users may make informed decisions and give their full consent (or whether someone can consent on their behalf). Informed consent is particularly important if one considers the capacities of these groups as they are spelled out in law.

Conclusion

Research is the combination of systematic inquiry and a personal journey. The personal interests and style of each researcher and practitioner influences the questions asked and the approaches taken.

It is hoped the chapter will generate ideas for the reader about the approaches and findings used for the study of community nursing and public health care and their application to practice. In particular, it identifies the knowledge base for primary health care and the topics and methodologies of relevance to the field. Reflective practice and research mindedness are described as part of the primary care practitioner's tool kit for recognising and drawing on experience which in turn contributes to the evidence base which informs research and practice. The world wide web (www) plays an important part in making a wide range of materials electronically accessible as part of the policy, practice and research base. Issues such as ethics, proposal writing and funding are also raised to further assist primary care practitioners to apply and use research.

Research, in its various guises, is no longer an optional extra in the modern health service. Indeed, the current NHS agenda actively supports the development of a critical research culture. This chapter aimed to assist primary care and public health practitioners to shape a role for themselves within that culture in order to meet their own professional and personal needs and those of patients and clients. See Box 6.4 for suggested further reading.

Box 6.4   Further reading

- Audit Commission Reports – www.audit-commission.gov.uk
- Cochrane database – www.cochrane.org/reviews/
- The 2001 Census – www.statistics.gov.uk/census2001
- Department of Health – www.dh.gov.uk
- Eppi-Centre – http://eppi.ioe.ac.uk
- Health Impact Assessment – www.hiagateway.org.uk
- National Institute of Clinical Excellence (NICE) – www.nice.org.uk
- National electronic Library for Health (NeLH) – www.library.nhs.uk
- National Institute for Health Research – www.nihr.ac.uk
- Our Healthier Nation – www.webarchive.org.uk/pan/11052/20050218/www.ohn.gov.uk/index.html
- The National Library for Public Health – www.library.nhs.uk/publichealth/
- York Centre for Systematic Reviews and Dissemination – www.york.ac.uk/inst/crd/

Journals

- Links Page – www.sciencekomm.at/journals/medicine/nurse.html
- *Nursing Standard* – www.nursing-standard.co.uk
- *Journal of Advanced Nursing* – www.journalofadvancednursing.com/
- *Nursing Times* – www.nursingtimes.net/
- The Sociology of Health and Illness – www.blackwellpublishing.com/shil_enhanced/

Ethics

- National Research Ethics Service – www.nres.npsa.nhs.uk/
- The Human Rights Act 1998 – www.gov.uk/acts/1998/htm

Funding

- Foundation of Nursing Studies – www.fons.org
- Florence Nightingale Foundation – www.florence-nightingale-foundation.org.uk
- The Association of Medical Research Charities – www.amrc.org.uk
- Directory of Grant Making Trusts – www.trustfunding.org.uk
- The NHS Service Delivery and Organisation (SDO) Research and Development programme – www.sdo.lshtm.ac.uk

Networks

- Communication, help, advice and information network (CHAIN) – http://chain.ulcc.ac.uk/chain/
- The Developing Practice Network – www.dpnetwork.org.uk/
- The Public Health Network – public-health@jiscmail.ac.uk

Statutory body
- Nursing and Midwifery Council – www.nmc-uk.org
(All websites accessed in November 2008.)

References

Abramson, J.H. & Abramson, Z.H. (1999) *Survey Methods in Community Medicine.* Churchill Livingstone, Edinburgh.

Association of Medical Research Charities (2004) *The Association of Medical Research Charities.* Available at: www.amrc.org.uk (accessed 24 November 2008).

Association for Research in the Voluntary and Community Sector (2000) *Code of Good Practice for Researching in the Voluntary Sector.* ARVAC, London. Available at: www.arvac.org.uk (accessed 24 November 2008).

Atkinson, P. (1995) Some perils of paradigms. *Qualitative Health Research,* **5,** 117–124.

Baum, F. (1995) Researching public health: behind the qualitative–quantitative methodological debate. *Social Science and Medicine,* **40,** 459–468.

Bell, J. (2005) *Doing your Research Project: A Guide for First Time Researchers in Education and Social Science,* 3rd edition. Open University Press, Buckingham.

Benner, P. (1984) *From Novice to Expert: Excellence and Power in Clinical Nursing Practice.* Addison Wesley, Menlo Park, California.

Black, N. (1994) Why we need qualitative research. *Journal of Epidemiology and Community Health,* **48,** 425–426.

Brink, P.J. & Wood, M.J. (1994) *Basic Steps in Planning Nursing Research: From Question to Proposal.* Jones & Bartlett, Boston.

British Broadcasting Corporation (BBC) (2008). *BBC Radio 4 News.* Broadcast 1 April 2008.

Bryman, A. (2007) Barriers to integrating quantitative and qualitative research. *Journal of Mixed Methods Research,* **1,** 1–18.

Bryman, A. (2008) *Social Research Methods,* 3rd edition. Oxford University Press, Oxford.

Clark, A., Reid, M., Morrison, C., Capewell, S., Murdoch, L. & McMurray, J. (2008) The complex nature of informal care in home-based heart failure management. *Journal of Advanced Nursing,* **61,** 373–383.

Coghlan, D. & Brannick, T. (2005) *Doing Action Research in Your Own Organization,* 2nd edition. SAGE, Thousand Oaks, California.

Cotter, A. & Smith, P. (1998) Epilogue: setting new research agendas. In: *Nursing Research: Setting New Agendas* (ed. P. Cowley Smith). Arnold, Hodder Headlines, London, pp. 212–228.

Crichton, N. (1990) The importance of statistics in research design. *Complementary Medical Research,* **4,** 42–49.

Czuber-Dochan, W., McBride, L. & Wilson, J. (1997) Exploring the concepts of research through the media. In: *Research Mindedness for Practice* (ed. P. Smith). Churchill Livingstone, Edinburgh.

Daly, J., Macdonald, I. & Willis, E. (1992) *Researching Health: Designs, Dilemmas, Disciplines.* Tavistock/Routledge, London. pp. 234–247.

Department of Department of Health (1992) *Health of the Nation: A Strategy for England.* Department of Health, London.

Department of Health (1997) *The NHS: Modern, Dependable.* Department of Health, London.

Department of Health (1999a) *Saving Lives: Our Healthier Nation.* Department of Health, London.

Department of Health (1999b) *Health Impact Assessment: Report of a Methodological Seminar.* The Stationery Office, London.

Department of Health (2001) *Research Governance Framework for Health and Social Care.* Department of Health, London.

Department of Health (2002) *Liberating the Talents: Helping Primary Care Trusts and Nurses to Deliver the NHS Plan.* Department of Health, London.

Department of Health (2003) *The Victoria Climbié Inquiry Report of an Inquiry by Lord Laming.* Department of Health. London. Available at: www.dh.gov.uk/en/Publicationsandstatistics/Publications/PublicationsPolicyAndGuidance/DH_4008654 (accessed 24 November 2008).

Department of Health (2003) *Supplementary Prescribing by Nurses and Pharmacists within the NHS in England: A Guide for Implementation.* Department of Health, London.

Department of Health (2004a) *Every Child Matters: Change for Children.* Department of Health, London.

Department of Health (2004b) *The Chief Nursing Officer's Review of the Nursing Midwifery and Health Visiting Contribution to Vulnerable Children and Young People.* Department of Health, London.

Department of Health (2004c) *Choosing Health: Making Healthy Choices Easier.* Department of Health, London.

Department of Health (2004d) *The NHS Improvement Plan: Putting People at the Heart of Public Services.* Department of Health, London. Available at: www.dh.gov.uk/en/Publicationsandstatistics/Publications/PublicationsPolicyAndGuidance/DH_4084476 (accessed 24 November 2008).

Department of Health (2004e) *NHS Improvement Plan: Putting People at the Heart of the Public Services.* Department of Health, London.

Department of Health (2005a) *Chronically Sick and Disabled Persons Act 1970: Research and Development Work Relating to Assistive Technology 2004–2005).*

Department of Health, London. Available at: www.dh.gov.uk/en/Publicationsandstatistics/ Publications/PublicationsPolicyAndGuidance (accessed 24 November 2008).

Department of Health (2005b) *Raising the Profile of Long Term Conditions Care: A Compendium of Information.* Department of Health, London. Available at: www.dh.gov.uk/en/Publicationsand statistics/Publications/PublicationsPolicyAnd Guidance/DH_082069 (accessed 24 November 2008).

Department of Health (2005c) *Supporting People with Long Term Conditions: An NHS and Social Care Model to Support Local Innovation and Integration.* Department of Health, London. Available at: www.dh.gov.uk/en/Publicationsandstatistics/ Publications/PublicationsPolicyAndGuidance/ DH_4100252 (accessed 24 November 2008).

Department of Health (2006a) *Our Health, Our Care, Our Say: A New Direction for Community Services.* Department of Health, London.

Department of Health (2006b) *Modernising Nursing Careers: Setting the Direction.* Department of Health, London.

Department of Health (2006c) *NHS Surges Ahead on Key Care Outside Hospitals Reform.* Department of Health, London. Available at: www.dh.gov (accessed 24 November 2008).

Department of Health (2006d) *Our Health, Our Care, Our Community – Investing in the Future of Community Hospitals and Services.* Department of Health, London.

Department of Health (2006e) *Strategic Review of Research and Development – Mental Health.* Department of Health, London. Available at: www.berr.gov. uk/dius/science/science-funding/framework/ next_steps/page28988.html (accessed 4 December 2008).

Department of Health (2007a) *Towards a Framework for Post Registration Nursing Careers (Consultation Document).* Department of Health, London.

Department of Health (2007b) *Facing the Future – Chair Ros Lowe.* Department of Health, London.

Department of Health (2007c) *Practice Based Commissioning News.* Available at: www.dh.gov.uk/ en/Managingyourorganisation/Commissioning/ Practice-basedcommissioning/DH_4131190 (accessed 4 April 2008).

Department of Health (2008a) Research and Development Map. Available at: www.dh.gov.uk/ en/Sitemap/Researchanddevelopmentmap/index. htm (accessed 4 April 2008).

Department of Health (2008b) *Research and Development A–Z: A Comprehensive List of Research and Development (R&D) Work in the DH and the NHS.* Available at: www.dh.gov.uk/en/Researchanddevelopment/ A-Z/Researchgovernance/DH_4002306 (accessed 4 December 2008).

Dingwall, R. & Fox, S. (1986) Health visitors' and social workers' perceptions of child care problems. In: *Research in Preventive Community Nursing Care: Fifteen Studies in Health Visiting* (ed. A. While). Wiley, Chichester.

Donaldson, L. (2006) *What Makes a Good Doctor?* Speech to the Joint Committee on Postgraduate Training for General Practice at the Royal College of General Practitioners, 21st February 2006. Available at: www. dh.gov.uk/en/Aboutus/MinistersandDepartment Leaders/ChiefMedicalOfficer/CMOPublications/ QuoteUnquote/DH_4102558 (accessed 4 December 2008).

Dunkley, R. & Baird, A. (2000) *Training Needs Analysis for Public Health.* Public Health Resource Unit. Oxford.

Everitt, A., Hardiker, P., Littlewood, J. & Mullender, A. (1992) *Applied Research for Better Practice.* Macmillan, Basingstoke. p. 4–5.

Field, P.A. & Morse, J.M. (1994) *Nursing Research: The Application of Qualitative Approaches.* Chapman Hall, London.

Fielding, N. & Schreier, M. (2001) Introduction: on the compatibility between qualitative and quantitative research methods, *Forum: Qualitative Social Research.* Available at: www.qualitative-research.net/index. php/fqs/issue/view/26 (accessed 4 December 2008).

Foss, C. & Ellefsen, B. (2002) Methodological issues in nursing research. *Journal of Advanced Nursing,* **40**, 242–248.

Foundation of Nursing Studies (FoNS) (1996) *Reflection for Action.* FoNS, London.

Franks, V. & Smith, P. (2002) *Context, Continuity and Change: Reassessing the Nursing Task.* Presentation to the Association for Psychoanalytic Psychotherapy in the NHS, Tavistock Clinic, London.

Freshwater, D. & Bishop, V. (2003) *Nursing Research: Appreciation, Critique and Uitilisation.* Palgrave, Basingstoke.

Gibbons, M., Limoges, C., Nowonty, H., Schwattzman, S., Scott, P. & Trow, M. (1994) *The New Production of Knowledge: The Dynamics of Science and Research in Contemporary Societies.* Sage, London.

Gilbert, N. (2001) *Researching Social Life,* 2nd edition. Sage, London.

Gomm, R., Needham, G. & Bellman, A. (2000) *Evaluating Research in Health and Social Care.* Sage and the Open University, London.

Greenfield, T. (ed.) (2002) *Research Methods for Postgraduates.* Arnold, London.

Greenhalgh, T. (2006) *How to Read a Paper: The Basics of Evidence-Based Medicine,* 3rd edition. Malden, Mass. BMJ Books/Blackwell, Oxford.

Guba, E.G. & Lincoln, Y.S. (1989) *Fourth Generation Evaluation.* Sage, Newbury Park.

Guba, E.G. & Lincoln, Y.S. (1994) Competing paradigms in qualitative research. In: *Handbook of Qualitative Research* (eds N.K. Denzin & Y.S. Lincoln). Sage, Thousand Oaks, California, pp. 105–117.

Hanlon, J. (1994) Ghost of the poll tax. *Red Pepper,* June: 33.

Harden, A. & Ogden, J. (1999) Young women's experiences of arranging and having abortions. *Sociology of Health and Illness,* **21**, 426–444.

Harris, A. (1993) Developing a research and development strategy for primary care. *British Medical Journal,* **306**, 189–192.

Health Visitors Association (HVA) (1994) *Mix and Match.* HVA, London.

Health Visitors Association (HVA) (1995) *Weights and Measures.* HVA, London.

Holloway, I. & Wheeler, S. (2002) *Qualitative Research in Nursing,* 2nd edition. Blackwell Publishing, Oxford.

Howson, A. (1999) Cervical screening, compliance and moral obligation. *Sociology of Health and Illness,* **21**, 401–425.

James, T., Smith, P. & Gray, B. (2004) Emotions, evidence and practice: the struggle for effectiveness. In: *Shaping the Facts: Evidence-Based Nursing and Health Care* (eds P. Smith, T. James, M. Lorentzon & R. Pope). Elsevier Science, Edinburgh, pp. 55–70.

Kendall, S. (1997) What do we mean by evidence? Implications for primary health care nursing. *Journal of Interprofessional Care,* **11**, 23–34.

Kelle U. (2001) Sociological explanations between micro and macro and the integration of qualitative and quantitative methods, [online]. *Forum: Qualitative Social Research.* Available at: www. qualitative-research.net/index.php/fqs/article/view/966 (accessed 4 December 2008).

Kitson, A. (2008) Approaches used to implement research findings into nursing practice: Report of a study tour to Australia and New Zealand. *International Journal of Nursing Practice,* **7**, 392–405.

Koch, T. (1994) Establishing rigour in qualitative research: the decision trail. *Journal of Advanced Nursing,* **19**, 976–986.

Kuhn, T. (1970) *The Structure of Scientific Revolutions,* 2nd edition. University of Chicago Press, Chicago.

Laming, H. (2003) *The Victoria Climbié Inquiry.* Report of an Inquiry, Departments of Health & Home Office, London.

Macaulay, A., Commanda, L., Freeman, W., Gibson, N., McCabe, M., Robbins, C. & Twohig, P. (1999) Participatory research maximises community and lay involvement. *British Medical Journal,* **319**, 774–778.

Macleod-Clark, J. & Hockey, L. (1989) *Further Research for Nursing.* Scutari Press, London.

Medawar, P. (1984) *The Limits of Science.* Oxford University Press, Oxford.

Melia, K. (1982) 'Tell it as it is': qualitative method ology and nursing research: understanding the student nurse's world. *Journal of Advanced Nursing,* **7**, 327–335.

Meyrick, J., Burke, S. & Speller, V. (2001) *Public Health Skills Audit 2001: A Short Report.* Health Development Agency, London.

Monkley-Poole, J. (1997) Research proposal writing and funding. In: *Research Mindedness for Practice* (ed. P. Smith). Churchill Livingstone, Edinburgh.

Moore, R.A. (1995) Helicobacter pylori *and Peptic Ulcer – A Systematic Review of Effectiveness and an Overview of the Economic Benefits of Implementing What is Known to be Effective.* Cortecs, Isleworth.

National Institute of Clinical Excellence (2002) Perspectives on evidence based practice. Available at: www.nice.org.uk/niceMedia/pdf/persp_evid_dmarks.pdf (accessed 7 May 2008).

National Institute for Health Research (2008) *About the National Institute for Health Research.* Available at: www.nihr.ac.uk/about.aspx (accessed 24 November 2008).

Neuman, W. (2006) *Social Research Methods: Qualitative and Quantitative Approaches,* 6th edition. Pearson/Allyn and Bacon, London.

Oakley, A. (1992) *Social Support and Motherhood: the Natural History of a Research Project.* Blackwell Publishers, Oxford.

Pain, R. & Francis, P. (2003) Reflections on participatory research. *Area,* **35**, 46–54.

Parahoo, K. (2006) *Nursing Research: Principles, Process and Issues,* 2nd edition. Palgrave Macmillan, Basingstoke.

Pearson, P. (2008) Public health and health promotion. In: *Community Public Health in Policy and Practice,* 2nd edition (ed. S. Cowley). Ballière Tindall Elsevier, Edinburgh, 46–60.

Polit, D. & Beck, T.C. (2008) *Nursing research.* Lippincott Williams & Wilkins. Philadelphia.

Popay, J., Rogers, A. & Williams, G. (1998) Rationale and standards for the systematic review of qualitative literature in health services research. *Qualitative Health Research*, **8**, 341–351.

Pope, C & Mays, N. (eds) (2000). *Qualitative Research in Health Care*. BMJ Books, London.

Pope, R., Graham, L. & Jones, P.C. (2004) Randomised controlled trials: illustrative case studies. In: *Shaping the Facts: Evidence-Based Nursing and Health Care* (eds P. Smith, T. James, M. Lorentzon & R. Pope). Elsevier Science, Edinburgh, pp. 89–110.

Pound, P., Bury, M., Gompertz, P. & Ebrahim, S. (1995) Stroke patients' views on their admission to hospital. *British Medical Journal*, **311**, 18–22.

Punch, K.F. (2000) *Developing Effective Research Proposals*. Sage, London.

Rees, C. (1992) Practising research based teaching. *Nursing Times*, **88**, 55–57.

Rogers, B.L. (2005) *Developing Nursing Knowledge: Philosophies, Traditions and Influences*. Lippincott Williams & Wilkins, Philadelphia.

Royal College of Nursing (1982) *Promoting Research Mindedness*. Royal College of Nursing, London.

Royal College of Nursing (1993) *Ethics Related to Research in Nursing*. Royal College of Nursing, London.

Sandelowski, M. (1993) Rigor or rigor mortis: the problem of rigor in qualitative research. *Advances in Nursing Sciences*, **16**, 1–8.

Sapsford, R. & Abbott, P. (1998) *Research Methods for Nurses and the Caring Professions*. Open University Press, Buckingham.

Scholes, J., Chellel, A., Scott-Smith, W., Volante, M., Coulter, M. & Colliety, P. (2008) *An Evaluation of an Educational Intervention (Physical Assessment Module) for the Non-Medical Workforce to Efficiently Provide Unscheduled Services Across the Primary and Secondary Sector in One SHA*. University of Brighton/University of Surrey.

Schön, D.A. (1987) *Educating the Reflective Practitioner*. Jossey Bass, San Francisco.

Silverman, D. (2005) *Doing Qualitative Research: A Practical Handbook*, 2nd edition. Sage, London.

Smith, P. (1987) The relationship between quality of nursing care and the ward as a learning environment: developing a methodology. *Journal of Advanced Nursing*, **12**, 413–420.

Smith, P. (1989) Nurses' emotional labour. *Nursing Times*, **85**, 49–51.

Smith, P. (1991) The nursing process: raising the profile of emotional care in nurse training. *Journal of Advanced Nursing*, **16**, 74–81.

Smith, P. (ed.) (1997) *Research Mindedness for Practice*. Churchill, Livingstone, Edinburgh.

Smith, P. (2004) Gathering evidence: the new production of knowledge. In: *Shaping the Facts: Evidence-based nursing and health care* (eds P. Smith, T. James, M. Lorentzon & R. Pope). Elsevier Science, Edinburgh, pp. 111–138.

Smith, P., James, T., Lorentzon, M. & Pope, R. (eds) (2004) *Shaping the Facts: Evidence-Based Nursing and Health Care*. Elsevier Science, Edinburgh.

Smithies, J. & Adams, L. (1993) Walking the tightrope: issues in evaluation and community participation for health for all. In: *Healthy Cities: Research and Practice* (eds J. Davis & M. Kelly). Routledge, London.

Social Enterprise Coalition (2008) *What is Social Enterprise?* Available at: www.socialenterprise.org.uk/pages/what-is-social-enterprise.html (accessed 4 December 2008).

Strachin, G., Wright, G. & Hancock, E. (2007) An evaluation of a community health intervention programme aimed at improving health and wellbeing. *Health Education Journal*, **66**, 277–285.

Strauss, A. & Corbin, J. (1994) Grounded theory methodology: an overview. In: *Handbook of Qualitative Research* (eds N.K. Denzin & Y.S. Lincoln). Sage, Thousand Oaks, California, pp. 273–285.

Taylor, L. & Blair-Stevens, C. (2002) *Introducing Health Impact Assessment (Hia): Informing the Decision-Making Process*. Health Development Agency, London.

The *Guardian*. (2008) *Devastating Report reveals Baby P Failings*. Report by J. Carvel, social affairs editor. 2 December 2008, pp. 1–2.

Upton, D.J. (1999) How can we achieve evidence-based practice if we have a theory-practice gap? *Journal of Advanced Nursing*, **29**, 549–555.

Vydelingum, V. (2000) South Asian patients' lived experience of acute care in an English hospital: a phenomenological study. *Journal of Advanced Nursing*, **32**, 100–107.

Vydelingum, V., Colliety, P., Hutchinson, K. & Smith, P. (2004) Mapping the Needs of the NHS Public Health Practitioner Workforce in PCTS. Surrey and Sussex Strategic Health Authority, unpublished report.

Walker, M.F., Gladman, J.R.F., Lincoln, N.B., Siemonsma, P. & Whiteley, T. (1999) Occupational therapy for stroke patients not admitted to hospital: a randomised controlled trial. *The Lancet*, **354**, 278–280.

Wanless, D. (2004) *Securing Good Health for the Whole Population, Population Health trends.* Treasury, London.

Watts, G. (1999) Cases in need of evaluations. *The Times Higher*, pp. 30–31.

Webb, C. (1992) The use of the first person in academic writing: objectivity, language and gate keeping. *Journal of Advanced Nursing*, **17**, 747–752.

Journals

Journal of Interprofessional Care (2000) Special Issue on the New Collaboration, **14**.

Nursing Ethics: An International Journal for Health Care Professionals. Hodder Headline, London.

Chapter 7 **Health Visiting**

Marion Frost and Sandra Horner

Introduction

As discussed in the previous edition of this book (Sines *et al.* 2005), the loss of separate registration for health visitors and the development of a new part of the Nursing and Midwifery Council (NMC) register for specialist community public health nurses in 2004 led to an uncertain future for the health visiting profession. However, a recent major review of the role of health visitors requested by the Secretary of State for Health (*Facing the Future*, Department of Health [DH] 2007a), has given health visiting a clearer direction and firmly established the profession's role in the public health arena.

This review recognises that health visitors have a key role to play in the strategy developed by the Labour Government to modernise the National Health Service (NHS). This aims to reduce inequalities in health and well-being by improving access to health and health care with services built around the needs of the public (DH 2002a, 2006a 2007b). The unique contribution expected from the health visiting profession is a focus on early intervention, prevention and health promotion for young children and families using public health skills and knowledge to improve both short- and long-term health outcomes.

Furthermore, demographic changes, technological advances, consumer demands and an increase in disorders related to lifestyle factors such as obesity have influenced the pattern of delivery of health and social care requiring a more efficient and effective way of working. Health visitors must respond to the changing health needs of the individuals, families, groups and communities they serve and take the opportunity to review and clarify their role within the context of the wider workforce. Primary care trusts (PCTs) will need to ensure there are sufficient public health nurses, including qualified health visitors, effectively trained to tackle the government's agenda.

The future for health visitors therefore appears to be within the developing children's workforce, leading teams and working collaboratively to plan and deliver services that improve the health and life chances of all children and families, while providing early intervention and intensive support to those most at risk (DH 2007b). This process involves a high level of expertise using best available evidence to work with the population to identify and raise awareness of health needs, influence policies affecting health and facilitate activities that promote health and well-being. The extent to which the profession of health visiting has historically adapted to change and is now able to respond to this new agenda will be examined.

The development of the profession

There is some debate about the nature of the work undertaken by the original practitioners who came to be known as health visitors (Dingwall 1977). While much of their early focus was on the provision of health advice and assistance to mothers of young infants in response to the high infant mortality rates and squalid living conditions that were witnessed in the late 1800s, some were prominent in influencing policy decisions that aimed to reduce inequalities in health. There was also a missionary aspect to the service which initially grew out of the philanthropic endeavours of the middle classes and only gradually became organised by the state.

In 1862, the Ladies Sanitary Reform Association was formed in Manchester and

Salford and is generally acknowledged to be the start of the health visiting profession (Mason 1995). Respectable working women were appointed to go from door-to-door among the poorer classes to teach individuals about hygiene and child welfare, mental and moral welfare, and provide social support with the aim of reducing inequalities in health. Alongside this, women sanitary inspectors carried out voluntary public health work, supervising housing, sanitation and structural defects. One of their members, Margaret Llewellyn-Davies, identified the effects of social and economic deprivation on the health and well-being of families. Her detailed accounts of the harrowing experiences of childbirth and parenting were instrumental in the introduction of maternity and child welfare benefits in the National Insurance Act of 1911 (Billingham *et al.* 1996).

Another example of sanitary inspectors seeking to influence the socio-economic environment of their clients was exemplified by the work of The Women's Public Health Officers Association (which later became the Health Visitors Association). The association moved a number of resolutions on the need for improved maternity services at the Trades Union Congress (TUC) in the 1920s and 1930s which led to the TUC working with the British Medical Association to draw up a scheme for a national maternity service in 1939 (TUC 1981).

While these activities could be described as evidence that health visiting is firmly rooted in a public health approach, there is little doubt that during the first half of the twentieth century, health visiting activity focused on maternal and child health from a more individualised perspective. Indeed, Blane (1989) argues that it was the assiduous work of the health visitors at this time which played a central role in reducing infant mortality. Ironically, although the dramatic reduction in infant and child deaths seemed to vindicate the work of health visitors it also raised questions about the continued need for the service which had, by 1918, become obligatory (Dingwall & Robinson 1993).

Under the NHS Act 1946, the scope of health visiting broadened to include working with all age groups although still retaining a major focus on mothers and children. The Jameson Report (Ministry of Health [MoH] 1956), in reviewing the sphere of work of the health visitor, proposed a generalist role as a 'family visitor' whose key function was primarily health education and social advice. However, many health visitors still felt they had a continued responsibility to raise public awareness of health needs during a time when public health and prevention became sidelined by medical care (Billingham *et al.* 1996, Council for the Education and Training of Health Visitors [CETHV] 1977).

Public health and health visiting – 1970s onwards

In 1977, the CETHV formulated principles of professional practice which reflected the process of health visiting in a public health context (since updated by Cowley & Frost 2006):

- The search for health needs
- The stimulation of an awareness of health needs
- The influence on policies affecting health
- The facilitation of health enhancing activities

The principles (Box 7.1) provided a framework for the new public health agenda that began to emerge in the mid-1970s as part of the World Health Organization's global strategy (Lalonde 1974). This in turn legitimised the broader public health approaches to which the profession had aspired over the years. However, in 1974, the health visiting service moved from the control of the local authority to be part of the NHS. General practitioners (GPs) remained outside this merger and the later introduction of 'GP fundholding' under the NHS and Community Care Act 1990 enabled them to contract for health visiting services which included a maximum 10% public health role (Poytrykus 1993). The focus of general practitioners on the medical model of service provision created tensions for health visitors and concerns arose about the emphasis placed on achieving measurable targets, such as the uptake of child development checks and immunisations. This was carried

---

Box 7.1 Principles of health visiting (Sources: CETHV 1977, Cowley & Frost 2006, Twinn & Cowley 1992)

- *The search for health needs*: searching for health needs is the fundamental basis for health visiting practice and is the starting point for tackling health inequalities. Health visitors work proactively in their search for *actual* and *potential* health needs of individuals, families, groups and communities using a partnership approach to collect both qualitative and quantitative data. The search for health needs is purposeful and non-stigmatising, focusing on health and well-being rather than illness or disease. The basic premise is that everyone has a right to the best possible state of health.
- *Stimulation of an awareness of health needs*: having identified the health needs of the population health visitors seek to stimulate an awareness of inequalities, such as poverty, among individuals, families, groups and communities. Awareness raising may involve work with the media, community groups, lay organisations, action, pressure and self-help groups. Targets for awareness raising include clients, families, communities, health service managers, PCT boards, politicians and policy-makers, and all those agencies whose activities impact on health.
- *Influence on policies affecting health*: health visitors with their knowledge of health needs participate in the public health policy process by contributing information and advice to policy proposals and consultation documents, thus acting as advocates at a local and national level. This may be achieved through the activities of individual health visitors, professional organisations or specialist interest groups. Targets for political pressure also include local councillors, Members of Parliament and PCTs.
- *The facilitation of health-enhancing activities*: Health visitors acknowledge that individuals may find it difficult to adopt a healthy lifestyle because of their socio-economic circumstances and therefore seek not only to promote health and well-being at the individual level but to contribute towards changing the environment in which people live. They will also assist the development of group or community activities that aim to develop personal confidence, knowledge and self-esteem in order to enable people to adopt health enhancing behaviours and to make informed lifestyle choices.

---

out at the expense of 'upstream' public health activities such as influencing policy developments and working collaboratively to improve the environments in which people live.

Whilst for many qualified health visitors the reality of practice meant limited time allocated for public health work, the now defunct United Kingdom Central Council for Nursing, Midwifery and Health Visiting (UKCC 1994) proposed that the title of health visiting be expanded to 'Public Health Nursing – Health Visiting' in the specialist practitioner training programmes which then led to separate registration as a health visitor. The publication of the Standing Nursing and Midwifery Advisory Committee report (SNMAC 1995) reaffirmed the contribution of health visitors in 'championing' public health approaches through individual and community health promotion. More recently, the Labour Government's modernisation agenda has supported both a family-centred and public health role for health visiting practice (DH 1999a,b, 2001).

Modernising the role of the health visitor – a public health approach

Health visiting has a strong tradition of working proactively with individuals, families, groups and communities (DH 2001). Yet it is the very nature of the way in which health visitors work that has often made it difficult to define their activities and measure the long-term health outcomes. In a political climate of limited resources and ever-increasing demands on the service, the management emphasis in the NHS has been on short-term identifiable outcomes and immediately measurable outputs which have failed to take account of the longer-term benefits of a public health approach to practice.

With the election of a Labour Government in 1997 this ethos appeared to have changed and the opportunity for health visitors to further develop their role in the promotion of health and prevention of ill-health for individuals, families and communities was acknowledged. The publication of a number of significant documents set out a new health agenda in which health visitors were identified as having a pivotal role (Acheson 1998, DH 1999a,b, 2001, Home Office 1998). Health visitors were encouraged to modernise their role in response to the government's strategy for health, with its focus on health promotion, preventive care and reducing inequalities in health, which placed public health and primary health care centre stage.

The Acheson report (1998) identified a need for high priority to be given to improve the health of families with children, reduce income inequalities and raise the living standards of poor households. It specifically recommended that health visitors should further develop their role in providing social and emotional support for parents and their children in disadvantaged circumstances. The report identified the need to target the least well off in society in order to reduce health inequalities. Subsequently, in line with the government's 'joined up thinking' policy, *Saving Lives: Our Healthier Nation* (DH 1999a) identified health visitors as public health practitioners who would be pivotal to the achievement of this strategy, working in collaboration with local agencies, local communities and PCTs. Health visitors were encouraged to respond effectively to the government's agenda through developing 'a family-centred public health role, working with individuals, families and communities to improve health and tackle health inequality' (DH 1999a, p. 132). The DH published a strategy for nursing, midwifery and health visiting to respond positively to the modernisation agenda (DH 1999b) which restated the components of the modern role for health visitors. In addition, greater emphasis was placed on a leadership role for health visitors leading teams of nurses, nursery nurses and community workers working in partnership with local communities and vulnerable groups.

It was evident from the above recommendations that while an important component of the health visitor's role would still be supporting families with young children, they would also be expected to seek opportunities to work with other groups in the community. The *Health Visitor Practice Development Resource Pack* (DH 2001) offered a framework and guidance for practitioners, their colleagues and managers to develop the modern way of working with families and communities, and to work to common priorities such as national service frameworks. Furthermore, it recognised that health visitors had always been trained as public health workers and suggested that they needed to refocus their professional practice from routine task orientated activities to respond to priorities identified through community health needs assessment. However, starting from a perspective which is frequently based on an epidemiological approach to data collection may lead to professionals determining health care provision without proper consultation with service users, an integral aspect of public health work (Dingwall & Robinson 1993). Health visitors needed to combine the two approaches.

Delivering improvements in the health of the population has been at the core of the government's plan for modernising the NHS (DH 2002a, 2003a, 2004a). Health visitors, along with nurses and midwives, are required to be at the forefront of change in order to improve health and health care for their clients (DH 2002b, 2003a). Achieving the national targets to reduce the gap in infant mortality across social groups and raise life expectancy in the most disadvantaged areas faster than elsewhere, required coordination at government level, local strategic partnerships, participation of local people and innovation by frontline staff (DH 2003b). The *National Service Framework for Children, Young People and Maternity Services* challenged all those working with the public to deliver a high-quality service for children, young people their parents or carers (Department for Employment and Education [DfEE] & DH 2004).

As part of the modernisation programme, the government also recognised the need to secure public protection through improved professional self-regulation that is more open, responsive and accountable (DH 1999a). The professional body, the NMC, was required by law to develop a new simplified register as part of its function to protect the public. Following lengthy consultation, three parts were agreed to include nursing, midwifery and specialist community public health nursing (SCPHN). Commencing on 1 August 2004, all health visitors on part 11 of the UKCC register were automatically transferred to the new register with the title of Registered Specialist Community Public Health Nursing (Health Visiting) (NMC 2004).

This loss of separate registration for the health visiting profession was in direct conflict with the Labour Government's decision in 1999 to maintain separate registration for health visitors and had a hugely demoralising effect on the profession. While initially the unique and distinct nature of health visiting practice appeared to be endorsed by government policy, the subsequent Nursing and Midwifery Order 2001 removed all mention of health visiting, which is now subsumed under the umbrella of SCPHN. However, as Brocklehurst (2004a) suggested health visiting had the ability to respond and adapt to political and professional change. The way forward appeared to lie in recognising the opportunities available, forming strategic alliances with other agencies and supporting local communities in identifying and developing their own services (Brocklehurst 2004b).

Modernising nursing careers

In 2006, the government published *Modernising Nursing Careers* (DH 2006b), outlining how nursing roles and responsibilities needed to change to respond to reforms taking place in the structure of health care delivery which placed greater emphasis on care in the community and the home. New ways of working were required to provide quality services that put the needs of the public at the forefront, including integrated care based on best evidence and focused on prevention, health promotion and supported self-care. The development of new senior leadership roles such as modern matrons, community matrons and nurse consultants had given the

profession the opportunity to take on enhanced roles and develop entrepreneurial skills. Future careers were to be built around client pathways using competence and flexibility as the currency for personal development, with an increased number of assistants working as part of the multi-disciplinary teams.

Much of this strategy seemed to reflect the changes that had been required of health visiting practice in earlier government policy and in November 2006, as part of *Modernising Nursing Careers*, the government commissioned a specific review of health visiting practice in response to the lack of clarity and appreciation of the role which was threatening to undermine the profession (DH 2007b). A national consultation process followed with over 1000 health visitors and local leaders contributing to the debate plus a review group of stakeholders that brought together the expertise of professional bodies, academics, parenting organisations, commissioners, service providers practitioners and educationalists.

The health visiting review 2007

The purpose of the review, *Facing the Future*, was to make recommendations for a renewed role for health visitors within the changing context of public health and health care (DH 2007a). Factors identified as impacting on health visiting practice included:

- Cross-government policies on public health, children and social exclusion
- New evidence on the neurological development of young children, mental health promotion, the effectiveness of early intervention on prevention, parenting programmes and home visiting
- An increased emphasis on evidence-based practice
- 'Progressive universalism'
- Inequalities in health
- Changing public expectations and new technologies
- Changes in the workforce with new roles developing
- Integration of services, new commissioning arrangements and patterns of organisation

The consultation process revealed the uncertainty practitioners felt about the future of the profession and the current commissioning of services which had led to a loss of health visitor posts in some parts of the country. There was evidence of a marked variation in the health visiting interventions offered to service users in different PCTs, with home visiting at a minimum level in many areas. Parents, GPs and commissioners all appeared to have different expectations of the role.

A majority of those consulted recognised the need for change and the consensus view was that the future health visitor role should focus on working with others to improve the health of children and families. In particular, the future primary role of the health visitor was identified as:

- Leading and delivering the evidence-based Child Health Promotion Programme using a family-focused public health approach and
- Delivering intensive programmes for the most vulnerable children and families.

Depending on local demand and commissioning of services, health visitors were also considered able to provide wider public health programmes and primary care services for children and families. There was no agreement over whether health visiting services should be located within the new Sure Start Children's Centres or the primary health care team. Overall the review recognised the need to reform the existing health visiting service into 'a fully integrated preventative service for children and families within a public health context.'

Facing the future: the government response

The government's response to the review (DH 2007b) has been mainly supportive of the recommendations and acknowledged the unique contribution that health visitors can contribute to services for children and families. As frontline practitioners with public health skills and knowledge of local communities, health visitors are recognised as having expertise that could be used in the planning and commissioning of services

to ensure that those most disadvantaged receive extra support. The development of Sure Start programmes and their expansion into children's centres will continue to provide many health visitors with opportunities to work collaboratively and provide integrated services for children and families. Irrespective of how local services are commissioned, health visitors will be expected to maintain their links with both general practice and children's centres in order to maximise the reach of services and help support excluded families to access community-based services.

The government welcomes the leadership role for health visitors in the Child Health Promotion Programme (CHPP) but warns against a managerial role taking precedence over a participatory role. The CHPP is recognised as providing the overarching framework for universal preventive services for children. A model of progressive universalism will be recommended to ensure that all families receive support tailored to meet their specific needs, including home visits and community outreach.

Progressive universalism is:

'a universal service that is systematically planned and delivered to give a continuum of support according to need at neighbourhood and individual level in order to achieve greater equity of outcomes for all children. Those with greatest risks and needs receive more intensive support.'

(DH 2007a)

This level of service provision goes beyond a minimum core service provided by many PCTs where clients may only receive one assessment contact, frequently the new birth visit, with the expectation that clients then attend clinic based services for further support.

Family nurse partnership programme

In order to prevent social exclusion, the government is investing in a new intensive home visiting programme in ten pilot sites across England. Based on a model of support pioneered in the USA over the past 30 years by Professor David

Olds, the Family Nurse Partnership Programme (FNPP) provides health visitors and midwives with the opportunity to work with the most vulnerable families in society with the aim of achieving significant long-term benefits. The programme is focused on at risk young, first time parents, providing regular support visits during pregnancy and the first two years of a child's life which build on parent's strengths and use motivational interviewing techniques, therapeutic skills and specific programme materials. Long-term outcomes in America have included higher intellectual functioning in children and fewer behaviour problems, plus longer gaps between pregnancies (Olds *et al.* 2004). There is clear evidence from the US programme that it needs to be delivered by designated and specially trained practitioners (Olds *et al.* 2002). Overall, the government plans for more health visitors to work in disadvantaged areas, leading and delivering services that improve the health and life chances of children in these communities, are in line with the Children's Plan (Department for Children, Schools and Families [DCSF] 2007).

The updated CHPP (DH 2008)

Since the publication of the *National Service Framework for Children, Young People and Maternity Services* in 2004, there have been significant changes in parents' expectations, knowledge about neurological development, and in children's policy and services. The new programme aims to:

- Provide greater emphasis on promoting the health and well-being of children in the early stages – during pregnancy and the first five years of life
- Support a model of progressive universalism with a core programme for all children, and additional services for children and families with particular needs and risks
- Encourage partnership working between different agencies on local service developments
- Focus services on changing public health priorities such as obesity, breast-feeding, and social and emotional development

Delivery of the programme relies on a team approach that includes children's centre staff and members of the primary health care team, with an agreed and defined lead role for the health visitor. Effective leadership is required to ensure provision of a holistic and coordinated service tailored to meet local needs. The government has recommended that a health visitor takes responsibility for coordinating the CHPP as they have a public health nursing background, provide a service for a registered population of children from pregnancy to five years, have knowledge and understanding of child and family health and well-being, and skills in working with individuals and communities.

Challenges and opportunities for health visiting practice

The requirement for health visitors to work in new ways to respond to the changing context of health care has been clearly spelt out by the Department of Health (DH 2007b). However, there are a number of challenges for health visiting practice that need to be examined in relation to their contribution to supporting the developing agenda of working with children and families in a public health context.

Firstly, the uniqueness of health visiting practice has been recognised for its provision of a universal, non-stigmatising service to the well population, particularly families with children aged under five years (CETHV 1977; Home Office 1998). This has provided the opportunity to work with clients to identify and prioritise the health needs of a local population, taking into account the user perspective as required by current government policy (DH 2006b). However, with a steady decline in the health visiting workforce over the past 15 years, it is doubtful whether these policy expectations are continuing to be met (Cowley 2003; Craig & Adams 2007).

Targeting of services and selective home visiting may have led to a failure to identify vulnerable families who are least able to access services or fear being stigmatised. As Robinson (1999) suggested 'without universalist surveillance it is not possible to identify those in need of a greater health visiting input since the bulk of health and social problems occur in the large number of people who are not especially high risk rather than in the few who are high risk'.

(Robinson 1999, p. 18)

The concept of progressive universalism, which is to be welcomed, requires investment by government and service providers in a high-quality workforce appropriately trained and supported to identify and respond to those most at risk.

The government emphasis on targeting of services has also created dilemmas for the health visiting profession in relation to health promotion and health surveillance. Dingwall & Robinson (1993) argued that developing the health visiting service on a contractual basis in response to expressed need changes the nature of health surveillance with, for example, children being seen only at clinics where inadequacies of parenting may be difficult to identify and potential needs not identified. In order to reduce inequalities in health, home visiting should be viewed as a 'valid instrument of social policy', which advocates for those excluded from political decision-making through age or other factors. Opportunities for family health promotion have been eroded in areas where postal questionnaires have been used to review the developmental progress of children (Clarke *et al.* 2004). Hopefully, the government's support for developing children's services based on a model of progressive universalism will influence commissioners and managers to provide sufficient resources to enable the provision of robust evidence-based interventions.

The pressure for the provision of more cost-effective services has also led some PCTs to introduce screening tools in an attempt to identify those most at risk. While some practitioners may find these tools a useful aid, questions arise as to whether the level of risk is, or should be determined by professionals or clients, particularly where vulnerable people are involved. In addition, concerns have been expressed about the sensitivity of such tools in accurately identifying risk factors and the continuing relevance of identified factors which may change over time (Elkan *et al.* 2000). It is therefore crucial that health visitors and other practitioners use any such tool in conjunction with professional judgement, continually reviewing the factors identified and ensuring protection for children and vulnerable adults in line with government policy such as *Every Child Matters: Next Steps* (DH 2004b) and the *National Service Framework for Children, Young People and Maternity Services* (DfEE & DH 2004).

Nevertheless, the identification of actual and potential health needs is a cornerstone of the public health approach and remains fundamental to the planning of health care interventions in the modern NHS. In response to this, health visitors must continue to use their well-established skills in caseload analysis and community profiling to influence PCT decisions about the development of appropriate health care interventions and services, to meet the needs of the local population. Key issues may arise from the results of community profiling that could be in variance with central government targets and local health improvement plans.

Caseload analysis (Robotham 2005) provides health visitors with important information about the local population and the factors which impact on their lives, which may not be revealed in the local public health report. While mortality and morbidity rates provide a vital overview of the health of the community they may not identify those health issues which most concern individuals, nor do they necessarily identify relevant variables. For example, the Director of Public Health's Report may identify a high incidence of accidents among the under-5s. Yet it is the health visitor's records which could show the links between maternal depression and accidents or the fact that accidents occur most frequently where families are poorly accommodated or where there is a lack of play facilities. Health visitor records may also identify families who are becoming isolated because of racial harassment or fear of crime.

Furthermore, caseload and workload analysis provides an opportunity for health visitors to review work patterns to provide evidence for research-based practice and to evaluate their own practice. Information gathered should be critically analysed, acknowledging both its strengths and weaknesses, and used to support PCTs in commissioning relevant services and the implementation of local public service agreements (PSA). With a developing public health workforce, it is crucial that health visitors are clear about their role, using their knowledge of a community and robust data of the effectiveness of their interventions to market their service. However, the collection of these data is problematic, and where staffing shortages occur data collection and analysis may be incomplete.

At a time when the role of the health visitor has been validated as fundamental to advancing the public health agenda as well as supporting vulnerable families, questions must be asked about the extent to which the reality of practice reflects this expectation (DH 2007b).

Public health and health visiting practice

The professional practice of health visiting consists of identifying both actual and potential health needs and developing evidence-based interventions aimed at improving the physical, mental, social and emotional health of individuals, groups and communities. The emphasis is on a proactive approach to practice rather than merely responding to a demand for care, focusing on prevention and health promotion within a public health context.

Public health is defined by Wanless (2004, p. 3) as:

'the science and art of preventing disease, prolonging life and promoting health through the organised efforts and informed choices of society, organisations, public and private, communities and individuals.'

Public health is therefore considered to be the responsibility of everyone from the individual level to the societal level, although this may create tension between the role of the state in defining healthy choices for a population and the right of the individual to choose a particular lifestyle. Health visiting practice has always taken place within a political arena that changes its views on the role of the health service, the importance of the family and individual rights versus responsibilities. The adaptation of a typology proposed by Beattie (1991) and illustrated in Figure 7.1 provides a useful framework for identifying different aspects of the health visitor's role. In Beattie's typology, a basic premise is that effective public health interventions demand the application of an eclectic approach that combines activities at both the individual and collective level. These activities may be either expert-led (authoritative) or undertaken in partnership with clients (negotiated).

Twinn (1993) suggested that practitioners tended to adopt one paradigm rather than another. She argued that expert, authoritative advice giving at the individual level has been the more traditional approach to health visiting practice and focused on giving health education advice to parents about the care of their young children. This paternalistic approach suggests that the expert knows best and may lead to negative views of the service. A national web-based survey of mothers' views of the health visiting service carried out in 2006 found that some participants perceived practitioners as displaying judgemental attitudes based on a fixed set of values and/ or the pursuit of specific behaviours by parents (Russell & Drennan 2007). What parents valued was knowledgeable advice, support and reassurance, accessibility to the service, provision of group opportunities, and prompt referral to specialist services when their children had problems.

Negotiated partnership with clients to promote individual change is central to current government policy and requires the practitioner to take a more facilitative approach, where information is shared with clients to enable informed choices to be made. This approach values the client as knowledgeable but may do little to recognise the circumstances in the environment which also influence health. Much of health visiting work has been based on an individual approach to changing behaviour through advice and support and in a public health approach, collective activities need to become more central in everyday practice.

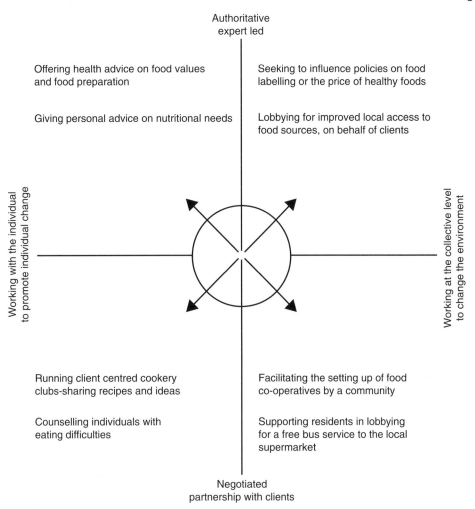

Figure 7.1   Beattie's (1991) typology. Ways of working with people with nutritional problems (adapted)

The concept of collective activities includes alerting politicians, policy makers, unions and PCTs to significant environmental influences and social circumstances which may make it difficult for individuals, families and communities to adopt or experience healthier lifestyles, despite health advice and client awareness. This collective response to changing the environment, in which individuals seek to achieve health, has been referred to as 'making the healthier choice the easier choice', a phrase coined by Milio in 1986 and used to develop more recent government policy: *Choosing*

Health: Making Healthy Choices Easier (DH 2004c). This reflects an acknowledgement that whilst individuals have a personal responsibility for maintaining their own health there maybe internal and/or external constraints which make this difficult or even impossible to achieve. Thus there is a need for interventions by government and other relevant agencies aimed at minimising these constraints and strengthening the resources of individuals, families and communities, so that they are better equipped to build social capital, resist breakdown and meet their own health needs.

In seeking to develop initiatives aimed at meeting health needs, the health visitor is expected to work in collaboration with other relevant agencies across the state, private and voluntary sectors. In their evaluation of a trailblazer SureStart, Northrop *et al.* (2008) found that co-location of health visitors with midwives and community mothers was effective in responding to needs identified by clients. Likewise Harris & Koukos (2007) describe a multi-agency structure for their SureStart work in Swansea. Community profiling was used to inform the process and, in particular, clients of all types were involved in the planning of services and the evaluation. Pritchard & de Verteuil (2007) argue that the ability to access health care equitably is significant in improving health outcomes. The links between poor health, access to health care and poverty are well-recognised. The use of a health equity audit tool can identify and redistribute resources according to need. In applying such a tool to a health visiting service, Pritchard & de Verteuil (2007) suggest that those clients who have the greatest need should have the greatest resources in terms of health visiting input. Services should be based on the health needs of a population and supported by notions of social justice.

A more recognisable community development approach is included in the *Health Visitor Practice Development Pack* (DH 2001). However, Forester (2004) suggested that in order to deliver a true public health agenda based on multi-agency collaboration and community participation, health visiting practice needs to develop further. It especially needs to gain strategic level support as well as ground-level enthusiasm. Recently trained specialist community public health nurses, including health visitors, are particularly well-equipped to tackle this role, having studied leadership and management and new paradigm public health and health promotion.

The way forward

There is an urgent need for health visitors to re-evaluate their contribution to the public health agenda and seek out new ways of working which more effectively support collective as well as individual approaches to health care (Box 7.2). The government has clearly identified that all nurses, midwives and health visitors are required to change existing practice and plan services, with others, in new ways looking at the whole system and the pathway of care (DH 2002b). Services are to be based on actual and potential need (DH 2008b) with service users and the public being central to the planning and development process. Working in isolation, as identified by Smith (2004), is no longer a viable option, and the development of children's centres should facilitate this process.

Box 7.2 A public health approach for health visiting practice

- Tackling the causes of ill-health, not just responding to the consequences
- Looking at health needs across the whole population as well as responding to the needs of the individuals, families or groups
- Planning work on the basis of local need, best available evidence and national health priorities
- Working collaboratively towards achieving public service agreements
- Using information collected about local community health needs to influence service development, promoting community involvement in the process
- Working with other agencies and sectors for health gain, planning services that promote and protect health and well-being
- Finding out which population groups have significant health needs and targeting resources to address these
- Taking action to make healthy choices easy choices, including supporting community development activities
- Leading partnership working for health
- Influencing policies that affect health locally and nationally
- Finding meaningful ways to evaluate the impact of health visiting practice

(*Health Visitor Practice Development Resource Pack*, DH 2001 & Royal College of Nursing [RCN] 2007).

Developing skills in partnership with the wider public health workforce and using opportunities to lead and influence change are essential components of SCPHN practice. Health visitors need to have the confidence to value their expertise and contribution to supporting families, mothers and children, a key theme of government policy outlined in *Tackling Health Inequalities: A Programme for Action* (DH 2003b) and endorsed in Facing the Future (DH 2007b). They must take the opportunity to plan and deliver quality children's services for the most vulnerable in society and the wider population, as identified in the updated CHPP 2008. Health visitors also need to consider how they may contribute to the development of community polyclinics, as outlined in the proposed Darzi plans for the NHS, recognising that clients living in London, in particular, need better access to health care which takes account of ethnicity and cultural issues (Darzi 2007). The rest of the country is also being consulted about local need and how the public can be partners in the decision-making (DH 2008a). Although there is no specific mention of a public health role, health visitors need to be assertive in raising their profile within these consultations because the specific areas of care being considered include children's health and staying healthy.

Health visitors and their teams need to work with consultants in public health medicine, school nurses, general practitioners, midwives, mental health services, social workers, community development workers, health promotion specialists, benefits advisers, nursery school workers and others from the state, voluntary and private sectors. The provision of innovative, accessible services that promote positive parenting, engaging communities as well as individuals, is vital for addressing the underlying determinants of health. The development of children's trusts, bringing together health, social and education services in order to secure integrated commissioning of services, has been designed to facilitate this process (DH 2004b).

Health visitors have much to contribute to an agenda that involves breaking down health and social care boundaries a task which, for many, is part of everyday practice. Dealing with the long-term underlying causes of health inequalities such as poverty and poor housing has always been part of health visiting practice. Health visitors have well-developed negotiation and advocacy skills that can be used in working with differing age groups to influence service provision, gain access to appropriate resources and make a difference to people's lives (Harrison & Lydon 2008; Rogers 2003). They need to develop their leadership role, embracing opportunities to become representatives on policy-making committees and acting on ideas based on best available evidence that meet the needs of local people.

The use of current best evidence to support health care decision-making underpins clinical governance and accountability in practice (NMC 2008). The systematic review of research evidence on the effectiveness of domiciliary health visiting is of significance in the move towards evidence-based practice and the consequence of health visiting practice on the health outcomes for clients and communities (Elkan *et al.* 2000). However, Wanless (2004) warned of the general lack of evidence about the cost effectiveness of public health work. Evaluation in situations where outcomes evolve over a period of time (such as public health work) is a complex process as it is difficult to prove that any change is due to a particular intervention (Houston 2003). A lack of commitment by the government to take forward public health in England in a systematic way, has led to the development of piecemeal initiatives leaving practitioners feeling undervalued (Wanless *et al.* 2007).

Health visitors must have access to databases, allocating time to search for good quality information. They must develop the skills and the will to change practice based on the findings of research, as in the development and evaluation of the Solihull Approach parenting group (Bateson *et al.* 2008). As the emphasis increases on health informatics and the application of information technology within the educational preparation of health visitors and the work setting, such challenges should be overcome. Education and training, including continuing professional development must prepare practitioners appropriately for their new roles to enable the future generation of health visitors to contribute effectively to the changing agenda for children and families in a public health context.

Conclusion

This chapter has explored the need for health visitors to participate proactively in public health provision at the individual, family, group and community level working collaboratively with public, private and non-statutory agencies to promote health and prevent ill-health in different settings. Valuing health and treating it as a positive resource has always been central to health visiting practice.

The requirement to focus the health visiting service on children and families in a public health context has been clearly identified in government policy. Health visitors must value their knowledge and skills, confront the dilemmas in practice, and have the confidence to seek opportunities to plan, develop and lead new approaches to practice in consultation with the public. To enable this process, supportive management and organisational structures need to be developed that facilitate practice.

More importantly, new ways of measuring the effectiveness of health visiting must be found, based on a realisation that public health initiatives aim to produce long-term benefits to society. Measuring the number of activities achieved excludes opportunities for developing imaginative and strategic public health approaches identified as essential for promoting the health of society. As the Office for Public Management (2000, p. 40) said, health visiting must be 'measured not by the activity it undertakes but by the difference it makes'.

References

Acheson, D. (1998) *Independent Inquiry into Inequalities in Health Report*. The Stationery Office, London.

Bateson, K., Delaney, J. & Pybus, R. (2008) Meeting expectations: the pilot evaluation of the Solihull Approach Parenting Group. *Community Practitioner*, **81**, 28–31.

Beattie, A. (1991) Knowledge and control in health promotion: a test case for social policy and social theory. In: *The Sociology of the Health Service* (eds J. Gabe, M. Calnan & M. Bury). Routledge, London.

Billingham, K., Morrell, J. & Billingham, C. (1996) Reflections on the history of health visiting. *British Journal of Community Health Care Nursing*, **1**, 468–476.

Blane, D. (1989) Preventive medicine and public health: England and Wales 1870–1914. In: *Readings for a New Public Health* (eds C. Martin & D. McQueen). Edinburgh University Press, Edinburgh.

Brocklehurst, N. (2004a) The new health visiting: thriving at the edge of chaos. *Community Practitioner*, **77**, 135–139.

Brocklehurst, N. (2004b) Is health visiting 'fully engaged' in its own future well-being? *Community Practitioner*, **77**, 214–218.

Council for the Education and Training of Health Visitors (1977) *An Investigation into the Principles of Health Visiting*. Council for the Education and Training of Health Visitors, London.

Clarke, M., Hague, D., Mortimer, B. & Thompson, S. (2004) Should every three year old receive a routine review? *Community Practitioner*, **77**, 101–104.

Cowley, S. (2003) Modernising health visiting education: potential, problems and progress. *Community Practitioner*, **76**, 418–422.

Cowley, S. & Frost, M. (2006) *The Principles of Health Visiting: Opening the Door to Public Health Practice in the 21st Century*. UKSC, Amicus & CPHVA, London.

Craig, J. & Adams, C. (2007) Survey shows ongoing crisis in health visiting. *Community Practitioner*, **80**, 50–53.

Darzi A, (2007) *Health Care for London: A Framework for Action*. NHS London.

Department for Children, Schools and Families (DCSF) (2007) *The Children's Plan Building Brighter Futures*. The Stationery Office, London.

Department of Health (1999a) *Saving Lives: Our Healthier Nation*. The Stationery Office, London.

Department of Health (1999b) *Making a Difference: A Strategy for Nursing Midwifery and Health Visiting*. The Stationery Office, London.

Department of Health (2001) *Health Visitor Development Resource Pack*. Department of Health, London.

Department of Health (2002a) *Delivering the NHS Plan: Next Steps on Investment, Next Steps on Reform*. The Stationery Office, London.

Department of Health (2002b) *Liberating the Talents Helping Primary Care Trusts and Nurses to Deliver the NHS Plan*. The Stationery Office, London.

Department of Health (2003a) *Liberating the Public Health Talents of Community Practitioners and Health Visitors*. Department of Health, London.

Department of Health (2003b) *Tackling Health Inequalities: A Programme for Action*. The Stationery Office, London.

Department of Health (2004a) *The NHS Improvement Plan*. The Stationery Office, London.

Department of Health (2004b) *Every Child Matters: Next Steps*. The Stationery Office, London.

Department of Health (2004c) *Choosing Health: Making Healthy Choices Easier*. The Stationery Office, London.

Department of Health (2006a) *Our Health, Our Care, Our Say: A New Direction for Community Services*. The Stationery Office, London.

Department of Health (2006b) *Modernising Nursing Careers: Setting the Direction*. The Stationery Office, London.

Department of Health (2007a) *Facing the Future: A Review of the Role of Health Visitors*. The Stationery Office, London.

Department of Health (2007b) *The Government Response to Facing the Future: A Review of the Role of the Health Visitor*. The Stationery Office, London.

Department of Health (2008a) *Our NHS Our Future. NHS Next Stage Review Leading Local Change*. The Stationery Office, London.

Department of Health (2008b) *The Child Health Promotion Programme Pregnancy and the First Five Years of Life*. The Stationery Office, London.

Department for Employment and Education & Department of Health (2004) *National Service Framework for Children, Young People and Maternity Services*. The Stationery Office, London.

Dingwall, R. (1977) *The Social Organisation of Health Visitor Training*. Croom, Helm.

Dingwall, R. & Robinson, K.M. (1993) Policing the family? Health visiting and the public surveillance of private behaviour. In: *Health & Wellbeing: A Reader Health & Wellbeing: A Reader* (eds A. Beattie, M. Gott, L. Jones & M. Sidell). MacMillan, London.

Elkan, R., Kendrick, D., Hewitt, M., Robinson, J.J., Tolley, K., Blair, M., Dewey, M., Williams, D. & Brummel, K. (2000) The effectiveness of domiciliary health visiting: a systematic review of international studies and a selective review of the British literature. *Health Technology Assessment*, **4**, 1–339.

Forester, S. (2004) Adopting community development approaches. *Community Practitioner*, **77**,140–145.

Harris, S. & Koukos, C. (2007) Sure start: delivering a needs-led service in Swansea.*Community Practitioner*, **80**, 24–27.

Harrison, S. & Lydon, J. (2008) Health visiting and community matrons: progress in partnership. *Community Practitioner*, **81**, 20–22.

Home Office (1998) *Supporting Families*. The Stationery Office, London.

Houston, A. (2003) Sure start: the example of one approach to evaluation. *Community Practitioner*, **76**, 294–298.

Lalonde, M. (1974) *A New Perspective on the Health of Canadians*. Minister of Supply and Services Information Canada, Ottawa.

Mason, C. 1995 Towards public health nursing. In: *Community Health Care Nursing*, 3rd edition (ed. D. Sines). Blackwell Science, Oxford.

Milio, N. (1986) *Promoting Health Through Public Policy*. Canadian Public Health Association, Ottawa.

Ministry of Health (1956) *An Inquiry Into Health Visiting (The Jameson Committee)*. HMSO, London.

Nursing and Midwifery Council (2004) *Standards of Proficiency for Specialist Community Public Health Nurses*. Nursing and Midwifery Council, London.

Nursing and Midwifery Council (2008) *The Code Standards of Conduct, Performance and Ethics for Nurses and Midwives*. Nursing and Midwifery Council, London.

Northrop, M., Pittam, G. & Caan, W. (2008) The expectations of families and patterns of participation in a Trailblazer Sure Start. *Community Practitioner*, **81**, 24–28.

Office for Public Management (2000) *Leading the Future*. T.G. Scott, London.

Olds, D., Robinson, J., O'Brien, R., Luckey, D.W., Pettitt, L.M., Henderson, C.R., Ng, R., Sheff, K.L., Korfmacher, J., Hiatt, S. & Talmi, A. (2002) Home visiting by paraprofessionals and by nurses: a randomised control trial. *Pediatrics*, 110, 486–96.

Olds, D., Kitzman, H., Cole, R., Robinson, J., Sidora, K., Luckey, D.W., Henderson, C.R., Hanks, C., Bondy, J. & Holmberg, J. (2004) Effects of nurse home visiting on maternal life course and child development: age 6 follow-up results of a randomised trial. *Pediatrics*, **114**, 1550–1559.

Poytrykus, C. (1993) Public health role cut as GP contracts start to bite. *Health Visitor*, **66**, 188–189.

Pritchard, C. & de Verteuil, B. (2007) Application of health equity audit to health visiting.*Community Practitioner*, **80**, 38–41.

Robinson, J. (1999) Domiciliary health visiting a systematic review. *Community Practitioner*, **72**, 15–18.

Robotham, A. (2005) Skills in specialist community public health nursing–health visiting: working with individuals and families In: *Health Visiting: Specialist*

Community Public Health Nursing (eds A. Robotham & M. Frost) Elsevier Churchill Livingstone, London.

Rogers, E. (2003) Health visitors and older people: 'thinking out of the box'. *Community Practitioner*, **76**, 381–385.

Royal College of Nursing (2007) *Nurses as Partners in Delivering Public Health*. Royal College of Nursing, London.

Russell, S. & Drennan, V. (2007) Mother's views of the health visiting service in the UK: a web-based survey. *Community Practitioner*, **80**, 22–26.

Sines, D., Appleby, F. & Frost, M. (2005) *Community Health Care Nursing*, 3rd edition. Blackwell, London.

Smith, M. (2004) Health visiting: the public health role. *Journal of Advanced Nursing*, **45**, 17–25.

Standing Nursing and Midwifery Advisory Committee (1995) *Making It Happen*. Department of Health, London.

Trades Union Congress (1981) *Women's Health at Risk*. Trades Union Congress, London.

Twinn, S. (1993) Principles in practice: a re-affirmation. *Community Practitioner*, **66**, 319–321.

Twinn, S. & Cowley, S. (1992) *The Principles of Health Visiting: A Re-examination*. Health Visitors Association, London.

United Kingdom Central Council (1994) *The Future of Professional Practice: The Council's Standards for Education and Practice Following Registration*. United Kingdom Central Council for Nursing, Midwifery and Health Visiting, London.

Wanless, D. (2004) *Securing Good Health for the Whole Population*. HMSO, London.

Wanless, D., Appleby, J., Harrison, A. & Patel, D. (2007) *Our Future Health Secured?* King's Fund, London.

Chapter 8 **General Practice Nursing**

Karol Selvey and Mary Saunders

Introduction

General practice nursing is the fastest growing community health care nursing discipline and since 1996 the full time equivalent workforce has grown by 23% (Drennan & Davis 2008). Practice nursing has emerged as a high-profile career opportunity and offers a range of opportunities for nurses who enjoy patient contact, wish to work autonomously but within a team, caring not just for individuals but also for families and communities within the wider primary and social care context. This chapter is divided into two sections, firstly exploring the context of general practice and practice nursing and the policy that has shaped it. The second section will discuss the role and functions of the practice nurse, illustrated by case scenarios.

Historical development of practice nursing

The first practice nurse was employed in 1913, however it was not until 1966 that changes in regulations in the doctor's charter enabled general practitioners (GPs) to employ nurses as part of their ancillary staff. This anomaly, in considering nurses as part of ancillary staff, had a detrimental effect on the development of the role as nurses were often denied opportunities for professional development through lack of funding and subsequently often led to relative professional isolation. The changes incorporated within the GP contract (Department of Health [DH] 1989) implemented in 1990 had a large impact on the numbers of practice nurses employed as the contract advocated a change from the focus of general practice as being curative and reactive to one of being preventive and

proactive. Practice nurses, throughout the 1990s, developed expertise in chronic disease management and health promotion. However, this rapid expansion highlighted the existence of a fragmented approach to education and training for the profession. Despite this, practice nurses developed their own informal networks to support and disseminate good practice and through the Royal College of Nursing (RCN) practice nurse forum lobbied for specialist practitioner recognition from the United Kingdom Central Council (UKCC), which was achieved in 1994.

A much wider range of continuing professional development programmes are now available for practice nurses and many gain experience of nursing within general practice before undertaking nurse practitioner programmes. The majority of practice nurses are employed by GPs who maintain independent contractor status, although more recent policies to review the provision of general practice have produced a range of models which have included awarding contracts to independent companies to provide general practice services. It is important, however, to recognise that the implication of contractor status means that practices operate as small businesses. This has both advantages and disadvantages. Freedom from a hierarchical nursing structure has allowed many nurses a significant level of autonomy, but alongside this is the potential for lack of professional supervision and development as well as participation in the network of support that usually comes from belonging to a larger organisation. Nurses looking to work in general practice should be aware that the direct employer/employee relationship might mean the practice nurses may have to negotiate their own contract, conditions of service and study time to meet professional development needs. However, with Social Enterprise models for care provision being advocated by the government as one of the options for care provision to fit with the concept of encouraging 'plurality of commissioning', the experiences of practice nurses may well be necessary for other staff working in such organisations (see Chapter 20).

The impact of policy and General Medical Services (GMS) contracting on practice nursing

The role of the practice nurse can be extremely broad and span the complete age range of the practice population. The variety of services provided by practice nurses can range from tasks such as dressings, suture removal and venepuncture through to nurse-led long-term condition management and first contact consultations where the nurse sees patients with minor illness and undifferentiated conditions. The degree of specialisation of the nurse will depend on the size of the practice, the support of the GP partners and the health needs of the practice population. However, current health policy (DH 2006, 2007a) supports expansion of nursing roles and many new services are being designed and developed with practice nurses adopting the lead role (Woodroffe 2006). All practice nurses need to be able to function as part of a team but also work autonomously, managing the nursing workload and governance aspects linked to their role. They are also required to work effectively on an interpersonal level with patients, members of the wider health care team and other agencies and therefore, are required to possess a broad range of clinical knowledge and skills as well as being cognisant of the context within which general practice and the primary care organisation (PCO) function.

Currently the predominant model of General practice is that of independent contractor status for GPs, with the practice run as a small business and therefore, it is important for any nurse to understand how the GMS (and other related contracts) influence how the practice functions.

This section aims to provide the background to the development of the current contract and consider how this influences the work of practice nurses.

Historically, GPs were contracted to the National Health Service (NHS) to provide medical services for a registered population according to non-negotiable terms defined within the 'Terms and Conditions of Service', which included 24-hour responsibility for patients 365 days per year. The recognition that this nationally negotiated system for contracting with GPs was inflexible and bureaucratic, instigated a radical modernisation of general practice that began in 1990 (DH 1989, 1990). Subsequent policy development sought to encourage the development of innovative schemes that enabled alternative service delivery models. Personal Medical Services (PMS) schemes introduced in 1997 (DH 1997), for example facilitated the emergence of a range of diverse service delivery systems more closely linked to population health needs. Other commissioned models include the less widely used Alternative Medical Provider Services (APMS) and Primary Care Trust Medical Services (PCTMS) contracts as the basis for service delivery. Further information about each of these models can be found on the DH website (www.dh.gov.uk/en/Healthcare/Primarycare/Primarycarecontracting/index.htm).

The providers of a PMS service could include individual GPs, a practice, a PCT or a group of practitioners, including GPs and nurses. These contracts enabled practices to exert greater control over their substantive budgets, provided they were able to demonstrate how resources would be utilised to improve services to meet the identified needs of the registered practice population and increase facilities for disadvantaged groups such as the homeless and individuals with mental health needs. The implementation of the PMS contract also provided significant opportunities to raise the profile of practice nurses who undertook the provision of a variety of nursing-led services that utilised a considerable diversity of advanced practitioner roles and competencies.

A qualitative evaluation of second wave PMS practices in south-east London undertaken in 2003, identified the critical success factors for PMS as being the provision of additional clinical staff, a cohesive communicative team with a visionary leader and good management systems (de Lusignan *et al.* 2003).

In 2003 the new GMS contract afforded PCOs greater flexibility over how and from whom services were commissioned and included for the first time the potential to utilise alternative providers such as the voluntary sector, commercial providers, NHS trusts, other PCTs, and allowed for direct PCT provision of services alongside GMS and PMS contracts. The new commissioning arrangements were intended to support an expansion of primary care capacity, incorporating delivery of a wider range of services. The underpinning concept was to introduce new mechanisms to afford practices greater control over the range of services that they provided in conjunction with a financial incentive linked to continuous improvement in the quality of the service they actively delivered.

The GMS contract (DH 2003) preserved the status of existing practices as incumbent providers who maintain an obligation to provide those core services deemed essential, such as the management of patients who are ill, or believe themselves to be ill and the management of individuals with chronic disease or terminal illnesses. Practices also had a preferential right to provide additional services, but were able to opt out of such provision in accordance with fixed UK-wide rules.

Additionally, enhanced services, that is, essential or additional services delivered to a higher standard, or services not provided through essential or additional services could also be commissioned by PCOs as appropriate to meet local health need. There are three types of enhanced service: directed, national and local enhanced services.

Directed enhanced services must be provided within each PCT for its population but will not always be provided by every practice. These services include childhood immunisations, influenza immunisations in the over 65 and 'at-risk groups', minor surgery above that

included as an additional service and services for disturbed and aggressive patients and are accompanied by nationally developed specifications and costs. National enhanced services are commissioned to meet local need and therefore may not be commissioned within every PCT area. Locally developed services designed to meet local health needs that were agreed with a practice or other provider are identified as local enhanced services.

The GMS contract was the biggest change to occur in NHS general practice since its inception (NHS confederation/BMA 2003). Although list-based general practice remained at the heart of the new contract, it remains an NHS contract between the PCO and the practice, not the individual GP. This radical shift allowed, for the first time, for nurses, and others, to become partners within a practice rather than just employees. A number of pioneering nurses have taken up partnerships and there are some nurse-led practices that employ GPs (see www.meadowfields-practice.co.uk). However, those who have entered into partnerships highlight the requisite range of skills necessary for personal and professional success (Greaseley 2007).

The framework of the GMS contract has an inbuilt duty of clinical governance, weaving through the quality and outcomes framework (QOF) based on current best available evidence. The QOF was intended to be a voluntary system that both encouraged and rewarded high-quality care and management through participation in an annual quality improvement cycle. The framework covers four domains: clinical, organisational, additional service and patient experience which contain a series of areas with quality standards defined by key indicators. Achievement against each indicator will earn the practice points, which convert into a monetary value. Additional points are available to reward improved access and breadth of care. However, in order to ensure that resources are targeted at areas where both morbidity and contractor achievement are greatest in order to assist in the reduction of health inequalities, QOF clinical domain payments are adjusted by practice disease prevalence as recorded by practice data and in turn then related to national prevalence norms. The aim of this adjustment is to deliver a more equitable distribution of quality rewards in the light of the different workloads that contractors will face in delivering the same amount of quality points. Verification of achievement is via the introduction of the Quality and Outcomes Framework Management and Analysis System (QMAS) and annual review visits undertaken by a team of assessors.

The disease categories incorporated within the clinical indicators are those previously identified as national priorities where evidence exists of the health benefits to be gained from enhancement of service provision and where the principal responsibility for ongoing management resides with the primary care team (see Box 8.1). However, it is on the shoulders of practice nurses that the demands of the contract fall. Already practice nurses provide, on the whole, the bulk of any long-term condition management within primary care and the complex needs of individuals with co-morbidities have been well documented (NatPaCt 2004). It is the intention that the focus within the

clinical standards of the contract on the active management of long-term conditions will demonstrate a significant benefit for such individuals who are often, but not always, older members of the practice population. The development of accurate registers of patients who experience chronic disease has, over time, allowed for an increasingly structured approach to be adopted to direct service provision. The range of indicators contained within the clinical domain of the contract is intended to ensure that consistent standards of appropriate intervention are provided across practice populations.

During 2007–8, the government has been negotiating with GPs to amend the current contract, primarily with the view to encouraging GPs to extend opening hours to facilitate improved access for patients. This has included a rearrangement of QOF in an attempt to incentivise GPs to offer these services (see www.nhsemployers.org/pay-conditions/primary-886.cfm).

Practice nurses are ideally placed to deliver the clinical standards cited within the clinical domain, by taking the lead on the management of the identified long-term condition areas. It is imperative, therefore, that practice nurses continue to develop specialist skills in these areas and ensure that they engage fully with the career opportunities currently being presented by the development of emerging positions such as specialist nurse in areas such as heart failure and diabetes and community matrons within PCOs.

The government has been developing policies that support the transfer of services from acute hospitals to primary care with policies focused on *Shifting the Balance of Power* (DH 2001a). One specific example of such changes related to the management of long-term conditions within the primary care sector through the development of new services, such as intermediate care teams, stroke rehabilitation schemes and other services which were provided to focus care outside of acute hospital settings. This ongoing process of review is continuing within the context of the *NHS Next Stage Review*, with the interim summary published in October 2007 (DH 2007a), underpinned by key points relating the government's vision for the NHS in so far as

---

Box 8.1   GMS contract Clinical Domain Disease Areas

- Coronary heart disease
- Heart failure (left ventricular systolic dysfunction)
- Atrial fibrillation
- Stroke and transient ischaemic attacks
- Hypertension
- Hypothyroidism
- Diabetes
- Mental health
- Chronic obstructive pulmonary disease
- Asthma
- Epilepsy
- Cancer
- Palliative care
- Dementia
- Depression
- Chronic kidney disease
- Obesity
- Learning disabilities

service should be fair, safe, personalised and effective.

The publication of national service frameworks (NSF), as part of the clinical governance strategy, enabled practice nurses to play a major role in ensuring that services were structured to meet not only the needs of patients, but also the clinical standards embedded in the NSFs. Public health priorities (cardiovascular disease, mental illness, cancer and accidents) were also highlighted with the effect that this strategy has influenced the way services are prioritised and delivered in general practice.

The NHS Plan (DH 2000) was very influential in the further development of general practice as it set access targets for the practice that exerted a major influence on performance. These targets advised that by 2004, patients could expect to see a health care professional within 24 hours or a GP within 48 hours of their request. Many practices have had to review their appointment systems to ensure they have been able to meet these targets. One impact has been that many practice nurses are fulfilling new roles such as triaging patients, undertaking telephone consultations or offering first contact services (see later section in this chapter on 'First Contact'). More recently the government has tasked Lord Ara Darzi to undertake a widespread review firstly in London and then in England. His national proposals will have a major impact on both general practice and the organisation and delivery of primary care services (DH 2008). Lord Darzi proposes setting up 'supersurgeries' (Royal College of General Practitioners [RCGP] 2008) or polyclinics/health care centres. This proposal aims to focus much more routine care and initial diagnostic care away from acute hospitals into the community by offering 'one-stop shops' for patients, with better choice and access and enabling a range of health and well-being needs to be provided in good premises. Although welcoming some aspects of the proposals the RCGP (2008) raises concerns that placing multiple services within polyclinics could end the unique relationship between patient and GP and suggests a federated model of caring for patients in primary care. This involves different GP practices working together in 'federations' or collaborations to deliver a more expansive range of health care services closer to home by health care teams known to the patients. Whatever model is adopted for future care provision it will incorporate the key concepts of moving care into the community, increasing access for patients and reducing the demand on acute and emergency services.

The opportunities for nurses to expand their roles have been strengthened by changes in legislation to allow nurses to become independent and supplementary prescribers. As practice nurses have developed their roles in general practice, the opportunity to become independent prescribers has also enhanced patient throughput, especially where patients are being seen on a 'first contact' basis or in out-of-hours services or where the nurse is an expert in key areas such as long-term condition management (for more information about this, see Chapter 18).

Practice nursing – roles and functions

As described earlier, the role of practice nurses can be very broad. The following section focuses on three key aspects of the role:

- First contact
- Public health
- Long-term condition management

First contact

On a typical day in the NHS, one million people contact their GP (DH/RCN 2003). In order to meet this demand, the service requires that care should be provided by the professional who is best able to deliver the required service as part of an integrated team. Consequently, clinical roles are being redesigned, and many practice nurses are now providing first contact services in general practice. This can take a variety of forms ranging from telephone triage to providing a nurse-led minor illness service. The level of clinical autonomy and the range and scope of clinical conditions individual practitioners are able to manage will continue to be dependent on their experience and the depth and breadth of their knowledge. In developing this area of professional practice, nurses must be cognisant of the legal and professional frameworks within which care is delivered and acutely aware of their accountability and acknowledge the limits of their competence (Nursing and Midwifery Council [NMC] 2008).

It has been suggested that as much as 70% of the work undertaken by doctors in primary care might be undertaken by appropriately trained nurses (Horrocks *et al.* 2002; Richardson *et al.* 1998). Evidence from a number of studies demonstrates that nurses are able to provide care to patients with minor illness or undifferentiated conditions at least as effectively as GPs, with the achievement of comparable health outcomes for patients (Laurent *et al.* 2005). Nurses also bring a different emphasis to the consultation as they tend to have a greater holistic focus and incorporate health promotion within the consultation to enable patients to self-manage their conditions in future.

Nurses who provide such services are required to develop expertise in advanced nursing practice including proficiency in consultation skills and accurate history taking alongside advanced clinical examination and decision-making skills. The case scenario in Box 8.2 highlights a typical 'first contact' consultation undertaken by the practice nurse and emphasises the importance of the history taking skills involved and the clinical decision-making necessary to ensure that this is simply a 'minor illness' that may be self-managed and not a symptom of a more serious problem.

Changes in health policy in the UK, such as the drive to reduce the length of hospital stay and the shift towards a primary care-led NHS, have led increasingly to the development of services that would traditionally have been the remit of secondary care (Cameron 2000) provided by health professionals in new roles (DH 1999).

Box 8.2   Case scenario: 22-year-old woman presents with four-day history of sore throat

Assessment of subjective presentation including:

- History – exposure to viral/other illnesses
- Past medical history – Is the patient immunocompromised? Are there known allergies to medications?
- Current medication – Use inhaled corticosteroid medication? Use of the contraceptive pill?

Objective findings through physical examination of head/neck/lungs/abdomen/neurological assessment. Possible differential diagnoses:

- Pharyngitis/laryngitis – viral/streptococcal/allergic/gonococcal/fungal/inhaled irritant
- Mononucleosis
- Gastro-oesophageal reflux disease
- Trauma
- Cancer
- Thyroiditis
- Angina/acute coronary syndrome

Possible investigations dependent on findings – full blood count; monospot.

Pharmacotherapeutics: dependent upon cause – treat symptomatically with hydration, decongestants, simple analgesia and rest. If antibiotics required – advice on dose/route/frequency/unwanted effects/possible need for additional barrier contraception.

Patient education: nature of illness/self-management

Re-assessment if failure to resolve/increase in symptoms (potential complications such as: thrombocytopenia, agranulocytosis, haemolytic anaemia, splenic rupture, myocarditis)

The current NHS review (DH 2007a) has highlighted the need to deliver accessible health care to individuals less equipped to engage with traditional general practice. It has been proposed that at least some of these services could be delivered through a health centre (or polyclinic) model offering a wide range of services previously supplied in secondary care. This increasing diversity in the function of primary care has required nurses to develop competence in a range of advanced nursing skills, such as those required to undertake first contact consultations, for which additional degree level training is required. This requirement is emphasised by the NMC definition of an advanced nurse practitioner, which explicitly identifies nurses practising at advanced levels as being highly experienced and educated (NMC 2006). As the development of advanced nursing practice has become central to the delivery of autonomous, professional, evidence-based, individualised, patient-centred health care, identification of standards for advanced nursing practice have been developed to provide protection for the public alongside a framework for development of expertise for advanced nurse practitioners (see Chapter 15).

Public health

Public health, and by implication enhancing the health status of the nation, has assumed increasing importance over the past ten years. The Faculty of Public Health (Three key domains of public health practice; www.fphm.org.uk/about_faculty/what_public_health/3key_areas_health_practice.asp) defines public health as: 'The science and art of preventing disease, prolonging life and promoting health through organised efforts of society' (Sir Donald Acheson). The public health approaches are that it is:

- Population based
- Emphasises collective responsibility for health, its protection and disease prevention
- Recognises the key role of the state, linked to a concern for the underlying socio-economic and wider determinants of health, as well as disease

- Emphasises partnerships with all those who contribute to the health of the population

The faculty identifies three domains in which public health specialists practice.

Health improvement
- Inequalities
- Education
- Housing
- Employment
- Family/community
- Lifestyles
- Surveillance and monitoring of specific diseases and risk factors

Improving services
- Clinical effectiveness
- Efficiency
- Service planning
- Audit and evaluation
- Clinical governance
- Equity

Health protection
- Infectious diseases
- Chemicals and poisons
- Radiation
- Emergency response
- Environmental health hazards

It can be seen that components of public health feature highly in practice nursing workloads. Practice nurses are involved in providing health protection services, such as immunisation programmes, working with patients and groups to enable them to understand their health needs and support them in self-management of care, case finding and screening, and a wide range of other activities aimed at improving both the health of individuals and that of the practice population. The Chief Medical Officer highlights progress towards public health issues in each of his annual reports and all PCTs have public health departments that are required to focus on how to tackle both national issues as well as those that have more local prominence. Another key government objective for public health policy is the reduction of health inequalities. This policy requirement is not just targeted at health but recognises additionally that there are many social determinants of health, not least those relating to education, housing and access to health services. The status report on the Programme for Action in Tackling Health Inequalities published in 2007 (DH 2007b) highlights some of the progress made in achieving the target: by 2010, to reduce inequalities in health outcomes by 10% as measured by infant mortality and life expectancy at birth. The report highlights some interesting statistics, although it acknowledges that many areas have been slow to change. Areas where practice nurses should have influence include:

- Teenage pregnancy – with a 13.3% drop in the rate of under-18 conceptions between 1998 and 2006
- Flu vaccinations – between 2002 and 2005 the percentage uptake of flu vaccinations

by older people increased (including for the most disadvantaged areas)
- Smoking – since 1998, smoking prevalence among adults including manual workers has decreased

Some topical areas with particular pertinence to practice nursing are influenza vaccination and protecting the most vulnerable patients, smoking cessation (to follow on from the smoking ban in public places that came into force in July 2007, which could be seen as a very influential public health measure), weight and obesity management (alongside a greater awareness of healthy eating, which will have a major impact on the development of some chronic diseases such as diabetes and coronary heart disease). An example of the practice nurse's involvement in public health is given in Box 8.3. The case scenario is about a consultation about preconceptual counselling and identifies the breadth of knowledge and

---

Box 8.3 Case scenario: 32-year-old woman attends practice requesting health advice prior to becoming pregnant

Health promotion advice and counselling can be offered opportunistically to all sexually active women who present for contraception, cervical cytology or other advice. Men should also be included in pre-conception counselling as their health will affect the quality of their sperm and fertility. Key elements for discussion are:

- Weight and nutrition – maintain body mass index (BMI) of 20–25. Healthy balanced diet for both partners, including increased intake of foods that contain folates, for at least three months prior to pregnancy and avoiding some foods, e.g. liver, unpasteurised foods, undercooked meat
- Folic acid supplementation – 400 mcg daily for first 12 weeks of pregnancy
- Exercise – encourage regular gentle exercise
- Rubella immunity – test and immunise as appropriate. Counsel and emphasise need to prevent conception for 1 month post-vaccination.
- Smoking – cessation advice emphasised
- Alcohol – both partners should avoid alcohol for four months prior to conception
- Sexual history – offer screening if identified as being at risk of vaginal or sexually transmitted infections. Requires sensitive counselling
- Illicit drugs – offer support; referral to drugs service may be appropriate
- Management of long-term conditions – importance of adherence to treatments. Referral to specialist as required, e.g. if woman has epilepsy/diabetes
- Genetic disorders – follow local referral procedures for genetic counselling

All advice provided should be supplemented with written information/leaflets that reflect each individual's level of literacy and language

awareness needed by the practice nurse to offer appropriate advice and support to the client.

Consultation skills

In order to work effectively with both individuals and groups, practice nurses must possess a wide range of skills and competencies. These include many areas of discrete knowledge that are necessary in order to work successfully with patients to enable efficient and effective management of their conditions, including health promotion as a key skill. While there are many excellent textbooks that introduce the reader to theories and models of health promotion (e.g. Naidoo & Wills 2008), it is important to consider the application of health promotion to practice. Practice nurses who come directly from an acute nursing background may have to adapt both their consultation skills and their approach to health promotion. Due to time constraints in acute settings, health promotion may only have been practised as a peripheral activity, for example providing a leaflet for the patient as he or she leaves the ward. In general practice much of the practice nurse's role will focus on asserting health promoting activities. This may entail working with the patient in primary prevention, for example administering childhood immunisations or travel vaccinations and health advice. In secondary prevention, the role may involve screening for cervical cancer or hypertension. In tertiary prevention, many practice nurses are involved with helping patients to manage their long-term conditions and activity is focused on assisting patients to attain the best quality of life within the constraints of the disease and its presentational states. In addition, practice nurses need to consistently utilise health promotion opportunities effectively, although some evidence suggests this could be improved (Douglas *et al.* 2006; Duaso & Cheung 2002). In order to do this they need to have an understanding of how to influence patient attitudes and behaviour at an individual level. This requires nurses to possess an awareness of cognitive psychological theories if attitudes and changes in behaviour are to be addressed and achieved. However, such approaches need to be applied within the context of other structural factors such as poverty, socio-economic status, inequalities and opportunities which may significantly limit an individual's ability to make an informed, healthy choice. Becker's health belief model (1974 cited in Naidoo & Wills 2008) provides a useful framework to assist in the identification of various factors that influence health beliefs. The model identifies that behavioural change will follow when the person has evaluated the feasibility and benefits of change against the costs. This evaluation may include their susceptibility to the disease, illness or injury and the severity of its impact. These individual perceptions may also be influenced by modifying factors such as demographic variables (age, gender, ethnicity), socio-psychological variables (personality, social class, peer and reference pressure) and structural variables (knowledge of the disease and prior contact with the disease). Patients may also be prompted to seek advice following 'cues to action' which may range from reading newspaper reports (e.g. prompting them to seek help following 'contraceptive pill scare stories') to direct action following personal experience of the illness of a family member or friend. Some idea of these influences elicited during the consultation will help the nurse to see how the patient may assess the positive and negative outcomes of behaviour change. Becker's model has also been expanded to include Bandura's (1977, cited in Naidoo & Wills 2008) concept of self-efficacy, which suggests that for behavioural change to take place, an individual must:

- Have an incentive to change
- Feel threatened by their current behaviour
- Feel a change would be beneficial in some way and have few adverse consequences.
- Feel competent to carry out the change

During consultations it is often helpful to use a problem-solving approach, working with the patient to assess their health needs, prioritising with them the issues that they perceive to be most important to them. It is here that the nurse is likely to introduce information that may challenge preconceived beliefs, although care must be taken that the information provided is tailored to that particular patient. Prochaska & Diclemente's (1984) trans-theoretical model of change may be useful in trying to understand how 'ready' or perceptible a patient may be to accept change at any given time. However, one limitation of this approach is that it focuses on psychological factors, whereas a person's ability to change is also influenced by social factors. The ability to integrate such disparate factors/concepts before negotiating an agreed plan demonstrates the possession and application of significant nursing expertise. Practice nurses also have the advantage of often being able to implement health-promoting activities over a period of time and therefore knowledge and experience of the implementation of a staged educational approach is essential.

Models such as that described by Ewles & Simnett (2003) help to structure such an approach, although it is essential that this is accompanied by robust record keeping that clearly articulates the process employed and measures the progress made for evaluation purposes. Maintaining records that chart progress in a patient's management plan may demand the deployment of more sophisticated IT skills now that the majority of practices operate a paperless electronic patient record system. An example of patients who might benefit from this staged approach are those who have been newly diagnosed with a long-term condition such as asthma. Occasionally concern or anxiety experienced at the time of diagnosis may limit the patient's ability to assimilate information and the nurse must prioritise the delivery of essential information and subsequently build on this to encourage patient self-management over the ensuing weeks and months. Accordingly, practice nurses need a thorough understanding of health promotion, health psychology and how to support behavioural change in order to accomplish effective health promoting outcomes with their patients.

Health needs assessment

Needs assessment has been an integral part of government policy since 1990 (DH 1990). Practices therefore need to develop collaborative strategies to assist in the production of their local practice profile. This will require analysis of collected patient and demographic data in order to target particular health issues within the practice and to inform the formulation of local practice development and business plans. Practice nurses are an integral part of the practice team and require a range of knowledge and skills to participate in developing the practice profile (for further information see Chapters 5 and 7). The practice profile will also need to reflect a range of key targets identified at national and local levels, which will be integrated to inform local PCT and strategic health authority delivery/commissioning plans, with the aim of providing the 'bigger picture'. PCT public health reports provide detailed information relating to local authority ward profiles, which may be helpful to practices when analysing data to make informed links between local demographic data and the health status of their local communities. Part of the practice nurse's role will be to collaborate in the development of practice profiles and to develop presentation and influencing skills in order to articulate the resultant, identified needs. This will enable the practice nurse's voice to be heard at PCT and professional executive committee levels where decision-making about strategy and deployment of resources takes place, forming a purposeful conduit for information sharing and decision-making between the trust board and its clinical workforce. A challenge to this system in the future will be the split between the commissioning role of the PCT and its provider functions. Practice nurses therefore need to understand the commissioning role of the PCT as they fulfil their function to 'procure' a range of effective and responsive health care services to meet national targets and to respond to local needs. However, this role is also changing as PCTs delegate an increasing share of commissioning decisions to practice-based commissioning (PBC) groups (Rhea 2008). PBC was introduced by the government in 2005 to devolve responsibility for commissioning services from PCTs to local GP practices with the aim of giving local clinicians greater control over resources, thus enabling them to respond more effectively to local, individual need. The benefits are perceived to be:

- The provision of greater variety of services from a greater variety of providers in a range of settings that are closer to home and more convenient to patients
- Bringing the decision-making process closer to communities, e.g. eliminating unnecessary hospital stays
- Greater involvement of frontline doctors and nurses in commissioning decisions

As yet, PBC has not really taken off in the way it was envisaged and opportunities for nurses and other health care professionals to engage in this process have been very limited. There has also been poor engagement of GPs in some areas and this has not been assisted by the restructuring of many PCTs in recent years. However, PBC offers great opportunities for practice staff to influence what is commissioned and provides opportunities to restructure services to respond more effectively to local identified needs. Health needs assessment must precede the commissioning of health care and one of the challenges that this will pose will be the extent to which users are truly engaged in the commissioning process as informed service users. Many practices will have a number of mechanisms for involving service users and commissioners of new services will now always wish to see how service development is underpinned by robust service user involvement strategies (for more information,

see Chapter 23). The inclusion of patient experience in the quality framework of the GMS contract represents an opportunity for practices to obtain systematic feedback from their patients about the quality of services they provide, as well as information about how effectively they are provided. These data can subsequently be used to inform practice service development plans and service redesign. However, achieving integration of patients' perspectives in a general practice setting will be challenging, not least that patients may fear being critical of a service on which they may profoundly depend. This challenge should encourage and stimulate practice staff to think creatively about how patients' views can be better represented.

Long-term conditions management

Managing chronic disease (or longer-term conditions) is a key component of the practice nurse's workload in general practice, and this is likely to increase since chronic disease is regarded as the biggest problem facing the health care system, with 60% of adults in England reporting a chronic health problem (NatPaCT 2004). It is estimated that, due to an ageing population, this figure will rise by 23% over the next 25 years. Chronic disease can be described as those which current medical interventions can only control and not cure. The data in Box 8.4 gives some indication of the size and spread of chronic disease.

Box 8.4   The scale of long-term conditions in the UK (NatPaCT 2004)

- 17.5 million adults in the UK may be living with a chronic health problem
- Up to 75% of people over 75 have a long-term condition
- 45% of people over 75 have more than one long-term condition
- 80% of primary care consultations are for chronic health problems
- Current estimates put the number of people with diabetes at 1.3 million with potentially another million undiagnosed
- Chronic obstructive pulmonary disease – affecting 600 000 people
- Asthma – affecting 3.7 million adults and 1.5 million children
- Arthritis – affecting 8.5 million individuals in the UK
- Epilepsy – affecting 400 000 people in England and Wales (1998)
- Mental ill-health – affecting one in six of the population including one in ten children
- 8.8 million people have a long-term illness that severely limits their day-to-day ability to cope

---

Box 8.5   Case scenario: A 64-year-old South Asian man with type 2 diabetes

- Management should be individualised, holistic, patient-centred, empowering, contextualised, culturally sensitive
- Patient education – starting point and lynchpin of management of disease and lifestyle adjustment. It should include: weight loss (0.5–1 kg/week) where appropriate; healthy eating plan – regular meals/low fat /low glycaemic index foods; regulation of alcohol intake; smoking – *vigorously discourage*; and tailored exercise
- Effective glycaemic control – education on factors that affect control, e.g. food, illness, stress, medication
- Effective pharmacotherapy – may include: hypoglycaemic agents, insulin, antihypertensives, analgesia, vitamin B_{12}, lipid-lowering therapies, aspirin, anti-obesity therapies, smoking cessation therapies
- Reduction of potential complications: microvascular (e.g. retinopathy, peripheral neuropathy, nephropathy) and macrovascular (e.g. atherosclerotic vascular disease)
- Comprehensive consistent and systematic review

The practice nurse will utilise the consultation skills described earlier in the chapter but tailor them to meet individual patient needs to ensure his management is culturally sensitive and takes into account the patient's personal beliefs with the ultimate aim of building a mutual understanding through a process of regular consultations, until the patient demonstrates sufficient understanding to manage his disease effectively. Figure 8.1 shows the three levels of care for people with chronic illness/longer-term conditions.

Many people with chronic illness have more than one long-term condition and 26% of these individuals in the UK have three or more problems. Most of these people are cared for by the primary health care team. However, health care professionals need to be aware that such individuals often have complex medication regimens and may supported by a number of different specialists as well as their GP. Alongside this, the burden of their disease may impact on their ability to function independently and they may have many associated social needs which may isolate them from their family or other support networks. Often the problems caused by the non-life threatening aspects of their illness cause people the greatest problems; frequently the psychological aspects of their care are poorly understood and they may have significant co-morbidities, such as depression.

Box 8.5 identifies a case scenario characteristic of the type of consultation for long-term conditions undertaken by a practice nurse. It highlights the key areas that the nurse should be knowledgeable about in order to monitor such patients and assist them to improve their self-management and prevent future complications.

Figure 8.1 shows the three levels of care for people with chronic illness/longer-term conditions. Most practice nurses will be involved with patients at levels 1 and 2. There is interesting evidence to suggest that supported self-care can be a highly effective means of improving the care of chronic disease (NatPaCT 2004). However, self-management encompasses more than the provision of information to patients, and the future will see a range of strategies designed to support patients and their carers in the ongoing management of their illness. Practice nurses are likely to be one of the key health care professionals involved in the education of patients and carers regarding self-management of their illness, supporting them in developing an understanding of the disease process and its potential impact, how to manage medication and other treatments and advising them how and when to seek health care. In order to do this, practice nurses need to be knowledgeable about common chronic diseases, the psychological impact these can have on patients and families and how to take this into account when planning a learning programme with the patient as well as possessing

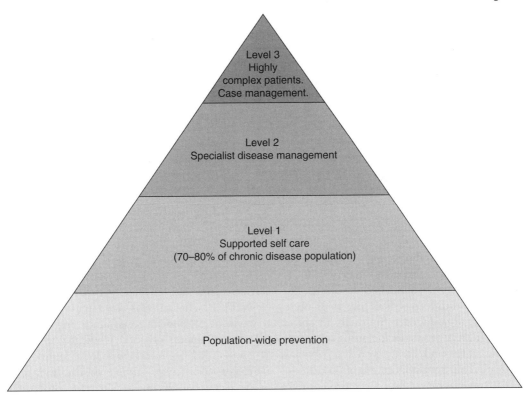

Figure 8.1 Diagram from *Chronic Disease Management: a Compendium of Information* (NatPact 2004). Reproduced under the terms of the Click-Use Licence.

awareness of the range of other support services available. The Expert Patient Programme (DH 2001b) is one example of an initiative aimed at empowering patients to take control of their disease and their lives (see Chapter 23).

The main provider of supported care is the primary care team, but this is wider than just general practice and includes, among others, community nurses, physiotherapists, opticians, pharmacists, dieticians and podiatrists. In order for care to be coordinated and evidence based, primary care teams will need to work in partnership with patients to ensure that there is:

- Registration of a population of patients for whom primary care teams identify problems, coordinate care and help support their condition – this will be achieved more effectively when electronic patient records allow for better information management linked in with the requirements of the QOF

- Recall of people to ensure they receive the care they need through the use of prompts and reminders
- Regular reviews of patients to ensure they receive the best evidence-based care and are supported to effectively manage their care

The standards established within the NSFs have started the process of ensuring an evidence-based approach to the care and management of conditions such as coronary heart disease and diabetes. The QOF included in the new GMS/PMS contracts is intended to influence significantly the continuous improvement of both the process and outcomes of management of long-term conditions.

Some practice nurses will be involved in disease-specific case management and may run designated disease clinics within general practice. However, for a minority of patients with severe or unstable forms of disease there is evidence that specialist input can make a difference especially with respect to reducing hospital admissions. Practice nurses therefore need to have strong links with specialist services to ensure patients are referred appropriately, although many patients will make their own contact if they are sufficiently aware of signs of deterioration in their condition. Examples of responsive specialist services that have been shown to improve patient outcomes are for chronic obstructive pulmonary disease, asthma, heart failure, depression and diabetes (NatPaCT 2004).

Individuals with long-term conditions are intensive users of health care services, utilising an estimated 69% of the primary and acute care budget in England (DH 2008) and account for 49% of all inpatient hospital bed days. Incidence of long-term conditions is most prevalent among the most disadvantaged individuals in society due to a plurality of factors including age, socio-economic status and lifestyle choices. As individuals develop multiple long-term conditions, their care requirements become more complex, often involving an intricate mix of health and social care needs, whereby simple problems can cause rapid deterioration in their condition, necessitating unplanned hospital admissions. Strategies such as the Patient At Risk of Re-hospitalisation case finding tool (PARR+) (Billings *et al.* 2006) or the Combined Predictive Model, which enable evaluation of data relating to frequent attendances at emergency departments or admission to hospital (so-called 'upstream' care), are being utilised to identify those individuals in a general practice population that may be most at risk. Active case management of these individuals by an advanced nurse practitioner, working proactively within a systematic, integrated care system, has been identified as central in improving both health outcomes and quality of life for patients, (DH 2004a, 2005). These 'community matrons' are intended to work in partnership with the patient, the wider health care team and local agencies to ensure a coordinated team approach to care. An underlying principle of this role is the intention to support and empower patients and their carers

by providing appropriate information to facilitate informed choice regarding options for care and to educate individuals to enable them to identify changes in their condition that may precipitate exacerbations of underlying problems and result in admission to hospital. Evaluation of targeted case management pilot schemes appear to demonstrate improved outcomes in both terms of reduced admission rates and patient satisfaction (National Primary Care Research and Development Centre 2005).

Providing quality care in general practice

All nurses working within general practice need to be aware of their accountability and responsibility as they may not necessarily have access to the hierarchical and governance support structures that are part of other sections of the NHS. Practice nurses need to understand the concept of clinical governance and its application to general practice. Clinical governance is an overarching framework for a number of different approaches aimed at improving quality (see Chapter 17). McSherry & Pearce (2007) summarise it as a system or systems that manage risk and monitor clinical quality through an organisation. These systems are underpinned by a drive towards increased collaborative working matched by an increased emphasis on individual accountability. There are three main areas within the clinical governance framework:

- Quality improvement
- Risk management/management of performance
- Systems for accountability and responsibility

Practice nurses need to possess a sound understanding of these key areas. They will be involved in a range of quality improvement mechanisms such as auditing and collecting data to demonstrate achievement of standards cited in the NSFs and QOF.

A key challenge in general practice is the introduction of skill mix into practice nursing teams, requiring a subsequent renegotiation of professional roles. The development of specialist practitioner and senior practice nurse roles alongside the expansion of other nursing and care roles has meant that practices are employing a wider range of staff with a diversity of qualifications and skill. This has included the introduction of health care assistants (HCA) into general practice to fill the void created by the metamorphosis of professional practitioners, many of whom are now performing more advanced roles. It is estimated that there are more than 350 000 HCAs employed within the NHS with 6500 of these working within general practice (Andrews & Vaughn 2007).

The Working in Partnership Programme (WiPP) was charged with creating capacity in general practice in England and has overseen a project to increase the number of HCAs employed in general practice (WiPP 2006). This is in common with the NHS generally, where there is a national drive to increase the number of HCAs. It has been suggested that HCAs could cover 12.5% of nurses' current workload and, subsequently current structures of health care provision are under examination. Consultation regarding the regulation of this expanding and highly varied role has been undertaken across the UK (DH 2004b). Currently a range of educational programmes are provided to support the development of unqualified staff and these include the acquisition of NVQ awards and Foundation Degrees. However, the uptake of these initiatives is very patchy across general practice and often depends on the willingness of employers to support the development of their staff. This progressive level of skill mix developed within the primary care team, which includes HCAs and less skilled nurses, raises issues of accountability. All practice nurses need to possess leadership and team management skills to ensure that staff to whom work is delegated are both competent to undertake the work and recognise their own accountability. All nurses must constantly review their practice against the principles set out in the NMC's *Code of Professional Conduct: Standards for Conduct, Performance and Ethics* (NMC 2008).

However a general practice team study undertaken by Savage & Moore (2004) found the meaning of accountability to be both elusive and ambiguous. This raises concerns of risk as patient safety must be paramount. Ongoing programmes of continuing professional development need to be in place to ensure competence, safety and evidence-based practice, but team leaders must also assume responsibility for the ongoing assessment of competence which, as Hatchett (2003) identifies, is an area that has been poorly addressed in nursing. All staff are required to have personal development plans (PDPs) and therefore appraisal skills are essential for those in team leader roles. *Agenda for Change* is not widely operationalised in general practice (see www.nhsemployers.org/pay-conditions/agenda-for-change.cfm), but aspects of staff development are identified in the GP contract. The development of protocols and care pathways, provided this is undertaken as a collaborative activity, is one way of guiding and standardising practice and ensuring clarity for all staff involved in providing care. This process is supported by the use and application of national guidelines sponsored by the National Institute for Health and Clinical Excellence and other organisations such as the Scottish Intercollegiate Guidelines Network, British Hypertension Society, etc. A range of decision-making tools (such as Clinical Knowledge Summaries [formerly Prodigy]; http://cks.library. nhs.uk/home) are also available online which can easily be accessed in practices. Electronic learning and support is a very rapidly growing area and ideally suited to general practice, and it is likely that many more web-based packages will be utilised in practices and their teams in the future. Recent examples include such packages such as Telehealth (see for example the telehealth systems being piloted in Kent (www.kent. gov.uk/SocialCare/health-and-wellbeing/ telehealth/ and www.telehealthsolutions.co.uk/). These will either be used to enhance the effectiveness of face-to-face consultations or may be applied to enhance the use of telemedicine and video-conferencing, enabling the practice to communicate directly with off-site specialists, diagnosticians and therapists.

The future

The pace of change in the health service is so rapid that it is difficult to predict what the future holds for practice nursing. However, services provided in primary care settings are bound to increase and the future will see more nurses and other health care professionals and ancillary staff working in these settings, often employed or working within a range of different organisations to support new service developments. Currently the NMC is consulting on the future for advanced practice and the DH is reviewing the findings of a consultation exercise on post-registration nursing. This consultation has set out options for a new careers framework for post-registration nursing. It fulfils a commitment in *Modernising Nursing Careers: Setting the Direction* (DH 2006) to align nursing careers with the NHS Careers Framework and develop new career paths for nursing. It proposes a framework built around patient care pathways. At the time of writing (April 2008) the implications for practice nursing remain unclear as NMC recordable specialist practitioner programmes are currently only in existence until 2010 and it is unknown if this level of qualification will remain in the future. However, what is clear is that practice nurses of the future are likely to need an excellent understanding and application of leadership and management skills to support a changing skill mix to provide opportunities for service redesign and the implementation of innovative approaches to service delivery. Such developments will be introduced alongside patient focused management initiatives relating to a broad range of long-term conditions and the expansion of roles into first contact services which may overlap with services provided by nurse practitioners. New models of service provision both in general practice and in primary care, will require the employment of nurses who are flexible and able to follow and support patients through a range of settings in their health care journey.

References

Andrews, H. & Vaughn, P. (2007) Skill mix evolution: HCAs in general practice. *Practice Nursing*, **12**, 619–624.

Billings, J., Mijanovich, T., Dixon, J., Curry, N., Wennberg, D., Dain, B. & Steinart, K. (2006) *Case Finding Algorithms for Patients at Risk of Rehospitalisation.* King's Fund, London.

Cameron, A. (2000) New role developments in context. In: *Developing New Clinical Roles: A Guide for Health Professionals* (eds D. Humphris & A. Masterson). Churchill Livingstone, London.

De Lusignan, S., Shaw, A., Wells, S. & Odunaiya, V. (2003) *Evaluation of Second Wave Personal Medical Services Pilots in South East London – A Qualitative Study.* Lambeth Southwark and Lewisham Health Authority. Available at: www.gpinformatics.org/download/publications/pmssummary.pdf (accessed 25 November 2008).

Department of Health (1989) *General Practice in the National Health Service: the 1990 GP Contract.* The Stationery Office, London.

Department of Health (1990) *NHS and Community Care Act.* Department of Health, London.

Department of Health (1997) *NHS (Primary Care) Act.* The Stationary Office, London.

Department of Health (1999) *Making a Difference: Strengthening the Nursing, Midwifery and Health Visiting Contribution to Health and Healthcare.* The Stationery Office, London.

Department of Health (2000) *The NHS Plan.* Department of Health, London.

Department of Health (2001a) *Shifting the Balance of Power within the NHS – Securing Delivery.* Department of Health, London.

Department of Health (2001b) *The Expert Patient – A New Approach to Chronic Disease Management for the 21st Century.* Department of Health, London.

Department of Health (2003) *Investing in General Practice. The New General medical Services Contract.* The Stationery Office, London.

Department of Health (2004a) *The NHS Improvement Plan: Putting People at the Heart of Public Services.* Department of Health, London.

Department of Health (2004b) *Enhancing Public Protection: Proposals for the Statutory Regulation of Health Care Support Staff in England and Wales.* Department of Health, London.

Department of Health (2005) *Supporting People with Long Term Conditions: Liberating the Talents of Nurses Who Care for People with Long Term Conditions.* Department of Health, London.

Department of Health (2006) *Modernising Nursing Careers.* The Stationery Office, London.

Department of Health (2007a) *Our NHS Our Future: NHS Next Stage Review – Interim Report Summary.* The Stationery Office, London.

Department of Health (2007b) *Tackling Health Inequalities: 2007 Status Report on the Programme for Action.* The Stationery Office, London.

Department of Health (2008) *NHS and Social Care Long Term Conditions Model.* Available at: www.dh.gov. uk/en/Healthcare/Longtermconditions/DH_ 084296 (accessed 20 May 2008).

Department of Health (2008) *High Quality Care for All: NHS Next Stage Review.* Final Report – Lord Ara Darzi, July, Cm7432). Department of Health, London.

Department of Health/Royal College of Nursing (2003) *Freedom to Practice: Dispelling the Myths.* Department of Health, London.

Douglas, F., van Teijlingen, E., Torrance, N., Fearn, P., Kerr, A. & Meloni, S. (2006) Promoting physical activity in primary care settings: health visitors' and practice nurses' views and experiences. *Journal of Advanced Nursing*, **55**, 159–168.

Drennan, V. & Davis, K. (2008) *Trends over Ten Years in the Primary Care and Community Nurse Workforce in England.* Commissioned by the Department of Health.

Duaso, M.J. & Cheung, P. (2002) Health promotion and lifestyle advice in a general practice: what do patients think? *Journal of Advanced Nursing*, **39**, 472–479.

Ewles, L. & Simnett, I. (2003) *Promoting Health – A Practical Guide*, 5th edition. Ballière Tindall, New York.

Greaseley, J. (2007) Essential Business Skills for New Nurse Partners. Available at: www.healthcarerepublic.com/news/Nurse/765974/Essential-business-skills-new-nurse-partners/ (accessed 5 May 2008).

Hatchett, R. (2003) *Nurse Led Clinic – Practice Issues.* Routledge, London.

Horrocks, S., Anderson, E. & Salisbury, C. (2002) Systematic review of whether nurse practitioners working in primary care can provide equivalent care to doctors. *British Medical Journal*, **324**, 819–823.

Laurent, M., Reeves, D., Hermens, R., Braspenning, J., Grol, R. & Sibbald, B. (2005) Substitution of doctors by nurses in primary care [review]. *Cochrane Database of Systematic Reviews*, **2**, Art No: CD001271.

McSherry, R. & Pearce, P. (eds) (2007) *Clinical Governance: A Guide to Implementation for Health Care Professionals.* Blackwell Science, Oxford.

Naidoo, J. & Wills, J. (2008) *Health Promotion: Foundations for Practice*, 3rd edition. Ballière Tindall, London.

National Primary Research and Development Centre (2005) *Evercare Evaluation Interim Report: Implications for Supporting People with Long Term Conditions.* National Primary Research and Development Centre, Manchester.

NatPaCT (2004) Chronic Disease Management – a Compendium of Information. Available at: www.natpact.nhs.uk (accessed 25 November 2008).

Nursing and Midwifery Council (2008) *Code of Professional Conduct: Standards for Conduct, Performance and Ethics.* Nursing and Midwifery Council, London.

Nursing and Midwifery Council (2006) *The Proposed Framework for the Standard of Post Registration Nursing.* Nursing and Midwifery Council, London.

Rhea, S. (2008) *Practice Based Commissioning. GP Practice Survey: Wave 3 results.* Department of Health, London.

Richardson, G., Maynard, A., Cullum, N. & Kindig, D. (1998) Skill mix changes: substitution or service development? *Health Policy*, **45**, 119–132.

Royal College of General Practitioners (2008) *The RCGP and Lord Darzi's review of the NHS.* Available at: www.rcgp.org.uk/pdf/factsheet.pdf (accessed 5 May 2008).

Savage, J. & Moore, L. (2004) *Interpreting Accountability – An Ethnographic Study of Practice Nurses, Accountability and Multidisciplinary Team Decision-Making in the Context of Clinical Governance.* Royal College Nursing Institute, London.

Woodroffe, E. (2006) Nurse led general practice: the changing face of general practice. *British Journal of General Practice*, **56**, 632–633.

Working in Partnership Programme (2006) *Healthcare Assistants Toolkit, NHS.* Available at: www.wipp.nhs.uk (accessed 5 May 2008).

Chapter 9 Contemporary Issues in District Nursing

Sue Boran

Introduction

It remains a changing and challenging time to be working in primary care with a relentless stream of policy documents from the Department of Health (DH) modernising the National Health Service (NHS) and nursing careers and outlining future care provision (DH 2006a, 2007a). These will continue to have a profound effect on community nursing and the role of the district nurse. What is clear, is that the shift of secondary care services to primary care will continue and now more so than ever there needs to be a nursing workforce with strong clinical leadership, committed to embracing the changes and leading teams of multi-skilled professionals ready to accept the challenges of designing and delivering services in primary care.

In keeping with contemporary thinking, primary care can be considered to be care that is provided outside acute hospitals and can be provided in a variety of settings that can include homes, general practice settings, clinics, community hospitals, diagnostic centres, primary care centres, intermediate care teams and mobile settings to accommodate the increasing diversity of service provision in primary care. More than 80% of NHS patient contact takes place in primary care and most secondary and tertiary care is accessed through primary care (NHS 2007).

This chapter is written at a time of some uncertainty about the future of the familiar title 'district nurse', and yet also with a determination that the modern district nurse can deliver an even more flexible, high-quality and forward thinking service, which works in partnership with diverse communities to place the patient at the centre of care delivery.

Historical origins

We have just celebrated the sixtieth anniversary of the NHS. In order to look forward it is important that we remember that district nurses can trace the origins of their role back to the nineteenth century. The earliest mention of nurses being specifically prepared to work in the community was in 1848, although the person attributed as being the founder of district nursing was William Rathbone, who provided the first fully trained hospital nurse, Mrs Robinson, to work with the sick poor in Liverpool in 1859 (Murray & Irven 1948). In a pamphlet written by Florence Nightingale, part of which was contained in a letter addressed to *The Times* and subsequently published on April 14 1876, there was some detail of her expectations of a district nurse, the manner of her training and the organisation of her life with the ultimate objective being to nurse all sick at home. The intention of this letter was to heighten public awareness for the need to train nurses to care for the sick poor, and to secure support for the nurses' training.

The sick nurse, as she was called, was concerned not only with the immediate nursing needs of the patient but also with the wider issues affecting patients and their families' or carers' health and welfare, within the context of contemporary issues. In 1859 some of those issues were poor sanitation, unemployment, overcrowding and a lack of education (Ridgely & Seymer 1954, p. 313).

Thus it can be seen that from their earliest origins, district nurses have been concerned with meeting not only the nursing needs of the individual, but also with caring for the whole person and for the carer's needs. Furthermore, district nurses acknowledge the significance of the environment in which the individual lives as well as acquiring an awareness of the wider factors influencing that individual's well-being, not simply their physical and nursing care needs, but also their psychological, environmental, financial and social care needs.

At the present time district nurses and community nursing teams remain the main providers of professional nursing care in peoples' homes. From such humble beginnings in the service to the 'sick poor', the contemporary district nurse has become firmly established in the role as leader of a team of nurses who provide a home-based universal nursing service.

The changing primary care workforce

The NHS has undergone a period of intense change, particularly over the past ten years. A range of modernisation initiatives and service redesigns have resulted in new ways of working within the NHS. This has impacted on health care professionals with the development of new roles, specifically within areas of clinical practice, with the principal aim of improving patient services, tackling staff shortages and increasing job satisfaction. New job roles arising from this process cross traditional, professional and organisational boundaries. Changes to the primary care workforce have been particularly rapid and have included:

- Community matron roles to implement case management approaches to support patients with the most complex health needs
- New and existing community specialist nurse roles to improve specific areas of disease management and prevention, for example in chronic obstructive pulmonary disease and coronary heart disease
- New nursing roles to support the expanding out of hours and unscheduled service provision and the growth in walk-in centres, minor illness services and expected polyclinics
- New roles to develop rapid response and intermediate care services to facilitate better demand management of acute services

Alongside this social enterprise, initiatives are being developed which may change the face of primary care nursing due to the influence of a range of different providers needing nurses skilled to work in a range of primary care settings.

The adult community nursing resource has also grown over the past ten years. Since 1996 there has been a 47% overall growth in the full time equivalent resource of qualified nurses and nursing support staff. The health care assistant resource has also grown over this period, while numbers of those nurses with a district nurse qualification have decreased in part from a decline in NHS employer commission and sponsorship in the district nursing programme (Drennan & Davis 2008). These figures may appear alarming when set in the context of changing demographics for the same time period that show an increase of 486 000 persons aged 65 and over in England. These changes mean that new opportunities are being offered to less-experienced nurses. The skills and competencies required of nurses in bands 5, 6 and 7 could be seen as broadly similar, however, the context in which these skills are delivered in primary care settings is different and this needs to be recognised in the preparation of nurses to work in these settings.

Practitioners are often working alone in environments that are not set up as health care environments and they need to be highly skilled in adapting and transferring their skills and in dealing with the highly complex collaborative relationships with both clients and families, as well as with health, social and voluntary agencies. This means that staff working in primary care across a range of different employers develop an enhanced awareness of the richness and diversity of primary care. Programmes of preparation for working in primary care need to reflect these key differences and prepare nurses for the professional and interpersonal skills that acknowledge that patients and their families are much more in control of their decisions and often responsible for the majority of care. Nurses working in primary care settings also need to be able to make more autonomous decisions as they are often physically distant from support or colleagues, although improved mobile phone technology often means they are no more that a phone call away from advice or support.

Depending on their responsibilities, nurses working in primary care will all need to be able to (NHS Employers Briefing 2006, www. nhsemployers.org/):

- Be involved in monitoring the health of the wider community and adapt and redesign services to target those most in need
- Have a greater involvement in promoting health and enabling self-care
- Be the first point of contact for some patients needing support or advice in primary care settings
- Have a greater understanding of the impact on patients and families and the appropriate ongoing care and management of long-term conditions
- Be aware of the impact of poor housing, low income, and social isolation and collaborate with others in strategies to address these issues
- Be confident in assessing and managing risks associated with patients and carers making their own decisions
- Understand and influence PCT and practice-based commissioning and the delivery of services that use resources effectively
- Demonstrate the nursing contribution to integrated health and social care services.

Given these changes it is crucial that these highly developed teams of nurses working in primary care settings are led and managed by appropriately trained, confident and knowledgeable practitioners who have a recognised qualification that can be benchmarked against a set of standards for practice. This is a role for the district nurse and this is the reason that many educational establishments have retained the specialist practice qualification for district nursing, but with programmes that have undergone major review. Students supported to undertake these programmes are likely to already be employed in staff nurse positions in primary care settings, but are selected by their employer as having the capability to lead primary care nursing teams and who start the programme with a body of underpinning clinical expertise in community nursing. This can be equated to a situation in an acute hospital ward where no ward manager would be appointed unless they were able to demonstrate clinical competencies and expertise in the appropriate clinical field. The district nursing programme would then build on this body of clinical expertise and prepare the practitioner to expand and deepen their knowledge and competence, and also be prepared to lead the nursing team and have the skills to innovate and develop the team's capabilities to respond to the rapidly changing context of primary care.

Gaining a specialist qualification is a benchmark of quality and the programme outcomes for district nursing preparation must be designed to equip practitioners with the knowledge and competencies necessary for the challenging role of leading a range of nursing service provision in order to sustain stability in ever-changing environments and to feel confident to take on the challenges this presents. The Standards for Specialist Education and Practice (Nursing and Midwifery Council [NMC] 2002) remain for now as the sole regulations for district nursing programmes in England. Specialist practice is the exercising of higher levels of judgement, discretion and clinical decision-making in clinical care to enable the monitoring and improvement of standards of care through supervision of practice, clinical audit, the development of practice through research and teaching, the support of professional colleagues and the provision of skilled professional leadership. This has been focused on four broad areas – clinical nursing practice; care and programme management; clinical practice leadership; and clinical practice development. Educational providers also build in additional aims that enable the students to (London South Bank University 2007):

- Build on a body of clinical expertise consolidated at post qualifying level
- Develop further clinical assessment, analytical and clinical decision-making skills

- Utilise their leadership and management skills to negotiate and influence creative service improvements
- Work with a range of professionals and agencies across health and social care, local authority, voluntary and independent sectors
- Articulate the complexities of working in primary care and strategies to manage the uncertainties of care and service provision managed by a range of health and social care professionals
- Demonstrate that they are capable of challenging professional boundaries using sound rationale
- Develop some specific competencies to enable progression towards the standards for an advanced nurse practitioner level proposed by the NMC (2006)

The aims of the district nurse are multi-faceted: to lead community nursing teams to prevent ill-health and to keep people healthy, thus avoiding the need for medical care; to provide support for those living with long-term conditions so that they are able to remain at home; to treat curable problems and to provide nursing care to those whose needs are acute and complex; and to offer palliative and terminal care to those who require it so that they may die in accordance with their wishes. The fulfilment of these aims represents a major task and one that makes complex demands on the role of the district nurse. To meet such demands the role needs to be reviewed and the educational preparation needs to be more flexible and responsive to shifting patterns of care delivery.

The changing role of the district nurse

Since the 1970s, the role of the district nurse has continued to receive attention. A number of policy documents have been issued which emphasise the valuable contribution made by community nurses in the delivery of health and social care in the community and in improving peoples' health (DH 1992a, 1997, 1999a,b).

Additionally, *The NHS Plan* (DH 2000), *Liberating the Talents* (DH 2002), *The NHS Improvement Plan* (DH 2004a), clearly place district nurses in new flexible roles that are critical in enabling individuals to be supported at home and in spearheading community based health provision to improve the public's health. As part of the primary health care team, the district nurse can be seen to be at the interface of health and social care delivery, undertaking a vital and increasingly complex role. More recently, the White Paper *Our Health, Our Care, Our Say* (DH 2006b) and Lord Darzi's report on London NHS (NHS 2007) and his final report of his overall review of the NHS (DH 2008) clearly set a new direction for community nursing, bringing health and social care services 'closer to home', a shift away from traditional hospital-based acute services towards enhanced primary care provision with multi-purpose clinics (polyclinics) housing a broad range of both medical and social care services. A greater emphasis on preventive care and 'patient-centred pathways' would also mean a paradigm shift in the way that people use health care services, away from a curative approach with an over reliance on health care services, treating people only after they had become ill to a preventive approach focusing on independence and healthier lifestyles, from a 'sickness service to a wellbeing service' (NHS 2007, p. 37).

Community nursing has been constantly developing and changing in response to government policy and to the changing needs of the communities served. In line with these changes the role of the district nurse will need to evolve and expand still further. Traditionally, the caseload of the district nurse has been the care of patients with long-term conditions, older people and those who are terminally ill. However, this does not take account of the work required when caring for people with complex and multiple needs. The present workload of the district nurse encompasses a whole range of activities that involve taking professional and managerial responsibility for the provision of appropriate pathways of nursing care and treatment through acute, long-term and terminal illness.

The district nurse provides a service which is accessible and meets both highly individual and complex needs of patients and carers in an effective and responsive way (DH 1999b; English National Board 1991). Advanced nursing care is formulated within a holistic framework to be delivered in the home setting and is based on knowledge of the individual's physical, psychological and social needs, which may involve the application of both technical and specialist skills. They remain professionally responsible and accountable for the quality of care that they provide and are pivotal in assessing the needs of individuals and their carers. They also lead and manage a multi-skilled team of nurses, able to work collaboratively with a multiplicity of agencies (statutory, voluntary and private) in order to deliver care to a defined population. However, in the future they will need to further broaden their scope of practice to manage long-term conditions and to fulfil the public health role of maintaining people at home. This will require them to think and work proactively and identify people before they become patients and anticipate problems before they arise. It is therefore essential that district nurses accept and discharge their role as experts in the assessment and identification of nursing and health-related needs.

However, it is the context of care in which the district nurse functions which has changed significantly in the past two decades. It will continue to change as government policy emphasises the provision of care either in the community, at home or as close as possible to people's homes (DH 2002, 2004a; NHS 2007). The shift from secondary to primary care has changed the emphasis of nursing need in the community. This change is reflected in the increasing number of frail older people and those with chronic disability and complex needs and terminal illness, who are now being cared for at home. The district nurse must, therefore, create opportunities to expand and further develop the role by building on the considerable body of knowledge and skill derived from the experience of many years of caring for individuals in the community.

While it is clear that the district nurse has the necessary knowledge and skills to lead a team of nurses who are able to deliver the government's modernisation agenda, it is evident that traditional methods of working will need to change. Nevertheless, it is important to have a professional identity. The more flexible approach to meeting the needs of the community will require a balance of skills between those of the generic primary care nurse and those of the primary care workers. The full range of skills offered by the primary workforce will continue to be needed to provide competent and effective care. In this way the needs of the patient will be met and there will be continuing motivation to recruit and retain district nurses and other community nursing staff all of whom have a role that is meaningful to the public.

There are also concerns that the numbers of district nurses are not increasing sufficiently to meet the demands made on them. The public at large is now better informed. Patients want to have more care at home and spend less time in hospital particularly in the light of increasing prevalence of hospital-acquired infections. This adds to the demands on the district nursing team. District nurses will be obliged to change their practice, but they will need the support of their organisation to do so effectively. The challenge for them is how to make their voices heard so that they can be part of the implementation of future change. This can be achieved by:

- Taking the initiative and informing their organisations of the needs and priorities of their communities rather than waiting to be told what to do
- Seizing this opportunity to redefine their role as district nurses of the future
- Obtaining more user involvement
- Organising a service that is responsive to the needs of the people for whom it is intended

The goal for the district nurse should be to provide services at a point that maximises access for people and provides greater flexibility (DH 2004a) so that being able to access a district nurse or a pharmacist directly rather than a GP is a viable and sustainable option.

Practice-based commissioning

Commissioning community services is a key element within NHS reforms and having a vision to shape future services is fundamental to its success. It is therefore essential that community nurses have an appreciation of the concept of commissioning and engage actively with it to improve services for their patients (Norman & Old 2007). Involvement from clinicians who have extensive knowledge of local populations is invaluable in the process of health needs assessment of their communities (Nutbrown 2006) and practitioners need to know how to contact relevant people engaged in the commissioning process to find out how they can be involved in the planning of services. Any new developments result in change, and support for this will be essential to encourage individuals to develop their knowledge and skills in taking on new and wider roles, supported by creative practice and innovative ideas (Martin *et al.* 2007). Entrepreneurial practice should be encouraged and ideas listened to. Being actively involved in the commissioning of services utilises nurses' knowledge about the community in order to inform and influence services that are needed to provide quality care to patients, which is fundamentally what nursing is about (Norman & Old 2007).

Earlier Cain *et al.* (1995) supported the notion that commissioning of health care is dependent on detailed information of the local community, which should include data on both health and social needs for effective planning and financial distribution. In this process it is the duty of the district nurse to inform commissioners of services about local health needs by providing a practice profile that acts as an indicator to identify health deficits. This involvement with service represents a key part of the district nurse's role as an advocate for patients' needs. Additionally, district nurses should draw on their skills of population profiling in order to identify the nature of the populations with whom they work. Their concern must be not just with the health needs but with the constituents of a given population, such as its ethnicity and diversity in terms of age range and gender.

Equally important are public health concerns such as housing, unemployment and the numbers of people with a long-term condition.

While the assessment of an individual's nursing needs remains central to the work of the district nurse a consideration of the needs of the wider population is of equal importance. District nurses find themselves in a unique position, working in partnership with patients in their environments on a day-to-day basis, which enables them to advise the service commissioners of the needs of both patients and carers (Wall 1998). The close relationships that develop over weeks or even years between district nurses and patients and their families builds a confidence and trust that enables patients to express their needs.

Clinical governance

Further advances in clinical practice have placed greater demands upon nurses to provide safe, effective care. While this may be exciting and challenging, district nurses need to be supported to ensure that they remain clinically competent and confident in the care they are providing as well as being accountable for their practice. As a team leader the district nurse has prime responsibility for the care carried out by all members of the district nursing team.

In order to ensure the success of clinical governance and provide an environment in which clinical excellence may be vigorously adopted, professionals will be required to sustain their professional development and professional practice. Within this context, clinical supervision is a necessary and important element in providing the support needed by district nurses not only to maintain their clinical standards but also to uphold them in their role as leaders of a team (DH 1999b).

Evidence-based practice demands that patients' care is based on the most up-to-date evidence of what is known to be effective (DH 1999b, p. 44). It requires that practitioners need continuously to develop their information and research appraisal skills so they can use the best available evidence to support their practice (DH 1999b). Within this context the district nurse needs to consider three elements: that practice is based on the best evidence available that will meet the patients' needs; that practice operates within a framework of reflection, evaluation and audit of outcomes; and that knowledge of achieved effectiveness is disseminated to other practitioners. These elements together reflect the duty of the nurse under the code (Standards of Conduct, Performance and Ethics for Nurses and Midwives), to ensure that each individual receives care based on the best available evidence or best practice (NMC 2008).

What is equally clear from the literature is that patients as the recipients of care, are integral to the clinical decision-making process. When the district nurse makes a decision regarding a patients' clinical care, not only should that decision be based on the best evidence available but it should also be made in consultation with the patient and the carers, so that it best suits the patient and the carers' needs. Patients who have a long-term condition, such as diabetes or multiple sclerosis, accrue a wealth of expertise in managing their own condition. The inclusion of the patients' and carers' experience will ensure that the expertise of the district nursing team and of other involved professionals is complemented by the expertise of the patients and the carers. The active involvement of patients in this process is central to the whole endeavour of clinical effectiveness, patient empowerment and evidence-based practice.

Risk management is another key aspect of clinical governance that district nurses must make integral to their work. It comprises the management of all aspects of clinical risk by ensuring that there are mechanisms in place to establish safe practice, which in turn safeguards the patients (DH 1999b). Risk may be defined as the potential for an unwanted or unexpected outcome, for example, injury to a patient or patient dissatisfaction and unhappiness in the form of a complaint. Risk management by definition is the systematic identification, assessment and reduction of risk to patients and staff. For risk management to operate successfully there needs to be a culture of openness, where incidents can be reported without fear of associated disciplinary action and where lessons can be learned from

mistakes and problems such as poor clinical performance can be dealt with constructively.

Adverse incident reporting or significant event auditing systems are fundamental to the clinical risk management process. They offer the opportunity to review incidents at an early stage. Where trends and similarities from incidents can be identified there may be opportunities to highlight organisational and communication problems which permit remedial action to be taken to prevent reoccurrence.

Managing long-term conditions through population management and a geographical perspective

In Great Britain, 17.5 million adults may be living with a long-term condition. It is also likely that up to 75% of those people aged over 75 years have a long-term condition, and this figure continues to rise (DH 2004a). Older people, in particular, often have multiple pathology, so a general principles approach to long-term conditions management would be more appropriate than a single disease approach. Patients need access to a wide range of services in primary care, with more care provided in the home or as close to home as possible. Appropriate support could enable many people to learn how to be active participants in their own care, permitting them to live with and manage their condition as an expert patient. With regular monitoring of the condition and support to make any necessary changes to lifestyle, complications may be avoided, deterioration slowed and the development of further complications might even be prevented.

Patients considered to be at a higher risk are provided with proactive support from a multidisciplinary team under the leadership of a district nurse. The aim is that patients will be enabled to make use of evidence-based protocols and pathways to manage their diseases themselves and avoid complications. To achieve this, good information technology will be required with patient registers, shared electronic health records and care planning. For people with more than one long-term condition, there is the potential for care to be complex, involving integrated health and social care agencies, working together. Such situations require a personalised case management approach, which would be entirely suited to a district nurse in the role as key worker actively managing and coordinating the care.

People with complex long-term conditions are also supported locally by a 'community matron' and many of these posts have been filled by district nurses who have the specialist knowledge to support these patients in such a way that they would be able to minimise the impact of the disease on their lives. The community matron helps them to manage their condition in a way that suits them, anticipating problems and helping to avoid complications in order to maximise their health and assist them to live longer. The illnesses that people live with for the rest of their lives, such as diabetes, asthma, arthritis or heart disease, can be controlled but not cured.

Case management has always been a major part of the district nurse's role. However, district nurses are now required to extend their physical and clinical assessment skills and include independent prescribing as part of their continuing professional development portfolio in order to provide more comprehensive care in the community. The outcome is fewer emergency admissions to hospital and the consequent trauma for patients and families. Teaching people to cope and to manage their diseases is a more productive use of resources and enables them to take greater control of their own treatment. In this way they are able to spend more time at home with their families and friends and have an enhanced quality of life. District nurses are expert at assessing nursing care needs and have much experience of collaborating with local GPs and other members of the wider primary care team. They already occupy a familiar point of contact for other health care professionals so that they are ideally placed to instigate joint responsibility for developing personal care plans. In this way, the best possible care would be delivered to patients and their families and problems for the patients could be anticipated

or managed before reaching a deterioration in health and hospitalisation.

By 2008, the Department of Health anticipated that there would be 3000 community matrons (district nurses) using case management techniques to care for around 250 000 patients with complex needs. The reality is that this target has not yet been reached for a variety of reasons: either the role has not been clearly defined or that the job is seen as an isolated role and not integrated into a team and not attracting district nurses because of this. There has also been a reduction of district nurses and commissioned places on district nurse training programmes and there has also not been the anticipated movement of nurses from acute settings moving into primary care (CHAI 2007). Many educational providers are actively promoting the enhanced and modern role of the district nurse as a leader of a complex team and are designing much more flexible, fit-for-purpose courses to include enhanced physical clinical assessment skills, illness monitoring and pharmacology, which are enabling students to exit courses and apply for a wider variety of senior nurse positions in primary care.

The application of single assessment process and better care coordination is essential for effective case management. Effective working between health and social care services is of critical importance when meeting the needs of people with long-term conditions. For such people who are often frail and old, it may be difficult to be at home coping with medication and trying to keep warm, well nourished and hydrated without support, particularly if they are alone, under stress, recently bereaved or have lost confidence in their ability to manage on their own. It is in such cases that district nurses are so effective in targeting resources and coordinating community based personalised health and social care so that stressful and disruptive admission to hospital can be prevented (DH 2004a). Effective communication skills also remain critical for engagement with patients and their families and liaison with patient support teams. An ability to facilitate and coordinate care is therefore essential together with the ability to develop service networks. The aim is to ensure that the care thus provided is patient-centred and is focused on attaining maximum independence, comfort and quality of life in the least invasive manner in the most appropriate setting.

Key workers or community matrons, many of whom are district nurses, together with a number of nurses from the acute sector, are responsible for the coordination of the service and the care of the patients. Many existing district nurses have expanded their physical and clinical assessment skills in order to provide care within this model and also to expand their scope of practice to include prescribing. District nurses who possess specialist community nursing knowledge are able to take the lead to identify 'high-risk' patients in their communities and manage and monitor caseloads appropriately to prevent acute exacerbations or problems that put patients at risk of admission or readmission to hospital. This approach should effectively reduce the number of people needing to be admitted to care homes for the older person (Evercare 2003). The Evercare model, which informed the development of the community matron role, has been evaluated extensively (Gravelle *et al.* 2007), but further local evaluation is required as funding for the future will be dependent on community matrons' success in meeting measurable clinical and patient-focused outcomes, such as the number of emergency visits, unplanned admissions, out-of-hours calls and GP home visits (Masterson 2007).

The era of the patient as the passive recipient of care has changed. It has been replaced by a partnership approach in which patients are empowered through information to contribute ideas that can help in their treatment and care.

Linked to this is the Expert Patient Programme (DH 2001). These expert patients are people with the confidence, skills, information and knowledge to be able to play a central role in the management of living with a long-term condition and to minimise the impact of the disease on their lives. The programme is designed to empower patients to manage their own health care and to listen to themselves and their symptoms. With the support of a district nursing team and a range of other health and social care professionals in the community as appropriate, the programme has been made effective. The rationale for the programme is that patients understand their disease better than health care professionals because they have acquired skills from their experiences of coping with their own long-term condition.

Non-medical prescribing

There have been huge developments in prescribing by non-medical practitioners within the past ten years. The inclusion of non-medical prescribing in the future district nurse's role makes Chapter 18 compulsory reading. The *Report of the Advisory Group on Nurse Prescribing* (DH 1989) recommended that the district nurse would be eligible to prescribe from a limited nursing formulary following the successful completion of a specific education programme. The legal framework for nurse prescribing came into being, with the passing of the Medicinal Products: Prescribing by Nurses, Act 1992 (DH 1992b). However it has not taken effect in isolation from other professional and service developments. The implementation of nurse prescribing has involved the collaborative efforts by community trusts, health authorities and primary care trusts to develop local systems and structures for its long-term support, monitoring and development.

For the district nurse, it is just the beginning of a learning process that will enhance the care and treatment of patients. Nurse prescribing has already had a significant impact on the district nurse's workload by speeding up the commencement of treatment as prescribed items are obtained more efficiently. The legal independence of nurse prescribing has brought with it additional accountability for practice: it is the responsibility for each prescribing district nurse to ensure that practice and prescribing is underpinned by current evidence and demonstrated competence. The extension of prescribing rights of community nurses requires them to build on the skills, knowledge and competencies developed in the early stages of nurse prescribing (Anderson 1999). District nurses have also increased their skills and knowledge with regard to clinical assessment which has enabled them to exclude abnormal pathophysiology, enhance their diagnostic skills, and build on their pharmacology knowledge base (Banning 1999; May 1998; Luker *et al.* 1998; Scowen 1995). Future progress in extending non-medical prescribing to other nurses will undoubtedly see further increases in the number of nurse prescribers and in the range of medicines available to them, with electronic prescribing improving the efficiency and quality of prescribing (DH 2004a).

Non-medical prescribing forms an integral part of the care and treatment provided by the district nurse and is an essential element of professional practice. It forms a key component of the district nurse's continuous professional development portfolio (DH 1998, 1999b).

Continuous professional development – lifelong learning

Change within the NHS is an ongoing and continuous process, demanding major investment in educational development for the workforce. As such there has been a considerable shift, both within professional organisations and in the higher education sector towards a culture that supports lifelong learning. For professional organisations the dilemma will be how to guide district nurses away from a defensive stance where change is always seen as a threat, towards the adoption of a more creative and proactive approach.

Despite preparing for change, engagement with the 'traditional' work of a district nursing team will still be required, but alongside this will also be the need to develop new proactive approaches to the management of long-term conditions and to develop public health aspects of their work with the aim of preventing people becoming 'dependant' patients. Collaboration with general practice nurses and nurses in the acute care setting will also be imperative as more complex care is devolved to primary care settings. Although patients should be encouraged to attend GP practices and other primary care facilities, there will still be significant numbers who will need to be managed in the home environment.

This chapter has only touched on the role of the district nursing team in the support of those patients and families requiring palliative and terminal care. The uncomfortable fact is that everyone will die. There is a need to ensure that all people at the end of their life, regardless of diagnosis, will be given a choice of where they wish to die and how they wish to be treated. Doyle (1999) and Hudson (2002) determined that 90% of patients with palliative care needs spend 90% of their final year at home. This shows that the care of patients who are dying constitutes a significant part of a district nurse's caseload, requiring advanced communication and assessment skills to determine what care would be beneficial to maintain patient and family control of the situation with the district nursing and palliative care team support. The district nurse will need to liaise with and refer to a wide range of practitioners from the multi-disciplinary team to support these patients and families at home and to communicate with the GP to ensure that the Gold Standards Framework is appropriately adhered to for the patient who is dying (Thomas 2001).

Responding to the changing policy context

As well as these changes governing professional regulation there have been a range of government imperatives relating to reform and modernisation of the NHS and social care services that require significant change in the way that health and social care services are designed and delivered. Since 1997 and Labour Party revival, policies have been developed to facilitate major reform and modernisation of the NHS. This started with a ten-year plan entitled *The New NHS: Modern, Dependable* (DH 1997) which was further developed to *The NHS Plan* (DH 2000). Key policies emanating from or related to this plan have been major drivers for a programme of unprecedented reform. These policies include *Choosing Health* (DH 2004b); *National Standards, Local Action* (DH 2004d); *Investing in General Practice. The New General Medical Services (GMS) Contract* (DH 2004c); *Liberating the Talents* (DH 2002); *Commissioning a Patient Led NHS* (DH 2005); *Supporting People with Long Term*

Conditions (DH 2006d); *Our Health, Our Care. Our Say* (DH 2006b) and a more recent consultation document *A Commissioning Framework for Health and Wellbeing* (DH 2007b). In 2006, the DH published *Modernising Nursing Careers: Setting the Direction* (DH 2006a), which highlights the ways in which careers in nursing and midwifery professions are set to become much more flexible and innovative in order that role development can respond appropriately to the ways in which services in the NHS and Social Care are developing and integrating and which focus on helping people to stay healthy and independent. Additionally, the DH published a consultation document *Towards a Framework for Post Registration Nursing Careers* (DH 2007a) that takes forward recommendations made in *Modernising Nursing Careers: Setting the Direction* (DH 2006a) to align nursing careers with the National Careers Framework and develop new career pathways for nurses.

The DH in its document *The NHS in England: the Operating Framework for 2007/8* (2006c) sets key targets for improving the health and wellbeing of the population. Nurses working in primary care have a pivotal role to play in working with members of the public and others to achieve these health targets in order to promote health and well-being and reduce inequalities in health. Of the 13 key targets, all of which have relevance for practitioners working in primary care, arguably the priorities for district nursing teams are:

- Older people – by improving the quality of life and independence of vulnerable older people by supporting them to live in their own homes where possible
- Supporting people with long-term conditions – by offering a personalised care plan for the most at risk vulnerable people through improved care in primary care and community settings
- Smoking – by reducing adult smoking rates to 21% or less by 2010
- Patient experience – to ensure that individuals are fully involved in decisions about their health care

- There is also an emphasis within the document on care close to home to:
  — Promote health and emotional well-being with stronger local services and support to reduce the prevalence of physical and mental illness
  — Develop services to support people in maintaining independent lives in their own homes reducing avoidable hospital admissions
  — Provide for timely hospital discharge with support from appropriate community services
  — Increase community capacity to support the shift of appropriate services from acute hospitals to convenient and safe local facilities

These developments and changes in both professional regulation and NHS requirements have provided us with the opportunity to review primary care educational preparation to ensure that programmes are fit for purpose and practice and that they offer a more flexible model of delivery based on the strengths of current primary and social care programmes, while also reflecting the need for more interprofessional education and facilitate the movement of staff and transfer of learning from acute to primary care settings.

In response to these policy demands, universities such as London South Bank University have focused their community nursing provision on the development of specialist practitioners by introducing new flexible educational pathways that focus on the needs of service providers and their clients. New emergent courses, while still retaining the specialist practice qualification for district nursing, also focus on the educational development of band 5 and 6 practitioners who may not wish to follow this pathway (preferring to practice in more generalist roles in primary care).

Universities have also introduced new educational programmes, aimed at enhancing the skills, knowledge and competencies of the support staff workforce. For example, since 2004, London South Bank University has offered Foundation Degrees in a range of subject areas for health care staff working to support registered practitioners. They are funded through the Higher Education Funding Council for England. The first cohort of primary care assistant practitioners qualified in 2006 and are trained to fulfil the requirements of a member of staff working at band 4. As Foundation Degrees are a relatively new development within health and social care, employers supporting these programmes will need to develop a workforce strategy that encompasses these new roles. In developing innovative and flexible solutions to prepare the primary care workforce, such assistant practitioners are likely to need continuing professional development and should be able to access additional learning opportunities to meet their own development needs and those of a rapidly changing service.

Conclusion

Uncertainty remains about whether there is a future for district nursing and no doubt this will be explored further in the DH consultation *Towards a Framework for Post Registration Nursing Careers* (DH 2007a). However, no matter what the outcome of this exercise is, changes in primary care service provision are going to need strong clinical leadership. This appears to be in line with DH thinking with respect to *Modernising Nursing Careers – Setting the Direction* (DH 2006a), which looks at national benchmarks for clinical leadership and advanced practice.

The government has established a challenging agenda for change in primary care, characterised by a multi-faceted role change for practitioners (epitomised by the gradual emergence of community matrons as clinical leaders). District nurses remain committed not only to helping people with long-term conditions live more satisfying lives, but also to being more actively involved in promoting the nation's health. The Wanless review *Our Future Health Secured* (King's Fund 2007) shows that the health of the population of England is not as good as that of comparable countries. The factors that contribute to poor health include relatively high levels of smoking (27% of the adult population) and obesity, in conjunction with low levels of

physical activity and low consumption of fresh fruit and vegetables (DH 2004a). Heart disease and strokes, mental illness, accidents, injuries and cancers have the greatest impact on the health of the population. In developed countries such as the UK the key risk factors for these diseases are smoking, high blood pressure, alcohol, high cholesterol and obesity. If we are to improve our standards of health, the focus must be not simply on treatment, but also on prevention and the prioritisation of preventive public health measures (DH 2004d). Balanced against this is the need to provide care at home for people with complex needs, frail older people, and those with acute needs as well as those requiring palliative and terminal care. All these challenges will lead to further changes to traditional ways of working but exciting opportunities lie ahead. Primary care trusts have to improve their respective population's health and for patients and this will be achieved through the knowledge and skills of district nurses and community nursing teams.

As the NHS becomes ever more patient focused with its emphasis on patient choice and involvement, district nurses need to respond to the challenges with creativity and enthusiasm. They should seize this opportunity to make a difference to people's lives and to become 'experts' in managing long-term conditions. Employers must consider the strategic purpose of district nursing and how it interfaces with other health and social services and in so doing clarify the services it provides. The development of quality standards and pathways of care within a community framework will ensure that these services are effective, evidence based and open to audit. It is important to appraise what is already being carried out effectively and what is still needed to enhance patient care. By becoming more vocal and assertive and by engaging purposefully in primary care reform, district nurses can be effective in the move for change.

Central to this vision of the future is the need for district nurses to retain that element of their role, which is held in such high esteem by patients and their carers, namely the trust and confidence and the value they place on being treated with humanity and kindness, under-pinned by effective teamwork, integration, collaboration and partnership (Audit Commission 1999; Hill 2000).

References

Anderson, P. (1999) Looking at the road ahead for nurse prescribing. *Nurse Prescriber Community*, 35–36.

Audit Commission (1999) *First Assessment: A Review of District Nursing Services in England and Wales*. Audit Commission Publications, London.

Banning, M. (1999) Nurse prescribing – education, education, education. In: *Nurse Prescribing – Politics to Practice* (ed. M. Jones, 1999). Baillière Tindal, Royal College of Nursing, London.

Cain, P., Hyde, V. & Howkins, E. (1995) *Community Nursing, Dimensions and Dilemmas*. Arnold, London.

CHAI (2007) *A Life Like No Other*. CHAI, London.

Department of Health (1989) *Report of the Advisory Group on Nurse Prescribing*, (chair Dr J. Crown). Department of Health, London.

Department of Health (1992a) *The Health of the Nation: A Strategy of Health for England*. The Stationery Office, London.

Department of Health (1992b) *Medicinal Products: Prescribing by Nurses Act*. The Stationery Office, London.

Department of Health (1997) *The New NHS: Modern, Dependable*. The Stationery Office, London.

Department of Health (1998) *A First Class Service: Quality in the New NHS*. The Stationery Office, London.

Department of Health (1999a) *Saving Lives: Our Healthier Nation*. The Stationery Office, London.

Department of Health (1999b) *Making a Difference: Strengthening the Nursing, Midwifery and Health Visiting Contribution to Health and Healthcare*. The Stationery Office, London.

Department of Health (2000) *The NHS Plan. A Plan for Investment. A plan for Reform*. The Stationery Office, London.

Department of Health (2001) *The Expert Patient: A New Approach to Chronic Disease Management for the 21st Century*. Department of Health, London.

Department of Health (2002) *Liberating the Talents. Helping Primary Care Trusts and Nurses to Deliver the NHS Plan*. Department of Health, London.

Department of Health (2004a) *The NHS Improvement Plan. Putting People at the Heart of Public Services*. Department of Health, London.

Department of Health (2004b) *Choosing Health: Making Healthier Choices Easier*. Department of Health, London.

Department of Health (2004c) *Investing in General Practice. The New General Medical Services (GMS) Contract*. The Stationery Office, London.

Department of Health (2004d) *National Standards Local Action: Health and Social Care Standards and Planning Framework 2005/06 – 2007/08*. Department of Health, London.

Department of Health (2005) *Commissioning a Patient Led NHS*. Department of Health, London.

Department of Health (2006a) *Modernising Nursing Careers: Setting The Direction*. Department of Health, London.

Department of Health (2006b) *Our Health, Our Care, Our Say: A New Direction for Community Services*. Department of Health, London.

Department of Health (2006c) *The NHS in England: the Operating Framework for 2007/8*. Department of Health, London.

Department of Health (2006d) *Supporting People with Long Term Conditions: An NHS and Social Care Model to Support Local Innovation and Integration*. Department of Health, London.

Department of Health (2007a) *Towards a Framework for Post Registration Nursing Careers, Consultation Document*. Department of Health, London.

Department of Health (2007b) *Commissioning Framework for Health and Well-being*. Department of Health, London.

Department of Health (2008) *High Quality Care for All: NHS Next Stage Review* (Final Report – Lord Ara Darzi, July, Cm7432). Department of Health, London.

Doyle, D. (1999) The provision of palliative care. In: *The Oxford Book of Palliative Medicine* (eds D. Doyle, G. Hanks, & N. Macdonald). Oxford University Press, Oxford.

Drennan, V. & Davis, K. (2008) *Trends Over Ten Years in the Primary Care and Community Workforce in England*. Department of Health, London.

English National Board (1991) *Criteria and Guidelines for Taught Practice Placements for District Nurse Students*. Circular 1991/05/MB. English National Board, London.

Evercare (2003) *Adapting the Evercare Programme for the National Health Service*. Evercare, USA.

Gravelle, H., Dusheiko, M., Sheaff, R., Sargent, P., Boaden, R., Pikard, S., Parker, S. & Roland, M. (2007) Impact of case management (Evercare) on frail elderly patients controlled before and after analysis of quantitative outcome data. *British Medical Journal*, **334**, 31–34.

Hill, J. (2000) Many challenges. *Nursing Management*, **6**, 29.

Hudson (2002) Intervention development for enhanced lay palliative caregiver support. *European Journal of Cancer Care*, **11**, 262–270.

King's Fund (2007) *Our Future Health Secured*. King's Fund, London.

London South Bank University (2007) *Programme Specification for District Nursing Awards in Primary Care*. London South Bank University, London.

Luker, K., Hogg, C., Austin, L., Ferguson, B. & Smith, K. (1998) Decision-making: the context of nurse prescribing. *Journal of Advanced Nursing*, **27**, 657–665.

Martin, J., Black, G., Cleverdon, S., Kelly, D., Shanahan, H., Kinnair, D., Southon, S. & Webb, S. (2007) Developing service provision for patients in primary care. *Nursing Standard*, **21**, 43–48.

Masterson, A. (2007) Community matrons: documenting the specialist contribution of the role. *Nursing Older People*, **9**, 37–40.

May, V. (1998) Nurse prescribing – ready or not. *Journal of Community Nursing*, **12**.

Murray, E.J. & Irven, I.D. (1948) *District Nursing*. Baillière Tindall and Cox, London.

NHS Employers Briefing (2006) *From Hospital to Home*. Available at http://ww.nhsemployers.org/ (accessed 24 November 2008).

NHS (2007) *Our NHS Our Future. Interim Report NHS Next Stage Review*. Department of Health, London.

NHS (2007) *Healthcare for London: A Framework for Action*. NHS, London.

Nursing and Midwifery Council (2002) *Standards for Specialist Community Education and Practice*. Nursing and Midwifery Council, London.

Nursing and Midwifery Council (2006) *Advanced Nurse Practitioner Standards*. Nursing and Midwifery Council, London.

Nursing and Midwifery Council (2008) *The Code: Standards of Conduct, Performance and Ethics for Nurses and Midwives*. Nursing and Midwifery Council, London.

Norman, K. & Old, C. (2007) PCT commissioning: how community nurse involvement can be encouraged. *British Journal of Community Nursing*, **12**, 518–520.

Nutbrown, S. (2006) New world of primary care. *Practice Nurse*, **32**, 70.

Ridgely Seymer, L. (1954) *Selected Writings of Florence Nightingale*. Macmillan, New York.

Scowen, P. (1995) Why community nurses need to know their pharmacology. *Professional Care of Mother and Child*, **5**, 2–4.

Thomas, K. (2001) *The Gold Standards Framework in Palliative Care. A Handbook for Practice*. Macmillan Publications, London.

Wall, A. (1998) From paper to practice. *Health Service Journal*, **108**, 28–29.

Chapter 10 **Community Children's Nursing**

Mark Whiting, Joan Myers and David Widdas

Introduction

In 1994, as the first edition of this text was being prepared for publication, the provision of community children's nursing (CCN) services in the UK was very different from the situation which is to be found as this fourth edition of the text is being written, in 2008. In 1994, almost two-thirds of the children in the UK lived in an area where there was no CCN service at all. Although some parts of the UK were relatively well provided for, with a range of both generalist and specialist CCN services, in other areas, particularly those whose populations were quite widely dispersed, community children's nurses were a 'rare breed'. The whole of South Western England NHS Region, for instance, contained only two generalist CCNs. A total of five nurses were employed (all in specialist roles) to provide a community nursing service for children in Wales. There was not a single CCN in the whole of Northern Ireland (Royal College of Nursing [RCN] 1994). This situation lead the 1997 House of Commons Health Select Committee to conclude:

'It is a cause for serious concern that only 50% of health authorities purchase CCN services

and that only 10% of the Country's children have access to a 24-hour CCN service'.

(para 48)

In the past ten years, however, there has been a dramatic expansion in CCN provision, with the most recent version of the RCN Directory of Community Children's Nursing Services (RCN 2008a; (www.rcn.org.uk/development/communities/specialisms/community_childrens_nursing/directory) listing a total of 243 CCN services throughout the UK. This is a remarkable achievement, for a workforce which in 1988 was made up of a total of 67 nurses based in only 27 teams in the whole of the UK (Whiting 1988) (Figure 10.1).

This expansion in the provision of CCN services has occurred during a period of quite dramatic transformation in health services provision for children. This began in the early 1990s, with three key publications, *The Welfare of Children in Hospital* (DH 1991), *Children First* (Audit Commission 1993) and *Child Health in the Community* (NHS Executive 1996). And this growth in CCN services has continued in the early years of the twenty-first century.

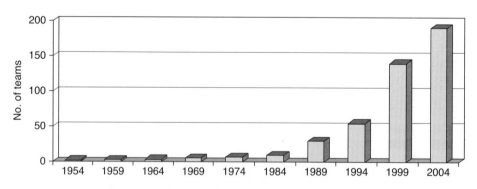

Figure 10.1 Community Children's Nursing Services UK provision 1954–2004.

In England, the major policy drivers within children's health and social care in the early years of the twenty-first century were crafted in direct response to two major reviews of children's services. The first was lead by Sir Ian Kennedy (The report of the public inquiry into children's heart surgery at the Bristol Royal Infirmary 1984–1995, 2001) and was focused on shortcomings in the care of children undergoing cardiac surgery at Bristol Royal Infirmary. The second review was that of Lord Laming (The Victoria Climbié Inquiry 2003), whose investigation was concerned primarily with the role of health and social care agencies in relation to the death of a 5-year-old girl, Victoria Climbié. These reports highlighted significant limitations in services provision for children, including poor communication and cooperation between agencies and inadequacies in leadership, coordination and management within and between services. The Laming inquiry was instrumental in guiding the development of a new over-arching strategy for children's services – *Every Child Matters*. In addition, the Kennedy and Laming inquiries have provided a significant guiding light in relation to several major policy initiatives (Box 10.1) each of which will be considered both in overall summary and also in respect of their specific relevance for the practice of CCN.

Box 10.1 Key policy strategy in children's health/social care 2004–8

- *Every Child Matters* (Department for Education and Skills [DfES] 2003, 2004)
- The *National Service Framework for Children, Young People and Maternity Services* (DH/DfES 2004a–f)
- *Our Health, Our Care Our Say* (DH 2006a)
- The Darzi Review, *Our NHS Our Future* (DH 2007) and *High Quality Care for All* (DH 2008a)
- *Better care: Better Lives. Improving Outcomes and Experiences for Children, Young People and Their Families Living With Life-limiting and Life-threatening Conditions* (DH 2008b)
- *Aiming High for Disabled Children* (Her Majesty's Treasury/DfES 2007)

Every Child Matters

Every Child Matters was initially published as a Green Paper in September 2003, the first stage in a process that was intended to transform the delivery of children's services. The Green Paper set out the principal aim of this transformation in the following statement:

> 'Our aim is to ensure that every child has the chance to fulfil their potential by reducing levels of educational failure, ill health, substance misuse, teenage pregnancy, abuse and neglect, crime and anti-social behaviour among children and young people'.

> (DfES 2003, p. 5)

As a result of an extensive consultation exercise, the Green Paper identified five outcomes which both 'mattered most to children and young people' (p. 5) and reflected clearly the government's own aspirations for the reform of children's services (Box 10.2).

Box 10.2 *Every Child Matters* – key outcomes (DfES 2003)

- *Being healthy*: enjoying good physical and mental health and living a healthy lifestyle
- *Staying safe*: being protected from harm and neglect
- *Enjoying and achieving*: getting the most out of life and developing the skills for adulthood
- *Making a positive contribution*: being involved with the community and society and not engaging in anti-social or offending behaviour
- *Economic well-being*: not being prevented by economic disadvantage from achieving their full potential in life.

The Green Paper, whose main target audience was those professional staff whose work was focused upon the provision of services to children, identified a need to focus action on four key areas:

- Supporting parents and carers
- Early intervention and effective protection
- Accountability and integration
- Workforce reform

The collective responses of health, social care and education professionals to the Green Paper consultation were largely supportive of its key proposals and more detailed guidance was published by the DfES in the spring of 2004 (DfES 2004) and in the subsequent Children Act 2004. Among a number of legislative changes introduced within the Act was the establishment of children's trusts whose work would be overseen by newly appointed Directors of Children's Services.

In respect specifically of the work of CCN services, *Every Child Matters* introduced a number of significant initiatives. The most important of these was the proposal to formally establish the role of *lead professional*, a practitioner who was expected to demonstrate a wide range of skills, including:

- The provision of psychological and emotional support to children and young people and their parents

- Achieving an appropriate balance between acting as an advocate on behalf of the child/family and empowering the child and family to take control of their own situation

- Networking and coordination between other members of the multi-agency support team

- Knowledge of local resources and sources of support for children and families

- A high level of expertise within their own practice discipline and awareness of the skills, knowledge and expertise of other members of the multi-agency team

Many elements of this role (Figure 10.2) correspond with those which have been identified as being central to the practice of community children's nursing (Cash *et al.* 1994, Proctor *et al.* 1998).

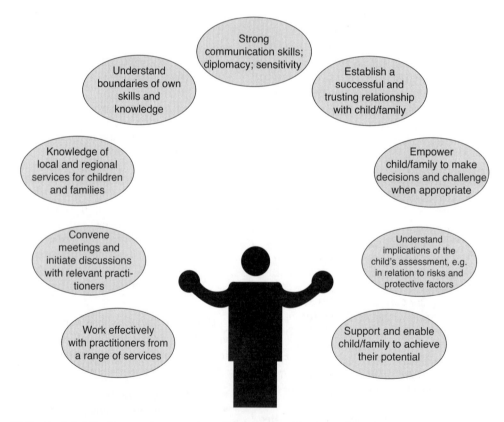

Figure 10.2   Useful skills for carrying out the role of lead professional (CWDC 2008). Reproduced under the terms of the Click-Use Licence.

National Service Framework for Children, Young People and Maternity Services

At around the same time as the *Every Child Matters* policy was being launched, the Kennedy (2001) and Laming (2003) reports were also providing a significant driver to the development of the *National Services Framework for Children, Young People and Maternity Services* (hereafter 'Children's NSF') (DH/DfES 2004a–f). National services frameworks were introduced in 1997 by the incoming Labour Government as a series of long-term overarching health strategies for improving specific areas of care. They key components of a national service framework are (DH 1997):

- Setting of national standards
- Identification of key interventions to improve health
- Provision of greater consistency in the availability and quality of services, right across the NHS

The Children's NSF was jointly published by the DH and the DfES. This in itself signalled a key commitment for inter-departmental working in relation to children – so called 'joined up Government' (Bogdanor 2005) It consists of ten over-arching standards for health services provision and was accompanied by a short series of exemplars (Box 10.3).

The Children's NSF incorporates a series of recommendations which relate specifically to community children's nursing provision and these are contained largely within Standards 6 and 8 with additional references within the 'asthma', 'acquired brain injury', 'long-term ventilation' and 'continence' exemplars. As a 'Marker of Good Practice' the framework requires that 'Community Children's Nursing Teams are available (as part of Children's Community Teams) in each locality' (DH/DfES 2004b, p. 5). The standard included a clear statement that additional funding was to be made available within the NHS to increase capacity in CCN teams, recognising that 'local organisation

---

Box 10.3   *National Service Framework for Children, Young People and Maternity Services*

Standard 1:   Promoting health and well-being, identifying needs and intervening early
Standard 2:   Supporting parents or carers
Standard 3:   Child, young person and family-centred services
Standard 4:   Growing up into adulthood
Standard 5:   Safeguarding and promoting the welfare of children and young people

All of the above included within a single 'core' standards document (DH/DfES 2004a)

Standard 6:   Children and Young People who are Ill (DH/DfES 2004b)
Standard 7:   Children in Hospital (DH/DfES 2004c)
Standard 8:   Disabled Child (subsequently re-titled 'Disabled Children and Young People and those who have complex health needs') (DH/DfES 2004d)
Standard 9:   The Mental Health and Psychological Wellbeing of Children and Young People (DH/DfES 2004e)
Standard 10:   Medicines for Children and Young People (DH/DfES 2004f)

Exemplars   Asthma (DH/DfES 2004g)
             Autism Spectrum Disorders (DH/DfES 2004h)
             Acquired Brain Injury (DH/DfES 2004i)
             Care pathway for the discharge and support of children requiring long term ventilation in the community (DH/DfES 2005)
             Continence (DH/DfES 2007)

is needed to allow efficient use of scarce staff'
(DH/DfES 2004b, p. 35). The standard recognised a diverse range of potential areas of activity for the CCN teams:

> 'Children's Community Teams including
> Community Children's Nursing Services need
> to provide appropriate support to children,
> young people and their families which responds
> to local needs and takes account of the need to
> prevent hospital admission, facilitate early
> discharge, and care for children with com-
> plex needs. Ideally, these should work across
> a number of settings, for example, hospital,
> home and school, improving continuity and
> maximising the available skills.'

> (DH/DfES 2004b, p. 33)

Our Health, Our Care, Our Say

In 2006, the White Paper *Our Health, Our Care,
Our Say* was published. Its key purpose was
to promote, principally through the vehicle
of practice-based commissioning, the necessary incentive to shift health services provision
from secondary to primary care under the ban-
ner heading 'Care closer to home'. This policy
directive was founded on several key principles
including:

- Hospital care is expensive and community
  care can often offer a less costly alternative
- Patients want greater choice and control –
  'They want a service that does not force
  them to plan their lives around multiple
  visits to large, hectic sites, or force them to
  present the same information to different
  professionals' (DH 2006a, p. 129).
- Technological change has allowed clinical activity that was previously exclusively
  available in hospital to be offered in a range
  of community settings
- A recognition that with an ageing population, hospital-focused models of care for the
  management of long-term disease are unsustainable and compare unfavourably with
  care models that are focused on prevention
  and supporting individual well-being in the
  community

The first three of these principles are clearly
relevant in the context of community children's
nursing practice and the White Paper offers the
following additional, specific advice to primary
care trusts (PCTs):

> 'For disabled children, children with com-
> plex health needs and those in need of pal-
> liative care, PCTs should ensure that the right
> model of service is developed by undertaking
> a review to audit capacity (including chil-
> dren's community nursing) and delivery of
> integrated care pathways against National
> Service Framework standards, agreeing
> service models, funding and commission-
> ing arrangements with their SHAs [strategic
> health authorities].'

> (DH 2006a, p. 104)

The Next Stage review

In July 2007, Alan Johnson, Secretary of
State for Health, announced a wide-ranging
review of the NHS, as it approached its sixtieth
year, to be led by Professor Ara Darzi. Within
three months, an interim report was published
by Lord Darzi (DH 2007a). The report challenged each of the NHS Regions in England
to establish a series of eight clinical pathway
groups (Box 10.4) whose work would focus
upon the central vision of delivering a 'fair,
personal, effective, safe and locally accountable
NHS' (DH 2007a, p. 8).

Almost all of the regional children's health
pathway groups identified particular roles that

**Box 10.4   Darzi pathway groups
(DH 2007a)**

- Maternity and newborn care
- Children's health
- Planned care
- Mental health
- Staying healthy
- Long-term conditions
- Acute care
- End-of-life care

were to be undertaken by CCN services in the future: Table 10.1 provides some illustrative examples from the regional review reports and illustrates the wide variation and diversity of practice within CCN services. Three key areas of work for CCNs are evident within the reviews:

- Supporting children with long-term conditions and disabilities and those requiring continuing care
- Care of children with life-limiting and life-threatening conditions including palliative and end-of life care

- Supporting new models of working, focused on ambulatory care, short stay/assessment units and urgent care centres

Each of these practice priorities feature prominently in the final Darzi report *High Quality Care for All* (DH 2008a) and provide a sense of the necessary direction of travel for CCN services in the coming years. However, as is evident in Table 10.1, there is considerable variation in the priorities identified by individual NHS Regions for CCN practice. This is perhaps unhelpful. If CCN services are to provide sustainable and

Table 10.1   Darzi regional pathway groups – children's health – Community Children's Nursing services

Region	CCN activity identified/highlighted
East Midlands	'The children's community nursing team should be available to support children with minor illnesses at home.' (p. 29)
East of England	'The multi-agency multi-disciplinary teams should work together and be located together, supported by a high quality information system to ensure better decision-making, audit and communication. In the longer term, Community Children's Nursing Teams will form the core of the larger multi-agency team.' (p. 68)
	'We therefore propose to review whether some hospitals should consider withdrawing from providing full inpatient children's services and instead develop their Children's Assessment Unit. In addition, PCTs would invest in additional children's community nurses.' (p. 70)
North East	Proposed model care pathway for ill/injured child: 'Discharged with appropriate follow up for self care hospital at home team, children's community nursing team, physiotherapy and social services etc' (p. 59)
North West	'There should be a "systematic" programme throughout the North West to reduce the need for inpatient care days, achieved through: better co-ordinated, team based and proactive care for children with long term conditions, involving the GP, children's community matrons and the team around the child' (p. 31)
South Central	'The first priority for children's services will be prevention, supported by excellent maternal care, school nurses, health visitors and community paediatric nurses. There will be access to a network of community-based palliative care teams of paediatric nurses and therapists for support and advice 24 hours a day. Community paediatric nursing teams with a variety of specialist and general paediatric skills will be available round the clock to give advice and practical support to families and children.' (p. 35)
West Midlands	'Each PCT should enable equitable access to a comprehensive community children's nursing service to cover acute/ambulatory care, respite care, palliative and continuing care, care of long term conditions and disability and 24 hour end of life care at home.' (p. 58)
Yorkshire and the Humber	End of life care. 'Families and children should be given choices about place of care based on clear information and a range of options, with 24/7 availability of support at home from Children's Community Nursing Teams.' (p. 86)

comprehensive coverage to local child populations, then potential conflicts in terms of the demands placed on such services by inconsistencies in regional prioritisation must be addressed as a matter of some urgency.

Better Care: Better Lives

The care of children with life-threatening illness featured significantly in the work of the Darzi children's health clinical pathways. This area has been the subject of quite detailed scrutiny in recent years. In May 2006, Patricia Hewitt, Secretary of State for Health, commissioned a review of children's palliative care to be led by Professor Sir Alan Craft. One of the main aims of the review was to 'find a more sustainable way of developing and funding services' (DH 2007b, p. 3). This comment stemmed in large part from the historical provision of a succession of short-term funding streams in children's palliative care dating back to the early 1990s. An earlier and comprehensive study undertaken by Hunt (1995) had identified significant variations in relation to both the provision and the practice of CCN working with children with cancer, particularly in respect of the influence/impact of the use of charity funding to pay nurses' salaries for that practice.

The DH *Palliative Care Review* (2007) was supported by additional work based upon detailed statistical (DH 2007c) and financial (DH 2007d) analysis. The financial analysis, which was undertaken by the Health Economics Consortium at the University of York, found wide variations in service size and capacity within many elements of children's palliative care services and in particular in CCN provision. The review evaluated each PCT's spend on services to children with a disability and concluded 'there is up to a 10 fold difference in funding levels, and it is likely that many PCTs are not providing sufficient services across the whole range of services for disabled children' (DH 2007d, p. 47). The economic review also demonstrated that most, if not all, of the costs of developing comprehensive community children's palliative care teams within England would be saved by

reductions in the demand for inpatient care (DH 2007d, p. 43).

In 2008, the Government published *Better Care: Better Lives*, a detailed response to the findings of the independent palliative care review. The review had identified three key funding priorities to improve the quality and experience of children's palliative care services and the Government response advised that 'Commissioners will want to take these into account when allocating the new Comprehensive Spending Review funding' (DH 2008, p. 19). The three priority funding areas are: CCN teams, short breaks and palliative care networks. In relation to CCN teams, the government advised:

> 'Commissioners will need to consider how this new funding can enable the development of children's community nursing services capable of providing an all-round care package, including end-of-life care, 24 hours a day, seven days a week in the location that the child and family prefer.'
>
> (DH 2008, p. 20)

In many parts of the UK, a focus on the needs of children with life-threatening and life-limiting illness particularly in relation to palliative and end-of-life care has significantly influenced the development of community children's nursing services during the course of the past 15 years. The availability of a number of short-term, pump-prime funding streams has undoubtedly allowed services to be introduced and developed where they might otherwise have never been established in the first place. However, the requirement for primary care organisations to identify the necessary revenue to maintain service funding beyond the initial investment has not always been realised and a number of services have not survived beyond the initial funding period.

It is to be hoped that the new arrangements based on comprehensive spending review investment and supported by both a Public Services Agreement indicator (HM Treasury 2008), and the NHS Operating Framework (DH 2007e) will ensure that for the first time in the development of CCN services a government has committed to sustainable 24/7 palliative care CCN services.

Aiming High for Disabled Children

In March 2007, the government published a detailed report setting out its overall priorities and aspirations for children in the context of the 2008–2011 Comprehensive Spending Review. *Aiming High for Disabled Children* (HM Treasury/ DfES 2007b) focused upon the need to sustain and build resilience within families, to provide increased personalisation in services delivery and to proactively support families in the greatest of need, with a particular emphasis on enabling families to break out of cyclical deprivation. The report indicated that a supplementary volume would be published which would focus on the particular needs of children with disabilities and, in May 2007, *Aiming High for Disabled Children: Better Support for Families* (HM Treasury/DfES 2007b) was published. This second report, which promised £340 million of new investment for children with disabilities, was warmly welcomed by a range of agencies which had been campaigning for improved services to this group of children. Francine Bates, Chief Executive of Contact-a-Family and a board member of the Every Disabled Child Matters (EDCM) campaign, observed:

> 'This new investment will start to transform the lives of families with disabled children all over the country. It shows that when the government says that every child matters, this really does mean every disabled child too. The campaign has lobbied hard to get this money, which is the reward for all the efforts by our coalition of organisations and families to get our issues higher up the agenda.'

> (EDCM 2007)

Aiming High for Disabled Children included a range of new initiatives intended to deliver significant improvements for children with disabilities and their families. The strategy includes a major commitment to improve the provision of short breaks for children and families including £280 million over the funding period allocated to local authorities with additional funding through the NHS settlement specifically intended to provide short breaks for children with disabilities and complex health needs. As noted above in the context of children's palliative care, this area of services provision has been further strengthened by the development of a formal indicator, the 'Disabled Children's Service Indicator within a Public Service Agreement published by the Treasury to support the Comprehensive Spending Review settlement.

PSA Delivery Agreement 12: Improve the health and well-being of children and young people

Indicator 5: Parents' experience of services for disabled children and the 'core offer'.

> 'A new indicator will be based on parents' experience of services and the "core offer" made in *Aiming High for Disabled Children*: clear information; transparency in how families can access services; integrated assessment; participation in shaping local services; and effective feedback. The measure will cover the families of all disabled children and ask about all services provided by their local authority and PCT. By 2011, disabled young people and their parents should be able to report a more favourable experience of these services: baseline and comparison data will drive best practice and improvements.'

> (HM Treasury 2008, p. 6)

The Public Service Agreement sets out a range of additional measures which are intended to ensure the delivery of 'joined-up' services for children: 3.56 Backed by an additional £370 million from Department for Children, Schools and Families (DCSF) and with additional DH funding for the NHS over the next three years, the two departments will act jointly to communicate the vision for supporting disabled children and issue guidance on making the 'core offer' a reality locally. In addition, delivery will include (HM Treasury 2008):

- Transforming short-breaks provision for disabled children and their parents and expanding accessible childcare
- Supporting development of a parents forum in each local authority
- Establishing a Transition Support Programme to ease the transition from childhood to adulthood
- Developing a national strategy on children's palliative care
- Piloting a national framework for children and young people's continuing care
- Developing a tool for transition planning for young people with neurodisabilities
- Improve accessibility to appropriate childcare for families with disabled children
- Scoping and delivering reform of community equipment and wheelchair provision

In addition the NHS Operating Framework for 2008/9 has clearly identified children with disabilities as a priority area against which PCT performance will be judged:

'disabled children: identifying actions and setting local targets on improving the experience of, and ranges of services for, children with disabilities and complex health needs and their families. This includes significantly increasing the range of short breaks, improving the quality and experience of palliative care services, improving access to therapies and supporting effective transition to adult services.'

(DH 2007e)

As discussed earlier, in the context of the Darzi review, CCN services are well placed to provide support to children with long-standing conditions, including disabilities, though it is important to be ensure that the CCN's work remains firmly focused in the provision of specific nursing care to those children, and to recognise that many children with disabilities do not require the services of a CCN. However, defining exactly what the work of a community children's nurse is may not be so straightforward. The nature of the work of CCN services is very diverse indeed, with no particular model dominating and significant variations in many aspects of the ways that services are organised and provided (Box 10.5).

In order to further explore a number of the issues raised both in the foregoing discussion and in relation to the diversity of practice within community children's nursing services, the remainder of this chapter will focus upon two broad themes: the CCN workforce and transitions from children's to adult services.

The community children's nursing workforce

How many CCNs do we need?
The question of how many community children's nurses might be required in order to meet

---

Box 10.5 CCN: role dimensions	
Hospital base	Community base
Managed within a hospital trust	Managed within a primary care organisation
Generalist nursing service	Specialist nursing service
Children with acute nursing needs	Children with long term conditions
Neonatal care	Transition to adult services
Focus upon avoiding unnecessary hospital admission	Focus on facilitation of 'early' hospital discharge
'Mainstream' NHS funding	Charity or 'pump-prime' funding

the needs of local child populations is not one to which there is a straightforward answer. There is, however considerable guidance relating to the expectations of what local CCN services might provide. The House of Commons Health Select Committee (1997) advised:

'The overall intention must be to introduce as soon as possible a home nursing service provided by appropriately qualified staff and available to all children requiring home nursing and their families. For many years there has been such a service available to all adults in their own homes. We consider that as a matter of principle, sick children need and deserve no less'.

(para 49)

In the children's NSF, there is an explicit commitment that 'Inequalities will be reduced, so that all children and young people have access to the services they need, no matter where they live or where they come from' (DH/DfES 2004a, p. 2). The 'Ill child' module of the NSF is very specific about the need for consistent CCN services provision:

'Primary Care Trusts ensure that Community Children's Nursing Teams are available in each locality (as part of the Children's Community Teams) and are based on local need. Services are developed in an integrated way across the local health economy'.

(DH/DfES 2004c, p. 35)

In its evidence to the Health Select Committee, the RCN (1996) estimated that in order to provide a full range of services to children, a ratio of one nurse per 10 000 child population was required. The rationale behind this estimate was based upon four major assumptions:

- The first consideration is that the skills required to confidently care for children with complex health needs at home are often quite sophisticated. In consequence the level of support required by parents who choose to care for their child in the community are considerable (DH 2000, Whiting 1995).

- Balanced against this is the second assumption, which is that parents will be taught to deliver much of the care to their own children – in particular to children with complex and continuing care needs – this obviates, in many instances, the need for nurses to themselves provide 'hands-on' care on a day-by-day basis and is very much aligned with the philosophy of 'partnership' (Taylor 2000).

- The third assumption is that the demand for care in the community will increase. This is a view supported within many of the regional Darzi reviews as well as by the Royal College of Paediatrics and Child Health (2007) and the RCN (2000, 2004a).

- The final strand of this argument establishes that there is an agreed range of nursing care needs for which CCNs might provide. This list draws on research undertaken by one of this chapter's authors in the late 1980s (Whiting 1988), was included in the RCN evidence to the Health Select Committee (RCN 1996) and appears in slightly modified form within the Committee's Report:
  — Neonatal (and post-neonatal) care
  — Caring for children with acute paediatric nursing needs
  — Supporting children undergoing planned surgery
  — Supporting children with long-term physical nursing needs
  — Follow-up of children who have required emergency treatment/care
  — Supporting the families of children with disability
  — Supporting families who are caring for children during the terminal phase of their lives

As noted previously, the regional Darzi reviews have indicated considerable variation in local priorities for CCN services, though it is not at all clear whether such prioritisation is to be achieved in the context of continuing to meet the all of diversity of needs endorsed by the Health

Select Committee or whether this is to be at the expense of one or more areas of need.

There are around 14 million children under the age of 16 in the UK. Based upon the RCN's suggested ratio of one nurse per 10 000 children, this would require a working population of around 1400 CCNs, almost three times as many as were identified by the RCN at the time of the Health Select Committee hearings. Although, as noted above, the CCN workforce has continued to expand since the mid-1990s, data about this workforce are not routinely collected by the DH. However, all indicators are that considerable variations remain in terms of both the size and composition of CCN teams as was recognised by the Children's NSF (DH/DfES 2004c). This has been further compounded by the evolution of the term community children's nurse which is being increasingly applied to a wide range of activities within different localities including:

- 'Traditional' CCN
- Disability Nursing
- Special School Nursing
- Palliative Care
- Diabetes Care
- Respiratory Care
- Community Oncology Nursing
- Continuing Care
- Advanced Practice
- Transitional Care

The numbers of CCNs who might be needed in a particular locality will clearly be dependent to some extent upon the range of services which are considered to fall within the context of that area of practice.

Band mix in the registered community children's nursing workforce

The range of skills required of a CCN team will vary considerably, depending upon the needs of the local child population and the areas of practice within which the team is engaged. The terms 'skill-mix' and 'grade-mix' are often used interchangeably, most commonly when a 'review of skill-mix' within a service is actually focused on the bands or pay scales of staff posts within a service rather than of the skills which are required either of the service as a whole or of individual posts. Several aspects of the particular 'skills' portfolio for a CCN team are considered elsewhere in this chapter. A brief consideration is therefore given at this point to the matter of grade/band mix within CCN services and of the composition within teams of registered children's nurses as it relates to the *Agenda for Change* bands 5, 6, 7 and 8.

Band 5 is the entry level to qualified nursing practice in CCN team. The Royal College of Nursing (2007b) identifies the following key activities within the role of a band 5 community staff nurse:

- Assess patients, plans, implement care in the community, provide advice
- Maintain associated records
- Carry out nursing procedures
- May provide clinical supervision to other staff, students

When appointing staff to Band 5 posts within CCN teams it may be appropriate to consider the need for staff to have already undergone a period of post-registration consolidation/preceptorship, perhaps in a hospital based post in advance of taking on potentially more autonomous roles within a CCN team. The Darzi review has recently recognised the value of a more robust approach to preceptorship in the context of post-registration nursing practice and suggests the need for:

'A foundation period of preceptorship for nurses at the start of their careers will help them begin the journey from novice to expert. This will enable them to apply knowledge, skills and competences acquired as students, into their area of practice, laying a solid foundation for life-long learning'.

(DH 2008e, pp. 19)

Band 6 is described by the Royal College of Nursing (2007b) as being appropriate to the profile of a nurse specialist or district nursing sister, identifying the following activities:

- Assess patients, plans and implements care in the community

- Provide advice to patients/clients; maintain associated records
- Carry out nursing procedures
- Coordinate nursing team workloads

Band 7 is considered by the RCN (2007b) as being appropriate for team manager posts within community nursing, though such a banding may also be appropriate for CCNs whose role also includes that of community specialist practitioner teacher or for a nurse whose specialist clinical skills might be considered as advanced practice (see below). The RCN (1997) identifies the following elements of the Band 7 role:

- Manages team of community nurse specialists and other staff covering a geographical area, including recruitment and appraisal
- Assesses patients and plans and implements care; maintains associated records
- Carries out nursing procedures

Many nurses within Bands 7 and 6 might have completed the Specialist Practitioner Qualification in CCN (see below). Band 8 may be appropriate for community matrons or consultant nurses. The RCN (2007b) identifies the following elements of the community matron's profile:

- Manages and provides leadership for managers, specialist nurses/midwives and other staff in a primary care setting
- Ensures patient/client/carer involvement in development of services and promotes better health, social care and medicines management
- Provides specialist education and training to other staff
- Maintains compliance with, and development of, policies, procedures and guidelines, including case management; coordinates care in a community setting

New ways of working

Community children's nurses provide nursing care and support to children and young people (CYP) and their families at home, school or other community setting (RCN 2000). Many CCNs have an enhanced level of knowledge and skills in a specialist area such as diabetes,

oncology or eczema management. Those who have completed programmes as specialist practitioners are able to:

'Assess, plan, provide and evaluate specialist clinical nursing care to meet care needs of acutely and chronically ill children at home and assess, diagnose and treat specific diseases in accordance with agreed medical/nursing protocols'.

(United Kingdom Central Council for Nursing, Midwifery and Health Visiting [UKCC] 2001, p. 21)

While in the past, the major focus of CCN work has been in the care of children with disabilities and long-term conditions (Myers 2005, Whiting 1988) in order to address the diverse needs of the local child populations, CCNs will need to change and adapt to new models of services delivery, taking on novel and emerging roles in order to ensure that all children with nursing needs are managed closer to home.

As the NHS responds to the challenges of twenty-first century health care, new models of community services are evolving (DH 2006, 2008c). This will require extended working hours and the development of urgent care or paediatric assessment units which may be co-located with emergency departments or aligned with GP surgeries or 'polyclinics' which the Darzi review has suggested will provide the infrastructure to shift hospital-based care into a more local setting and improve existing GP, community care and social care (DH 2007a).

The House of Commons Health Select Committee (1997) suggested that every GP should have access to a named community children's nurse. Ten years later, *A Framework for Action* (DH 2007f) highlighted the need to develop services closer to home with specialist nurses aligning themselves to GP practices to prevent hospital admission and provide outpatient services in the surgery. The Children's NSF (DH 2004c) stated that CCN services should be an integral part of the primary health care and community provision. The aim is to provide a greater range of services and to offer extended opening hours to enable a more accessible nursing and medical provision of care in the community to meet the local needs of the population. As noted above, CCNs are well placed to embrace the new model of community care and new ways of working that the Darzi review will demand of them.

Nurse-led care

One of the ways in which community children's nurses can support the new model of working in the community is by offering a more specialist service to children whom a GP would usually refer to secondary care. CCNs are well positioned to be able to embrace practice-based commissioning (DH 2005) where the local GP practices have the responsibility of commissioning services for the local population. In so doing, CCNs are able to support the delivery of care closer to home eliminating unnecessary hospital visits or admission by re-directing care that traditionally would have been held in secondary care into a range of primary care settings. For example outpatient's clinic, including nurse-led clinics, can be held in a range of out-of-hospital settings (Box 10.6).

Community matrons

As noted above, a major focus of CCN activity in recent years has been upon children's palliative care. The focus on long-term conditions and the management of complex care under the definition of palliative care has defined a significant proportion of CCN activity. Many elements of the core competencies of the community matron (Woodend 2006) will be familiar to a large number of CCNs.

- 'Act as a case manager for a maximum of 50 patients with long term conditions.
- Provide active care on a regular basis: at least monthly.
- Prevent hospital admissions by providing intensive home support.'

(Woodend 2006, p. 51)

In Walsall PCT, the role of the community matron in CCN services has recently been established. The post-holder is based with other community matrons but works closely with the local CCN team. The competencies of the community matron role have been a key feature of CCN practice since the 1980s, however the current focus on long-term conditions offers great opportunities to expand and develop this area.

Consultant nurses

Currently within the UK, there are approximately 37 consultant nurses within the field of children and young people's nursing (RCN Children's Consultant Nurse Forum, personal

---

Box 10.6 A nurse-led eczema clinic in Islington

The nurse consultant in CCN set up an eczema clinic based in two health centres in Islington PCT in 2006. The majority of children are referred to the clinic by GPs and health visitors although parents and other professionals can also refer. The clinic has led to improved health outcomes for children requiring eczema care through providing a seamless local community service. It has reduced the need for children to be referred to secondary care. The nurse consultant only refers to a dermatologist in secondary care if the eczema cannot be adequately managed in the community. As a result there is a more consistent approach to eczema support and education for families and greater compliance and understanding of practical advice given. The nurse consultant has completed the nurse independent prescribing course which has greatly enhanced her autonomous practice in the management of children with eczema. The nurse consultant is able to complete the whole process of assessing, diagnosing and prescribing treatment and giving follow-up advice. An important aspect of prescribing is checking the parents' understanding of how to use emollients or topical steroids prescribed and being able to provide explanation before writing a prescription.

communication 2008). Within CCN/complex care there are currently three posts with two more in the advanced stages of planning. Manley (1997) described the nurse consultant role in the terms of expert practitioner, educator and researcher. Guest and colleagues (Linter 2003, p. 83) argued that the consultant nurse role 'has resulted in improved systems, procedures and protocols and has improved the motivation and competence of staff, resulting in better patient services and patient care.'

CCN services have pioneered the community matron model. Long-term condition management has been a feature of CCN teams since the early 1980s (Whiting 1988). However, new roles such as those of nurse consultant and nurse practitioners and community matrons have much to offer CCN development in this time of significant change.

Advancing practice

The Royal College of Nursing (2008) has defined the advanced nurse practitioner as:

'a registered nurse who has undertaken a specific course of study of at least first degree (Honours) level and who... receives patients with undifferentiated and undiagnosed problems and makes an assessment of their health care needs, based on highly developed nursing knowledge and skills, including skills not usually exercised by nurses such as physical examination...'

(RCN 2008b, p. 3)

However, there has been much confusion and ambiguity over the definition of the advanced nursing practitioner role. Wilson & Bunnell (2007) argue that part of the difficulty in reaching a definition is that advanced nursing practice is an umbrella term for a range of different emerging nursing roles. Conversely it might be argued that the advanced nursing practitioner role is not so much based on different nursing roles but on an extension or expansion of the nursing roles to include skills and competencies that were once considered medical roles.

The Nursing and Midwifery Council (NMC 2005) in its consultation document on registration and regulation of the advanced nursing practitioner defines the role as:

'A registered nurse who has command of an expert knowledge base and clinical competence, is able to make complex clinical decisions using expert clinical judgement, is an essential member of an interdependent health care team and whose role is determined by the context in which she practices'

(NMC 2005, p. 8)

Bryant-Lukosius *et al.* (2004) stated that advanced practice nursing represents the future frontier for nursing practice and professional development. The advanced nursing practitioner role is a dynamic and evolving role which enables the expert clinical nurse to make professional autonomous decisions, from a wide range of competencies, knowledge and skill base. The development of the role has blurred the boundaries between medicine and nursing regarding tasks such as history taking, physical assessment, diagnosing and prescribing treatment, all of which have become more of a shared responsibility (Baid 2006).

The Royal College of Paediatrics and Child Health (RCPCH 2007) has recently highlighted that, as a result of the impact of the European Working Time Directive (EWTD), there will need to be a greater cooperation between professional and organisations in a geographical area. This will include rotating staff between services and joint training. One of the solutions to the challenges of acute and urgent care services identified by RCPCH (2007) is to recruit and develop the role of children's nurses to enable a reduction in attendance to emergency departments. The NMC (2005) confirms that many of the roles taken on by advanced nursing practitioners were previously preserved for doctors. Paton (2005) acknowledges that the EWTD has placed a restriction on junior doctors working hours, which in turn has led to nurses taking on medical responsibilities. Many other factors, such as government and other associated policies/reviews (DH 2007a, 2008a, NHS Institute for Innovation and Improvement 2008), increased emergency attendance (Audit Commission 2001, DH 2008d) and the need to reduce waiting times has been instrumental in the development of the advanced nursing practitioner role (Robinson & Inyang 1999).

Community Children's Nurses are ideally placed to provide first contact and acute assessment of needs. However, CCNs will need to further develop their acute care skills and develop advanced nurse practice skills, including nurse prescribing skills and physical assessment skills, if they are to be able to fully assess, diagnose and prescribe treatment. The development of these competencies will greatly enhance the CCN role to support the new model of care closer to home and will equip CCNs with the necessary preparation to allow them to work more closely with primary care staff in urgent care centres or paediatric assessment centres based with GP practices and in 'polyclinics'. This might be achieved by developing an advanced level of competence/skill in relation to the care of children with acute illness – possibly based upon a formal educational preparation in advanced nursing practice in addition to co-working with GPs in a range of primary care settings or with paediatric medical staff in ambulatory/short stay assessment/urgent care centres. The RCPCH (2007) has also recognised that through the development of an enhanced knowledge/skills-base within community children's nursing services many aspects of the care of children with a range of more long-term health care needs can be managed by the CCNs with significantly less input from paediatric medical staff.

The government has devolved responsibility for commissioning services from PCTs to local GP practices through practice-based commissioning (DH 2005). GPs will have the resources to provide services by identifying patient needs and designing effective and appropriate health service in response to local need. CCNs with advanced nurse practitioner skills working in partnership with GPs will be able to provide high-quality, joined-up service for children with both acute and long-term or life-threatening conditions. Service provision will be more accessible, convenient and appropriate if CCNs with advanced nurse practitioner skills worked more closely with GPs.

Non-medical prescribing

One of the key areas of development for CCNs is that of non-medical prescribing. Duxbury (2002) has argued that the boundaries between medicine and nursing are becoming increasingly blurred as the advanced nurse practitioner combines both medical and nursing models to develop consultation-style approaches, for instance in relation to patient history taking. A CCN with advanced practice nursing skills will also be competent in physical assessment skills, interpretation of test results and in prescribing medication (Barratt 2005). These skills are vitally important when prescribing for children in primary care setting such as GP practices, walk-in centres and urgent care centres and polyclinics, as well as when working with children and families in their own homes. CCNs who have completed nurse independent prescribing course have developed a range of competencies in non-medical prescribing (NMC 2006), including:

- Knowledge development
- Competence to assess a patient's clinical conditions
- Undertaking a thorough medical and medication history
- Diagnosis
- Decision-making relating to the management of a child's presenting condition
- Deciding whether or not to prescribe
- Identifying and prescribing appropriate medication,
- Advise the child and parents on side effects and risk
- Monitor the response to medication and advice given

The skills of non-medical prescribing will become an increasing necessity for CCNs if they are to effectively deliver new models of service.

Modernising Nursing Careers – educating a workforce that is fit for the future

Up until the mid-1990s, the community children's nursing workforce was made up in large part of children's nurses who had served fairly lengthy 'apprenticeships' as hospital staff nurses and ward sisters before making the transition to community practice. Prior to the introduction of the Specialist Practice Qualification (SPQ) programmes in the mid-1990s (UKCC 1994, 2001), those children's nurses who wished to undertake formal educational preparation for a post in community children's nursing had little choice other than to complete either the district nursing or health visiting programmes (Whiting 2005). The SPQ programmes were warmly embraced by the CCN workforce and between 1997 and 2006 a total of 596 nurses gained the SPQ Community Children's Nursing qualification (NMC New Registrations for Specialist Practitioner – CCN Programme 1997–2006, personal communication 2007, Figure 10.3).

Without doubt, the CCN SPQ programme has significantly enhanced its status, equipping the CCN workforce with a range of skills and knowledge that was hitherto unthinkable (Wint 2005). However in recent years, both the

number of universities (higher education institutions [HEIs]) offering the programme and the number of students entering the course have declined sharply. This has occurred in large part because of three factors. The first of these was the introduction, in 2004, of a new set of standards for education in Specialist Public Health Nursing (NMC 2004), which lead a number of HEIs to design new curricula for their health visiting (HV) and school nursing (SN) programmes. One unintended consequence of this was the loss of the opportunity for co-timetabling of 'core' teaching content between HV, SN and CCN programmes. A number of HEIs who had previously offered the CCN programme alongside a number of other SPQ programmes now no longer do so.

The second factor was the change in arrangements for the provision of 'back-fill' monies to PCTs. Between 1996 and 2005, Workforce Development funding had been made available through the NHS SHAs to PCTs as a contribution to replacement costs for staff seconded to undertake the SPQ programmes. These funding arrangements were discontinued at around the same time that the Specialise Public Health Nursing programmes were introduced. This has led to a significant reduction in recent years in the overall numbers of student numbers across the range of SPQ programmes.

The final issue relates to the content of the SPQ curriculum. As noted above, the nature of community children's nursing practice has evolved

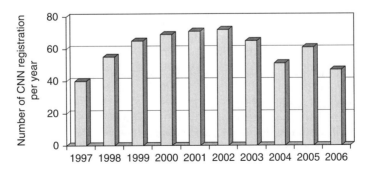

Figure 10.3 CCN New Registrations per year 1997–2006 (NMC 2007, personal communication).

at a rapid pace during the course of the past two decades in particular. It is clear that the original curriculum template for the CCN SPQ has failed to keep pace with the changing nature of that practice, particularly in terms of the diverse learning needs of potential programme entrants.

During the summer of 2007, one of the co-authors of this chapter (MW) made telephone contact with HEIs throughout the UK, who had previously offered the CCN SPQ programme. In total only five institutions reported that they intended to host the programme during the academic year 2007/8. The total number of student whom those HEIs anticipated would be undertaking the programme was 12, a significant reduction indeed from the peak of 72 student CCNs in 2002. So what does the future hold for the education of the CCN workforce?

In 2006, the four UK Chief Nursing Officers launched *Modernising Nursing Careers* (DH 2006c), a major review of post-registration nursing education at the heart of which was a recognition that in the future it will be necessary to:

- Develop a competent and flexible workforce
- Update career pathways and career choices
- Prepare nurses to lead in a changed health care system
- Modernise the image of nursing and nursing careers

At the heart of the document is the recognition that nursing needs to respond effectively to profound changes taking place both within the population and in the structures of health care delivery. The role of the CCN must continue to change in line with health reforms in order to ensure that children receive improved, quality care. This will include working in a range of settings crossing between hospital and community care and developing skills and competencies to prevent hospital admission and to promote care closer to home. These are exciting and challenging times for CCNs who are willing to embrace and influence change by developing their skills and competencies in line with the needs and of the population and with the NHS reforms. In 2007 as part of this ongoing review of post-registration nursing education the DH launched a major consultation: *Towards a Framework for Post-Registration Nursing Careers* (DH 2007g). The outcome of that consultation is eagerly awaited. It can not come soon enough for community children's nursing.

Support workers in the context of community children's nursing practice

In recent years the contribution of health care support workers has grown steadily within the NHS. The RCN had identified a number of roles which it considers may safely be delegated by qualified children's nurses to carers and support workers (Box 10.7).

Box 10.7   Managing children with health care needs: delegation of clinical procedures, training and accountability issues

The following procedures may be safely taught and delegated to non-health qualified staff following a child-specific assessment of clinical risk:

- Administering medicine in accordance with prescribed medicine in pre-measured dose via nasogastric tube, gastrostomy tube or orally
- Bolus or continuous feeds via a nasogastric tube
- Bolus or continuous feeds using a pump via a gastrostomy tube
- Tracheostomy care including suction using a suction catheter
- Emergency change of tracheostomy tube
- Oral suction with a yanker sucker
- Injections (intramuscular or subcutaneous). These may be single dose or multiple dose devices which are pre-assembled with pre-determined amounts of medication to be administered as documented

---

Box 10.7   (Continued)

in the individual child's care plan (pre-loaded devices should be marked when to be administered, e.g. for diabetes where the dose might be different in the morning and evening. In many circumstances there may be two different pens, one with short-acting insulin to be administered at specified times during the day and another for administration at night with long-acting insulin)

- Intermittent catheterisation and catheter care
- Care of Mitrofanoff: stoma care including maintenance of patency of a stoma in an emergency situation using, for example, the tip of a soft Foley's catheter and replacement of button devises once stoma has been well established for more than six months and there have been no problems with the stoma
- Inserting suppositories or pessaries with a pre-packaged dose of a prescribed medicine
- Rectal medication with a pre-packaged dose, i.e. rectal diazepam
- Rectal paraldehyde which is not pre-packaged and has to be prepared – permitted on a named child basis as agreed by the child's lead medical practitioner, i.e. GP or paediatrician
- Manual evacuation
- Administration of buccal or intra-nasal midazolam and Hypostat or GlucoGel.
- Emergency treatments covered in basic first aid training including airway management
- Assistance with inhalers, cartridges and nebulisers
- Assistance with prescribed oxygen administration including oxygen saturation monitoring where required
- Administration and care of liquid oxygen administration including filling of portable liquid oxygen cylinder from main tank
- Blood glucose monitoring as agreed by the child's lead nursing/medical practitioner, i.e. GP, paediatrician or paediatric diabetes nurse specialist
- Ventilation care for a child with a predictable medical condition and stable ventilation requirements (both invasive and non-invasive ventilation). NB: Stability of ventilation requirements should be determined by the child's respiratory physician and will include consideration of the predictability of the child's ventilation needs to enable the key tasks to be clearly learnt.

Source: Royal College of Nursing (2008d)

The expansion in both numbers of and the range of activities being undertaken by support workers has triggered a debate across the NHS: 'most striking has been the absence of explanations as to how and with what consequences support workers are used in the NHS.' (Kessler 2006, p. 1). It has been suggested that for a community children's nurse to take on the responsibility for delegation 'jeopardises their professional position' (Murphy 2001, p. 26). The NMC has recognised the concerns that may arise as a consequence of the delegation of clinical care roles by nurses to support workers and has addressed this in the two most recent versions of the Code of Professional Conduct. The 2008 code states:

- 'You must establish that anyone you delegate to is able to carry out instructions

- You must confirm that the outcome of any delegated task meets required standards
- You must make sure that everyone you are responsible for is supervised and supported'

(NMC 2008)

The focus within children's services upon inter-agency working set out in *Every Child Matters* (DfES 2003) and the Children's NSF (DH/DfES 2004a) have resulted in community children's nurses being required to train support workers across health, social care, education and the voluntary sectors making the legal and professional issues involved in delegation particularly pertinent to CCN practice. The RCN has provided significant input to a number of collaborative publications focused specifically on the training and delegation of support staff working in both social care (Lenehan *et al.* 2004, Rhodes *et al.* 1999) and education settings (Carlin 2005).

In 2005, the DfES provided funding to the Council for Disabled Children to support the development of a resource manual for health and education staff in supporting children with complex health needs within schools and early years settings (Carlin 2005). The guide brings together examples of good practice, including training materials and competency training systems, such as the Competency System from Coventry and Warwickshire Primary Care Trusts, consisting of PowerPoint presentations, teaching notes, workbooks and model answers and a competency document which includes a legal disclaimer to clarify responsibility (RCN 2007).

Delegation of clinical care tasks to support workers within the context of CCN practice is an area that is expanding at a rapid pace. Health care support workers are being employed in increasing numbers and the range of clinical tasks that they are undertaking is also expanding. Research to fully evaluate this development in terms of safety, clinical outcomes, quality and cost of care is, however, a neglected area and one that ought to be considered as a priority.

Transitions from children's to adult services

For many young people who form part of the CCN caseload, the transition from children's to adult services can be a time of significant challenges. Holistic and family-centred approaches to care are, in large part, well-established within children's services. This is not necessarily so in adult care provision where more disease-focused models of medical care predominate and the focus of professional attention shifts away from the family (with much information and care being delivered by professional staff working in partnership with child and parents together) towards the young person as an individual in their own right.

Transition has been defined as 'the purposeful, planned movement of adolescents and young adults from a child-centred to adult orientated health care systems' (Blum *et al.* 1993). Many children within CCN caseloads will make the transition to adult services (Cancelliere & Widdas 2005) including:

- Children with a range of long-term medical conditions such as diabetes, chronic renal disease, asthma, arthritis
- Children who are technology dependent, such as those with tracheostomies, gastrostomies, oxygen dependence, children who require assisted ventilation, etc.
- Children with life-limiting or life threatening conditions such as cancer, cystic fibrosis, muscular dystrophy
- Children with complex learning and physical disabilities

The numbers of children with long-standing and complex health needs who are surviving to adulthood is increasing (DH/DfES 2004c) and a growing number of these young people are reaching adulthood with significant dependence on supportive technology. Adult care services must be alerted well in advance to the complex needs of some of these young people. Close cooperative working between the CCN and their 'adult' counterparts is essential, and this may, at times, necessitate the provision by CCNs of formal training of adult nursing staff in some aspects of technical, clinical care.

In many ways, successful transition defines the relationship between adult and children's services. There is, however, a growing body of evidence of negative outcomes for young people when transition is not well planned and where the relationship between children's and adult services is poor. In a recent study by Watson (2000) of 20 young adults with renal disease who had received a transplant in children's services, eight transplants failed within 36 months of transfer to adult services and 35% of these were unexpected.

The transition from child-focused to adult-focused health services for children who have complex medical problems, including continuing dependence on medical technology, presents a range of significant and growing challenges for those who are charged with responsibility for providing health and social care services for this particular group of young adults. it is clearly a matter which is attracting growing attention – see for instance RCN 2004b, 2008d; DH/DfES 2006; Commission for Social Care Inspection 2007; Association for Children's Palliative Care [ACT] 2007; DCSF/DH 2007; DH/DCSF 2008)

While there is a growing consensus that transition is a process rather than an event, significant differences remain, within health, social care and education services in respect of the age at which young people make that transition. It is generally accepted that transition planning should begin at around the age of 14 (the Year 9 school review) with final transition occurring when the young person is ready and their future care pathway is in place (ACT 2007, DCSF/DH 2007, DH/DfES 2006).

The increasing policy profile of transition has led to groups being set up nationally, regionally and locally to develop transition services. Many local authorities now employ transition champions. For children with complex health needs community children's nurses have been identified as a key component of the transition process (DCSF/DH 2007), possibly in the role of lead professional. Health care plans can be another aid to achieving effective transition. A health plan will often comprise a self-assessment by the young person to identify their day-to-day needs and, in discussion with health professionals, an action plan to meet these needs in preparation for moving into adult health care provision (DH/DfES 2006). For many young people, this may be all that is required to ensure a 'good' transition. For those whose needs, particularly health needs, are more complex, more sophisticated multi-agency transition planning may be required.

Particular skill and sensitivity may be required when young people with life-threatening and life-limiting illness are making the transition to adult services, particularly where the young person has entered the palliative phase of care (Box 10.8).

Box 10.8 Palliative care in children

Palliative care in children has been defined as: 'an active and total approach to care, embracing physical, emotional, social and spiritual elements. It focuses on enhancement of quality of life for the child and support for the family and includes the management of distressing symptoms, provision of respite and care through death and bereavement' (ACT 2007).

The four palliative care modalities are:

- Young people with life-threatening conditions for which curative treatment may be feasible but can fail. Palliative care may be necessary during periods of prognostic uncertainty and when treatment fails. Examples include cancer, or irreversible organ failures such as heart, liver or kidney.
- Young people with conditions in which there may be long periods of intensive treatment aimed at prolonging life and allowing participation in normal activities, but where premature death is still possible or inevitable. Examples are cystic fibrosis, Duchenne's muscular dystrophy, human immunodeficiency virus (HIV)/acquired immune deficiency syndrome (AIDS).
- Young people with progressive conditions without curative treatment options, where treatment is exclusively palliative and may commonly extend over many years. Examples include Batten's disease, mucopolysaccharidosis, Creutzfeldt–Jakob disease.
- Young people with severe neurological disability, which may cause weakness and susceptibility to health complications leading to premature death. Deterioration may be unpredictable and not usually progressive. Examples are severe multiple disabilities following brain or spinal cord injuries, severe cerebral palsy.

Effective transition into adult services is a key aspect of a young person's care and is a quality indicator for CCN and adult services. For CCN, timely transition is essential to provide services to new referrals of children and families who require experienced child and family-focused care (Cancelliere & Widdas 2005).

Conclusion

This chapter provided a critical overview of CCN services provision at a time of great change in children's services. Major policy initiatives have been considered both in summary of the policy itself and with regard to the specific implications for CCN practice. Two major themes 'the community children's nursing workforce' and 'transitions from children's to adult services' were explored in particular detail in order to illustrate the many challenges and opportunities which lie ahead for CCN services.

References

Association for Children's Palliative Care (2007) *The Transition Care Pathway. A Framework for the Development of Integrated Multi-Agency Care Pathways for Young People with Life-Threatening and Life-Limiting Conditions.* Association for Children's Palliative Care, Bristol.

Audit Commission (1993) *Children First: A Study of Hospital Services.* The Audit Commission, London.

Audit Commission (2001) *Accident and Emergency: Review of National Findings (October 2001).* The Audit Commission, London.

Baid, H. (2006) Differential diagnosis in advanced nursing practice. *British Journal of Nursing*, **15**, 1007–1011.

Barratt, J. (2005) A case study of styles patient self-presentation in the nurse practitioner primary health care consultation. *Primary Health Care Research and Development*, **6**, 327–338.

Blum, R., Garell, D., Hodgman, C.H., Jorrissen, T.W., Okinow, N.A., Orr, P.D. & Slap, G.B. (1993) Transition from child-centred to adult health care systems for adolescents with chronic conditions. *Journal of Adolescent Health*, **14**, 570–576.

Bogdanor, V. (ed.) (2005) *Joined Up Government.* British Academy Occasional Papers. Oxford University Press, Oxford.

Bryant-Lukosius, D., DiCenso, A., Browne, G. & Pinelli, J. (2004) Advanced practice nursing roles: development, implementation and evaluation. *Journal of Advanced Nursing*, **48**, 519–529.

Cancelliere, L. & Widdas, D.J. (2005) Transition from children's to adult services. In: *Textbook of Community Children's Nursing*, 2nd edition (eds A. Sidey & D. Widdas). Elsevier, Edinburgh.

Carlin, C. (2005) *Including Me. Managing Complex Health Needs in Schools and Early Years Settings.* Council for Disabled Children, London.

Cash, C., Compston, H., Grant, J., Livesley, J., McAndrew, P. & Williams, G. (1994) *The Preparation of Sick Children's Nurses to Work in the Community P2000 Evaluation.* English National Board, London.

Children's Workforce Development Council (2008) *The Lead Professional: Practitioners' Guide. Integrated Working to Improve Outcomes for Children and Young People.* Children's Workforce Development Counci, Leeds.

Commission for Social Care Inspection (2007) *Growing Up Matters: Better Transition Planning for Young People with Complex Needs.* Commission for Social Care Inspection, London.

Department for Children, Schools and Families (2007) *The Children's Plan: Building Brighter Futures* (CMD 7280). The Stationery Office, London.

Department for Children, Schools and Families/ Department of Health (2007) *A Transition Guide for all Services.* The Stationery Office, London.

Department for Education and Skills (2003) *Every Child Matters.* The Stationery Office, London.

Department for Education and Skills (2004) *Every Child Matters: Change for Children.* The Stationery Office, London.

Department of Health (1991) *The Welfare of Children and Young People in Hospital.* HMSO, London.

Department of Health (1997) *The New NHS: Modern, Dependable.* The Stationery Office, London.

Department of Health (2000) *Shaping the Future NHS: Long Term Planning for Hospitals and Related Services.* Consultation Document on the Findings of the National Beds Enquiry – Supporting Analysis. The Stationery Office, London.

Department of Health (2005) *Practice Based Commissioning: Promoting Clinical Engagement.* The Stationery Office, London.

Department of Health (2006a) *Our Health, Our Care, Our Say: A New Direction for Community Services.* The Stationery Office, London.

Department of Health (2006b) *Extending Independent Nurse Prescribing Within the NHS in England: A Guide for Implementation.* The Stationery Office, London.

Department of Health (2006c) *Modernising Nursing Careers – Setting the Direction.* The Stationery Office, London.

Department of Health (2007a) *Our NHS, Our Future: NHS Next Stage Review, Interim Report.* The Stationery Office, London.

Department of Health (2007b) *Palliative Care Services for Children and Young People in England.* The Stationery Office, London.

Department of Health (2007c) *Palliative Care Statistics for Children and Young Adults.* Department of Health, London. Available at: www.dh.gov.uk/en/Publicationsandstatistics/Publications/PublicationsStatistics/DH_074701 (accessed 1 August 2008).

Department of Health (2007d) *Independent Review of Palliative Care Services for Children and Young People: Economic Study.* Health Economics Consortium, University of York, York.

Department of Health (2007e) *The Operating Framework for the NHS in England 2008/9.* The Stationery Office, London.

Department of Health (2007f) *A Framework for Action.* The Stationery Office, London.

Department of Health (2007g) *Towards a Framework for Post-Registration Nursing Careers.* The Stationery Office, London.

Department of Health (2008a) *High Quality Care for All.* The Stationery Office, London.

Department of Health (2008b) *Better Care: Better Lives. Improving Outcomes and Experiences for Children, Young People and their Families Living with Life-Limiting and Life-Threatening Conditions.* The Stationery Office, London.

Department of Health (2008c) *NHS Next Stage Review: Our Vision for Primary and Community Care.* The Stationery Office, London.

Department of Health (2008d) *Trends in Children and Young People's Care: Emergency Admission Statistics, 1996/97–2006/07, England.* The Stationery Office, London.

Department of Health (2008e) *A High Quality Workforce. NHS Next Stage Review.* The Stationery Office, London.

Department of Health/Department for Children, School and Families (2008) *Transition: Moving on Well.* The Stationery Office, London.

Department of Health/Department for Education and Skills (2004a) *National Service Framework for Children, Young People and Maternity Services: Core standards.* The Stationery Office, London.

Department of Health/Department for Education and Skills (2004b) *National Service Framework for Children, Young People and Maternity Services: Children and Young People who are Ill.* The Stationery Office, London.

Department of Health/Department for Education and Skills (2004c) *National Service Framework for Children, Young People and Maternity Services: Children in Hospital.* The Stationery Office, London.

Department of Health/Department for Education and Skills (2004d) *National Service Framework for Children, Young People and Maternity Services: Disabled Children and Young People and Those who have Complex Health Needs.* The Stationery Office, London.

Department of Health/Department for Education and Skills (2004e) *National Service Framework for Children, Young People and Maternity Services: The Mental Health and Psychological Wellbeing of Children and Young People.* The Stationery Office, London.

Department of Health/Department for Education and Skills (2004f) *National Service Framework for Children, Young People and Maternity Services: Medicines for Children and Young People.* The Stationery Office, London.

Department of Health/Department for Education and Skills (2004g) *National Service Framework for Children, Young People and Maternity Services: Asthma Exemplar.* The Stationery Office, London.

Department of Health/Department for Education and Skills (2004h) *National Service Framework for Children, Young People and Maternity Services: Autism Spectrum Disorder Exemplar.* The Stationery Office, London.

Department of Health/Department for Education and Skills (2004i) *National Service Framework for Children, Young People and Maternity Services: Acquired Brain Injury Exemplar.* The Stationery Office, London.

Department of Health/Department for Education and Skills (2005) *National Service Framework for Children, Young People and Maternity Services: Care Pathway for the Discharge and Support of Children Requiring Long Term Ventilation in the Community.* The Stationery Office, London.

Department of Health/Department for Education and Skills (2006) *Transition: Getting it Right for Children and Young People.* (National Service Framework for Children, Young People and Maternity Services). The Stationery Office, London.

Department of Health/Department for Education and Skills (2007) *National Service Framework for Children, Young People and Maternity Services: Continence Exemplar.* The Stationery Office, London.

Duxbury, J. (2002) Therapeutic communication and the nurse practitioner. In: *Nurse Practitioners: Clinical Skills and Professional Issues* (eds M. Walsh *et al.*) Butterworth & Heinnmann, Edinburgh.

East Midlands Strategic Health Authority (2008) *From Evidence to Excellence – Our Clinical Vision for Patient*

Care. East Midlands Strategic Health Authority, Nottingham.

East of England Strategic Health Authority (2008) *Towards the Best Together: A Clinical Vision for our NHS, Now and for the Next Decade*. East of England Strategic Health Authority, Cambridge.

Every Disabled Child Matters (2007) *Government Commits To Making Every Disabled Child Matter*. Press release 21 May 2007. Available at www.edcm.org.uk/ (accessed 1 July 2008).

Guest, D.E., Peccei, R., Rosenthal, P., Redfern, S., Wilson-Barnett, J., Dewe, P., Coster, S., Evans, A. & Sudbury, A. (2004) *An Evaluation of the Impact of Nurse, Midwife and Health Visitor Consultants*. King's College, University of London, London.

Her Majesty's Treasury (2008) *PSA Delivery Agreement 12: Improve the Health and Wellbeing of Children and Young People*. The Stationery Office, London.

Her Majesty's Treasury/Department for Education and Skills (2007a) *Aiming High for Disabled Children: Better Support for Families*. The Stationery Office, London.

Her Majesty's Treasury/Department for Education and Skills (2007b) *Aiming High for Children: Supporting Families*. The Stationery Office, London.

House of Commons Health Committee (1997) *Hospital Services for Children and Young People (Fifth Report)*. The Stationery Office, London.

Hunt, J. (1995) The paediatric oncology community nurse specialist: the influence of employment location and funders on models of practice. *Journal of Advanced Nursing*, **22**, 126–133.

Kessler, I. (2006) *Strategic Approaches to Support Workers in the NHS: A Shared Interest*. Picker Institute Europe and Oxford Said Business School, University of Oxford, Oxford.

Lenehan, C., Morrison, J. & Stanly, J. (2004) The dignity of risk. London. Council for Disabled Children – it is 2004 as cited *Managing Children with Health Care Needs: Delegation of Clinical Procedures, Training and Accountability Issues*. Council for Disabled Children, London.

Linter, S. (2003) Consultant Nurses in Children's Services. *Journal of Nursing Management*, **10**, 16–28.

Manley, K. (1997) Operationalising an advanced practice/consultant nurse role: an action research study. *Journal of Advanced Nursing*, **6**, 179–190.

Murphy, G. (2001) The technology-dependent child at home: part 2 – the need for respite. *Paediatric Nursing*, **13**, 24–27.

Myers, J. 2005 Community children's nursing services in the 21st century. *Paediatric Nursing*, **17**, 31–34.

National Health Service Executive (1996) *Child Health in the Community: A Guide to Good Practice*. The Stationery Office, London.

NHS Institute for Innovation and Improvement (2008) *Delivering Quality and Value. Focus On: Children and Young People Emergency and Urgent Care Pathway*. NHS Institute, Coventry.

North East Strategic Health Authority (2008) *Our Vision, Our Future Our North East NHS: A Strategic Vision for Transforming Health and Healthcare Services within the North East of England*. North East Strategic Health Authority, Newcastle upon Tyne.

North West Strategic Health Authority (2008) *Healthier Horizons for the North West: A New Vision for Health and Healthcare in the North West*. North West Strategic Health Authority, Manchester.

Nursing and Midwifery Council (2004) *Standards of Proficiency for Specialist Community Public Health Nurses*. Nursing and Midwifery Council, London.

Nursing and Midwifery Council (2005) *NMC Consultation on a Framework for the Standard for Post-registration Nursing*. Nursing and Midwifery Council, London.

Nursing and Midwifery Council (2006) *Standards of Proficiency for Nurse and Midwife Prescribers*. NMC, London.

Nursing and Midwifery Council (NMC) (2008) *The Code – Standards of Conduct, Performance and Ethics for Nurses and Midwives*. Nursing and Midwifery Council, London.

Proctor, S., Biott, C., Campbell, S. & Edward, S. (1998) *Preparation for the Developing Role of the Community Children's Nurse*. English National Board, London.

Rhodes, A., Lenehan, C. & Morrison, J. (1999) *Promoting Partnerships: Supporting Disabled Children Who Need Invasive Clinical Procedures*. Barnardos, Ilford.

Robinson, S. & Inyang, V. (1999) The nurse practitioners in accident and emergency departments: what do they do? *British Medical Journal*, **305**, 1466–1470.

Royal College of Nursing (1994) *Directory of Paediatric Community Nursing Services*, 11th edition. RCN, London.

Royal College of Nursing (2000) *Children's Community Nursing: Promoting Effective Team Working for Children and Their Families*. Royal College of Nursing, London.

Royal College of Nursing (2004a) *Services for Children and Young People; Preparing Nurses for Future Roles*. Royal College of Nursing, London.

Royal College of Nursing (2004b) *Adolescent Transition Care: Guidance for Nursing Staff*. Royal College of Nursing, London.

Royal College of Nursing (2007a) *The Regulation of Health Support Workers RCN Policy Unity*, Policy Briefing 11/2007.

Royal College of Nursing (2007b) *Job Profiles*. Available at: www.rcn.org.uk/support/pay_and_conditions/

agendaforchange/jobs/job_profiles (accessed 1 July 2008).

Royal College of Nursing (2008a) Directory of Community Children's Nursing Services. Available at: www.rcn.org.uk/development/communities/specialisms/community_childrens_nursing/directory (accessed 1 July 2008).

Royal College of Nursing (2008b) *Advanced Nurse Practitioners – An RCN Guide to the Advanced Nurse Practitioner Role, Competencies and Programme Accreditation*. RCN, London.

Royal College of Nursing (2008c) *Lost in Transition: Moving Young People Between Child and Adult Health Services*. RCN, London.

Royal College of Nursing (2008d) Managing Children with Health Care Needs: Delegation of Clinical Procedures, Training and Accountability Issues. Royal College of Nursing, London.

Royal College of Nursing/Paediatric Community Nurses Forum (1996) *Evidence Submitted to the House of Commons Health Select Committee*. Royal College of Nursing, London.

Royal College of Paediatricians and Child Health (2007) *Modelling the Future – A Consultation Paper on the Future of Children's Health Services*. Royal College of Paediatricians and Child Health, London.

South Central Strategic Health Authority (2008) *Towards a Healthier Future: A Ten Year Vision for Healthcare Across NHS South Central*. South Central Strategic Health Authority, Berkshire.

Taylor, J. (2000) Partnership in the hospital and community: a comparison. *Paediatric Nursing*, **12**, 28–30.

The Children Act (2004) Department of health, London.

The Report of the Public Inquiry into Children's Heart Surgery at the Bristol Royal Infirmary 1984–1995 (The Kennedy Report) (2001). The Stationery Office, London.

The Victoria Climbié Inquiry (The Lamming Report) (2003). The Stationery Office, London.

United Kingdom Central Council for Nursing, Midwifery and Health Visiting (1994) *The Future of Professional Practice – The Council's Standards for Education and Practice Following Registration*. United Kingdom Central Council for Nursing, Midwifery and Health Visiting, London.

United Kingdom Central Council for Nursing, Midwifery and Health Visiting (2001) *Standards for Specialist Education and Practice*. United Kingdom Central Council for Nursing, Midwifery and Health Visiting, London.

West Midlands Strategic Health Authority (2008) *Investing for Health. Step 2: Delivering Our Clinical Vision for a World Class Health Service*. West Midlands Strategic Health Authority, Birmingham.

Whiting, M. (1988) Community paediatric nursing in England in 1988. Unpublished MSc Thesis. University of London, London.

Whiting, M. (1995) Nursing children in the community. In: *Whaley and Wong's Children's Nursing* (eds S. Campbell & E.A. Glasper). Mosby, London.

Whiting, M. (2005) Educating community children's nurses: a historical perspective. In: *Textbook of Community Children's Nursing*, 2nd edition (eds A. Sidey & D. Widdas). Elsevier, Edinburgh.

Wilson, J. & Bunnell, T. (2007) A review of the nurse practitioner role. *Nursing Standard*, **21**, 35–40.

Wint, C. (2005) Setting the agenda for education. In: *Textbook of Community Children's Nursing*, 2nd edition (eds A. Sidey & D. Widdas). Elsevier, Edinburgh.

Woodend, K. (2006) The role of community matrons in supporting patients with long-term conditions. *Nursing Standard*, **20**, 51–54.

Yorkshire and the Humber Strategic Health Authority (2008) *Health Ambitions*. Yorkshire and the Humber Strategic Health Authority, Leeds.

Chapter 11 **School Nursing**

Maxine Jameson and Val Thurtle

Introduction

School nursing is at the forefront of policy change in the UK and school nurses are seen as pivotal to child-centred public health practice. The government aims to make 'this country the best place in the world for children to grow up' (Department for Children, Schools and Families [DCSF] 2007). School nurses have a vital role to play in leading strategic partnerships under Children's trust arrangements and to see that national priorities are translated into local delivery plans. Yet the challenge is enormous – in early 2007, Unicef published its first 'report card' of child health in affluent countries, using a multi-dimensional overview of childhood. Unicef found child health and well-being in the UK as the poorest among 21 industrialised nations (UNicef Innocenti Research Centre [UIRC] 2007).

This chapter seeks to examine some of the functions of school nursing and review its position in the twenty-first century. The government's renewed emphasis on public health, as well as the continued interest in children and young people, has provided all those who promote health in the school aged population with the potential to raise their profile. This opportunity requires all those involved in this field of employment to clarify the effectiveness of their work and make their interventions far more widely known.

Children as the future

Throughout recent history, children and young people have been recognised as a priority for investment with the aim of maximising the contribution that they can make to society and the wider economy. Their education has been

regarded as an area for investment for the workforce and the nation's security. Additionally, diseases of adulthood and emotional problems have increasingly been found to have their origins in early life (Blair *et al.* 2003; Townsend *et al.* 1992).

An alarmingly high number of young people grow up in unsupported families and in disruptive environments. Bullying of all kinds is a regular occurrence in many schools, gang membership and knife crimes regularly hit the headlines in the national press. The culture of binge drinking and the constant emphasis by the media of the desirability of early sexual activity result in a mixture of both physical and mental ill-health that often falls outwith the support systems provided by mainstream medical care. It is no exaggeration to say that the lives of young people are more blighted now by social and environmental issues than ever before. School nurses are confronted every day by these issues and are having to review the roles that they discharge in schools and the community. Professor David Hall (Debell 2006) suggests that a well-staffed and trained school nursing service could make a considerable contribution to addressing some of the problems experienced by young people in schools. However transformation in society can only be achieved by a coordinated and comprehensive inter-professional approach that is provided across all sectors.

Placing education high on the agenda

The education and promotion of positive health of children and young people has been given prominence in recent government agendas that span both health and education departments which, together with social services, are concerned with the welfare of children (DCSF 2007; Department for Education and Skills [DfES] 2003). The development of children's trusts (DfES 2003) integrating education, social services and health services, has taken this agenda further with the 2007 Children's Plan requiring a 'duty to co-operate' in which all local authorities and 'relevant partners' must have regard.

From the educational perspective, the development of the national curriculum, standard attainment tasks (SATs) (Education Reform Act 1988) and changes in the inspection system (Crown copyright 2005) have put the spotlight on the academic achievements of schools. All schools, including academies have a role to play in transacting the new agenda. Schools also have responsibility to contribute to and in turn be strongly supported by local health care trusts to ensure shared ownership of health-related outcomes for children and young people in the community. Schools must be able to help shape the planning and commissioning of services for young people and play a central role in the work of the Children's Trust Board. In return, the children's trusts must support individual schools in raising standards, and developing their vision and providing practical support to asset schools to promote the health and social well-being of all pupils.

Emphasis on public health for school health

Childhood is an important time for promoting public health as childhood disadvantage is thought to impact significantly on adult health (Graham & Power 2004). Public health approaches to working in schools aim to challenge disadvantage and social inequality, tackling health damaging behaviour, empowering children and their families and promoting good health.

Debell (2006) highlights the importance of the public health role undertaken by school nurses. Kuss *et al.* (1997) argues that public health nursing involves community empowerment, working with communities, families and individuals to achieve the prevention of illness, promotion

and protection of health and a developing concern with the environmental conditions surrounding a population. This involves working in partnership with children and young people and their families. The practical implication of this strategy requires that school nurses extend their practice beyond working with individual children and specific schools, and to work collaboratively with community groups and organisations. Primary care trusts (PCTs) strengthen opportunities to achieve this aim, enabling health care services to be delivered by a variety of health workers who are engaged with children and young people. Such an approach requires that health needs are assessed, both on an individual and group basis, and demands that steps are taken to encourage effective interprofessional and inter-agency working (DCSF 2007). Families, teachers and other professional staff should be involved in this process, but the school nurse for whom health is a priority, will often be the team leader and 'driver' in ensuring that health needs are identified and acted on.

Examples of such a coordinated approach can be seen in the Healthy Schools programme announced in the *National Healthy School Standard* (DfES 1999) and the *Healthy Living Blueprint for Schools* (DfES 2004). In particular positive action might be realised through the design and implementation of programmes that encourage physical activity, promote a positive diet and seek to reduce the incidence of smoking or stress among young people. The school nurse might also consider including risk reducing activities in health skills programmes as well as incorporating citizenship, personal and social education and health-related issues into the national curriculum. A key policy document, *Extended Schools and Health Services* (DfES/ Department of Health [DH] 2006) articulate health improvement as a joint community, family and school responsibility. The key reasons for focusing on the health of children and young people are:

(1) Health behaviours continue into adult life. This is a compelling reason for school nurses to develop targeted and specific

interventions for children and young people, such as smoking cessation groups.

(2) Immediate effect of health behaviours. Some health behaviours have a long term effect, i.e. alcohol consumption, others need to be addressed in a timely way, such as road safety.

(3) Worrying trends in morbidity and mortality. Statistics show patterns in the physical and mental health of children and young people related to suicide, sexual health and obesity.

(4) Developmental issues. Some children do not reach 'milestones' at the same time as their peers. Remedial action or support in achieving the best developmental progress for such children may be needed.

(5) Clustering of health risk. For example, those young people who smoke are also more likely to drink alcohol or use drugs. School nurses are ideally placed to be involved with public health promotion with these groups.

The focus of *Saving Lives* (DH 1999b) encouraged all schools to become 'healthy' schools, characterising the principle that 'good health and social behaviour underpin effective learning and academic achievement, which in turn promote long term health gain' (p. 46). The emphasis that *Saving Lives* placed on the promotion of the concept of community highlighted the school nurse's role within the wider neighbourhood, which also makes up a significant component of the young person's life. Public sector legislation since 1997 has promoted the concept of 'joined up thinking' through the development of partnerships between health-related agencies and government departments. Education and health staff need to liaise to develop a corporate agenda, which many are already doing at both school and strategic level. This is reflected in the document *Personal, Social and Health Education in Schools* (Ofsted 2005) and in associated links with government targets aimed at reducing heart disease and stroke, accidents, cancer, mental ill-health and child ill-health (DfES 2004).

Many would argue that school nurses have ideal opportunities to focus on public health as a primary responsibility. They have easy access to apply health promoting strategies to groups of school children, but also have a major role to play in working with individual children with specific health needs or disabilities. *School Nursing Within the Public Health Agenda* (DeBell & Jackson 2000), a shared document published by the three key professional organisations, outlined school nurses' responsibilities in promoting healthy lifestyles and healthy schools. The document also drew attention to school nurses' roles in promoting health in childhood and adolescence and managing chronic and complex health care needs in children and young people. The school nurse, as a specialist community public health nurse has multiple roles in seeking out health needs (individual and collective), promoting the health of children and young people, implementing health promoting strategies in school and in the community, encouraging activities that facilitate health as well as being a clinician.

Establishing the number of school nurses

We are frequently told that there are between 2500 and 3000 school nurses in the UK but no national registers exist to confirm this. Clarke et al. (2000) talked of 200 nurses providing a service to 2000 schools with around 490,000 school children in Wales, yet not a single school nurse trained in Wales between 1995 and 2000.

In 2005, the Royal College of Nursing (RCN) (Ball & Pike 2005) reported that 2211 of its members had 'school nurse' in their title, but 79% of those who responded to their survey worked part time and term time only, reducing significantly the conversion rate to whole time equivalents. The Nursing and Midwifery Council (NMC) register of Specialist Community Public Health Nurses (SCPHN) indicated there are 3009 registrants annotated as school nurses (NMC 2007), but not all of these will be actively practising school nurses. This number falls short of the actual number of 'school nurses' required to support the more than 11 million children of school age as identified in the 2001 census (National Statistics 2004).

Anecdotal reporting indicates big differences in the number of children or schools covered by school nurses. This came to the fore in the 2006 RCN Conference (attended by the Secretary of State for Health), when a school nurse from Cornwall announced that she was responsible for 28 schools and a further education college (BBC 2006). Numbers alone do not indicate the demands of the school age caseload, which are also influenced by the type of schools that make up the school nurse's workload, the socio-economic status of the area and the availability of other health workers.

Cotton *et al.* (2000) concluded that the allocation of resources between districts was not equitable and argued that the use of school nurse time was out of step with current evidence of need and effectiveness. In subsequent years, changes have occurred but in some areas improvements have been spasmodic, leaving primary care to focus largely on services centred on general practice. Bagnall & Dilloway (1996a) argued that increasing liaison with general practices was a way forward for the school health service. Work by Baptiste & Drennan (1999) in an inner city area indicated that primary care professionals were not fully aware of the role of the school nurse. General practitioners (GPs) in particular saw them concerned with problem-solving rather than health promotion. GPs and practice nurses saw little need for collaboration with school nurses and while they wished to increase their awareness of the school nursing service they felt the onus was on the school nurses to liaise with them. Richardson-Todd (2002) found, for example that GPs in Suffolk had a poor understanding of the school nurse's role and did not know how to contact the service. In many areas it would seem that school health and general practice services are running in parallel, with limited partnership working and there is limited evidence to suggest that practice-based commissioning will improve the situation (DH 2004a, 2008).

In the 1990s, school nurses very often practised outwith mainstream primary care services and some practitioners regarded them to have a lower status in the nursing hierarchy. For many their role was invisible and as such they were vulnerable as efficiency savings were sought (Cowley & Houston 1999; Community Practitioners' and Health Visitors' Association [CPHVA] 1998a). However school nurses themselves believed fervently in their role contribution and found the job to be a worthwhile and satisfying role (Thurtle 1996). Their age profile, in common with other nurses, was tilted, with a significant proportion approaching retirement age and in comparison with health visitors and district nurses were often paid at a lower grade than health visitors and district nurses. Formal educational training was the missing ingredient, having been at that time at a lower level in terms of length and academic value compared with health visitors and district nurses. These factors combined to encourage school nurses, and others with whom they worked, to see themselves as less valued than other community nurses. The advent of the SCPHN register (NMC 2004) finally addressed this perceptual, imbalance and placed school nurses on an equal level to their peers (Thurtle, Shifting identities. How specialist community public health nurses articulate their identity. Work in progress, 2009).

Education and training

In 1994 the United Kingdom Central Council for Nursing, Midwifery and Health Visiting (UKCC 1994) set a new standard for school nurse education and placed the profession within the context of a nurse specialist practice award at degree level. This change moved the status of this professional group forward, though limited provision was made in some higher education institutions, resulting in restricted access for some practitioners (DeBell 2000). DeBell & Tomkins (2006) found that some school nurses felt ill-prepared to respond to the range of needs they encountered. In particular some felt insufficiently trained to undertake essential counselling skills for 'children in need'.

The *Standards of Proficiency for Specialist Community Public Health Nurses* (NMC 2004) and

ensuing revalidated university education programmes has again emphasised the importance
of school nurse education, but the reduction in
sponsorship and secondment of school nurses
by their employers to undertake educational
preparation has meant that the number of school
nurses trained at this level has not risen as much
as might have been hoped for, despite the government aspiration that a trained school nurse
should be visible in every secondary school
(DfES 2004). However, while things may not be
perfect, studying alongside other public health
nurses has broadened school nurses' horizons
and has equipped them to undertake roles of
team leadership, providing them with the confidence to progress to senior management positions. The future of school nursing and public
health promotion among school aged children
depends on the proportion of leaders who are
able to influence the development of this specialist branch of nursing.

The future

School nursing is elusive in definition, since
practitioners work in a variety of settings and
within the context of a variety of contractual
obligations. School nursing also continues to
remain a service without legislative requirement
and without regulatory training, yet school
nursing is the only National Health Service
(NHS) professional group whose remit is to
entirely focus on the health needs of school age
children. *The Children's Plan* (DCFS 2007) set out
the aim of making the UK the best place in the
world for children to grow up, placing responsibility on local authorities to assume the vital
role of leading strategic partnerships under
children's trust (2007) arrangements (or as integral provider functions within local PCTs where
dedicated children's trusts do not exist). The
key deliverables arising from these collaborative
partnerships are translated into local PCT delivery plans. School nurses are well placed to work
with schools and the local PCT, working collaboratively between health education and the local
authority social services departments, sharing
in the planning and delivery of services. School
nurses should be at the heart of children's

trust arrangements, as both partners and drivers of frontline delivery, promoting well-being
through their full engagement with the work
of multi-agency partners. The NHS operating
framework 2008–09 (DCFS 2008) identifies child
health as a priority, but delivery of this agenda
requires strong multi-agency cooperation. An
important factor for delivering best outcomes
for children is the development and provision of
a world-class workforce, in which school nurses
are regarded as a vitally important component.
To achieve this level of exposure and prominence school nurses will need to share their
knowledge and skills with other community
leaders and managers, and raise the profile and
promote professional development opportunities for all local school nurses, irrespective of
their location or contractual status.

The public health role of the in school nurse

The NMC has defined the standards of proficiency to become a specialist community public
health nurse (SCPHN). These are underpinned
by ten public health principles, which are
grouped into four domains (NMC 2004):

- Search for health needs
- Stimulation of awareness of health needs
- Influence on policy affecting health
- Facilitation of health enhancing activities

These four domains were originally identified
as the principles of health visiting (Council for
the Education and Training of Health Visitors
[CETHV] 1977) and were adapted to form the
principles of school nursing (CPHVA). They
provide a useful framework to consider the
work of school nurses.

Search for health needs
Screening children's hearing, vision, height
and weight, is, in part, a key component of the
search for health needs. The Hall report (Hall &
Elliman 2003) led to a critical review of the
effectiveness of universal screening of school
children. Taking a population approach necessitates the identification of local priorities

and the specific needs of a school community to inform the design and implementation of delivery plans led by local needs. Health needs assessment (discussed elsewhere in this volume) should be central to the work of school health. Bagnall & Dilloway (1996b) comment that health need profiles provide a comprehensive record of the health and social needs of a school population and can reveal clear differences between schools, even if they are located in similar areas. Such data can inform local commissioning processes and can be used to negotiate service-led agreements, and inform school and wider policy developments. Profiling helps define where most effort should be focused, in accordance with national and local priorities and targets identified by PCTs. In turn, resultant data may be used to identify new concerns and assist in evaluating and resetting service goals. Establishing local priorities has reduced routine screening, and indicated the need to focus on health promotion and illness prevention. There is much discussion about profiling, but in some areas it is little more than an annual paper exercise that makes little impact on practice. Staff need to accept its relevance and utilise the views of service users, children and young people to form the basis for the design and implementation of local policies and delivery plans.

Stimulation of awareness of health needs
Graham *et al.* (2002) considered the improvements gained by teenagers' knowledge of emergency contraception through a teacher-led intervention. Whilst the resultant teaching sessions led to an improvement in young people knowledge about emergency contraception, it did not lead to a change in the pupils' sexual activity or actual use of emergency contraception. No doubt the same would hold true in terms of healthy eating, taking more exercise and even valuing self and each other. Raising awareness of health needs requires collaboration with individuals, schools and the wider community. This may involve working with an individual, for example to encourage them to participate in physical activity, or with school staff, parents and governors to improve facilities

for the provision of fresh drinking water, or with the local community to work towards the provision of safer roads and more play spaces. In so doing the school nurse should be actively influencing policies affecting health in the local school and its local external environment.

Current thinking on user empowerment and partnership supports the idea that the 'community' should play a central role in deciding upon how best to meet its own health needs. School nurses may be catalysts in this process, acting as coordinators or as participatory members of local action groups.

Influence on policies affecting health
School nursing teams should interact with teaching staff and their governing bodies to ensure that workable and realistic policies on personal and social education, nutrition and physical activity are designed and implemented. In so doing the promotion of health and lifestyle should be included in everyday activities transacted by the school. For examples the provision of special events, including health weeks, influencing what is included in a packed lunch, what is sold in the tuck shop and the condition of ablution areas.

Multi-agency working is seen to be most effective medium through which to change (DCFS 2008) knowledge, attitudes and risk behaviours at school and in the neighbouring community. It is also important for school nurses to identify and participate in addressing wider determinants of health such as poverty, poor educational attainment, social exclusion, poor housing and environmental factors (DH 1999a, 2004b, Social Exclusion Unit [SEU] 1999). Advocating for individuals and groups of children will underpin much of school nurses' activities. Providing a representative role for parents and young people on issues such as after school activities, play space and the provision of sexual health facilities is another example of their role.

Facilitation of health-enhancing activities
Schools remain an important setting within which to offer efficient and effective way support and guidance children and through

them, their families and the wider community (Department for Education and Employment [DfEE] 1999; European Network of Health Promoting Schools 2001, World Health Organization [WHO] 2001). Inequalities often start in childhood but all stages of childhood offer scope for improving health and preventing health risk behaviour among children, adolescents and young adults. Hence a healthy school setting can help children and adolescents attain their full educational and health potential now and as investment for the future.

The school nurse also has a clinical and therapeutic role and function. For example, as traditional childhood diseases diminish, new health problems and challenges have emerged which have a negative effect on child and adolescent development. These include an increase in chronic health conditions such as asthma, allergies, diabetes. Drug and alcohol misuse, teenage pregnancies and sexually transmitted diseases, suicides, accidents, injuries or deaths from child abuse are also indicative trends that require intervention from these practitioners. While the intensity of school health promotion (in its widest sense) varies from one school to another and between PCT areas, school nurses have a clear role to ensure that they are contributing actively to the development of local healthy schools (DH 2002). For example, the increased consumption of fruit and vegetables has been advocated as a preventive strategy (DH 2000a). Around two-thirds of the UK population is overweight (DfES 2004) and if the present pattern is not curbed the greatest cause of early death for the present generation of children will be obesity (House of Commons Health Committee 2004). Not surprisingly the children's national service framework (NSF) (DH 2003) linked childhood obesity with the need to promote a healthy diet and increase physical activity. School nurses promote healthy eating through direct teaching via the Personal Social and Health Education curriculum, by engaging with school health days and working in partnership with parents to discuss positively regarded food options, including provision of healthy lunch boxes (DH 1999c). School nurses therefore work closely within their schools to design and implement school policies that present informed messages about healthy eating. Encouraging schools to provide healthy options in vending machines, tuck shops and school meals is a component of this strategy.

Children and young people's sedentary lifestyle is another issue of concern to school nurses. The National Diet and Nutrition Survey (DH 2000b) found that 40% of boys and 60% of girls surveyed in Britain were failing to exercise adequately. While hopefully there has been an improvement in these statistics since 2001, it is not likely to be significant. Encouraging physical activity is an important focus for health promotion, helping to reduce excessive weight gain and chronic illnesses, and improving psychological well-being. School nurses working alongside community health project coordinators are becoming increasingly involved in the assessment and referral of children and young people who are overweight and are encouraging them eat healthily and to exercise regularly.

Health promotion activities may be discharged in different ways, and include provision of 'opportunistic drop in sessions' or young persons open access clinics. The latter have been implemented in many schools and have received positive evaluation (Osborne 2000). The school nursing service provides opportunities to maintain good health, to identify health problems, to offer appropriate advice or make referrals to specialist health and social care services and more generally to promote the health of younger people, their parents and at times, their teaching staff colleagues.

Another opportunity for school nurses to facilitate their health-enhancing role exists within the Extended Schools Initiative (DfES 2002a). The Education Act 2002 provided the legislative framework to enable schools to extend their facilities to pupils and the local community outside normal school operating hours. Examples of extra-mural services include parenting groups, performing arts and social club provision. School nurses can be also advise families on how to set up a range of health promotion and public health services, for example, healthy eating groups, accident prevention campaigns, smoking cessation groups, breakfast clubs, sexual health and contraception clinics, or through the organisation of a farmers' market in partnership with local businesses. The scope for health enhancing activities is vast, with the school nurse linking into national and local campaigns to promote the health of all children and young people. This is explored further in *Promoting the Health of School Age Children* (Thurtle & Wright 2008).

The emphasis on health-enhancing activities is not at the expense of working with those with specific health issues. Technology has led to more children who have complex health needs surviving through childhood and into adulthood (Hall & Elliman 2003). *Excellence in Schools* (DfEE 1997), and the Special Educational Needs and Disability Act 2001, set out rights for inclusion of children in mainstream education. If parents want a place for their child, the utmost should be done to facilitate this. This is fully supported in the *Special Educational Needs Code of Practice* (DfES 2002b). Around 1.45 million children were categorised as having some sort of special educational need (SEN) in England in 2005 – 18% of all pupils, of these around 242 500 pupils had statements of SEN; 2.9% of all pupils and the remaining 1.2 million pupils, were categorised as having SEN but did not were not in possession of a supporting statement, representing 15% of all school age pupils (House of Commons 2006). Not all children with special educational needs have a health problem and not all those with a diagnosed health difficulty require support with their education, but there is a strong overlap in the support needs required by the two groups. With the reduction of places in special schools and the government's commitment to the concept of inclusion, there are an increasing number of children with complex health and social needs attending mainstream schools.

The range of chronic complex needs varies; the most prevalent conditions include epilepsy, anaphylaxis, asthma, diabetes, sickle cell disease, hyperkinetic disorders, coordination difficulties, speech and language problems, enuresis, obesity, soiling and foot deformity (Meltzer *et al.* 2000). The majority of children presenting with these conditions cope well, gaining full education attainment and enriching the experience of their peers. The NSF for children states that:

'Children and young people who are disabled or who have complex health needs should receive co-ordinated, high quality child and family centred services which are based on assessed needs, which promote social inclusion and where possible enable them and their families to live ordinary lives as close to home as possible'.

(DH/DfES 2004, p. 7)

On many occasions support workers may attend to the day-to-day health care needs of these children but school nurses often assume either a direct care or leadership role in developing a care plan in partnership with parents, teachers, nurse specialists, support workers and the child. This ensures care is coordinated, information is shared between team members and agencies, medication or equipment is available and intimate or invasive treatments can be given effectively if necessary. Children needing invasive treatment remain in the minority but irrespective of the level of presenting need, school nurses always aim to promote the best outcomes for all children to afford them the opportunity to achieve their personal potential (DfES 2001a, 2002a).

Leadership and organisation

Leadership has been highlighted as important in the NHS (NHS III 2006) and particularly in school nursing as highlighted by DeBell (2000). As all health staff work in a changing context there is an additional need for leaders to work as change agents. There has been much discussion about leadership styles and transformational management as described by Burns (1978). Rosener (1990) claims that transformational leadership is essentially a woman leader's style. As school nursing remains predominately female, the use of charismatic leadership styles and well-developed interpersonal skills are very appropriate. In practical terms, being a leader in school health means building alliances within and outwith the team and ensuring that practice is rooted in research-based evidence. Creativity in outlook is also a key feature requiring readiness to take risks and, being prepared to advise others what has been achieved by disseminating best practice through the medium of publications, websites and by presenting at meetings and conferences.

Thinking creatively about the role of the school nursing service involves a division of labour. Different ways of working should be accompanied by a genuine skill mix, which will vary depending upon the needs of the local population. School nurses with different interests and expertise, perhaps in mental health, sexual health, behavioural or learning difficulties could, for example make up a local school health team. Qualified staff should work with those support staff who possess skills and interests in promoting health with children and young people. Leadership of such teams will raise the status of school nursing and provide the individuals involved with renewed personal and professional confidence. In so doing, the school nursing profession will be encouraged to grow to include practitioners with a variety of nursing and non-nursing skills and abilities, which in turn will promote richness and diversity.

Working in different ways will require school nurses to work in a variety of settings, other than educational establishments. By meeting with younger people in settings such as children's clubs and youth centres, young people may demonstrate personal motivation and readiness to assume responsibility for their own health care needs While educational settings are likely to remain the dominant area of practice, opportunities also exist for school nurses to undertake evening work and to engage in non-term-time public health promotional activity. This has been evidently effective in some areas (Madge & Franklin 2003).

Mental health – a specific issue

Promoting and maintaining positive mental health among the school age population is of crucial significance as it contributes to maintaining a good level of personal and social functioning, and influences future health behaviour. The Mental Health Foundation states that good mental health is characterised by a person's ability to learn; express and manage a range of positive and negative emotions; to form and maintain good relationships with others and to cope with, and manage, change and uncertainty. Having low self-esteem and being unfulfilled and stressed can result in mental distress, which is also a risk factor for the emergence of later physical health problems. This has a consequent impact on self-esteem, as well as on the selection of health choices, such as engaging in physical activity, healthy nutritional intake, valuing one's own image, substance misuse and avoiding risky sexual behaviour (Ramrakha *et al.* 2000).

Political commitment to place mental health at the forefront of health policy was presented in *The NHS Plan* (DH 2000c) and reiterated in later government policy, particularly in the *National Service Framework for Children, Young People and Their Families* (DH/DfES 2004). Standard 9 of the framework focuses specifically on mental health services and states that:

'All children and young people, from birth to their eighteenth birthday, who have mental health problems and disorders have access to timely, integrated, high quality, multi-disciplinary mental health services to ensure effective assessment, treatment and support, for them and their families'.

(DH/DfES 2004).

Young Minds, a children's mental health charity, cites challenging statistics to advise that one in ten children and young people aged between 5 and 16 have a diagnosable mental health disorder, which is around three in every school class (Office for National Statistics [ONS] 2004a). Between one in 12 and one in 15 children and young people deliberately self-harm (Mental Health Foundation 2006) and nearly 80 000 children and young people suffer from severe depression (ONS 2004a), with many of them presenting with the condition prior to the age of 10. Meltzer *et al.* (2003) indicate that many of these children are some of the most vulnerable young people in society, many of whom may be 'looked after' by local authorities as well as those who are homeless and young offenders (SEU 2004).

Mental illness has been identified as a barrier to learning, and strategies to promote mental health need to commence in early childhood (DfES 2001b). All regions are supported by children and adolescent mental health services (CAMHS). *Every Child Matters* (DfES 2003) and other government documents have advocated an expansion of this service. CAMHS frequently work with a four-tier model of service approach. First level staff, which would include school nurses, identify health problems, offer advice and treatment in less severe cases and promote good mental health. Clear routes need to be available for school nurses and others to refer young people to more specialised help in the other tiers and clinical supervision needs to be available for the practitioner. Many school nurses actually work at tier 2, where they might train others who (who might be within tier 1), work with those with more complex needs which require more specialist support, often when families are unwilling to use more specialist services. Tier 3 involves a specialist service for more severe, complex and persistent disorders and tier 4 relates specifically to tertiary-level services, such as day-units and highly specialised outpatient teams and inpatient units for older children and adolescents.

School nurses recognise that positive mental health is essential for academic success and that services that support prevention, early identification and treatment of mental illness are necessary to support pupils' achievement (DeBell & Jackson 2000). Practitioners provide mental health promotion activities within the school community, aiming to develop self-esteem, positive coping skills and stress management skills among young people. The profile of mental health promotion could be further raised through the national healthy schools standards. Mental health services should be comprehensive and coordinated effectively, providing easy access to their local populations, thus reducing the incidence of mental health problems among school children (DfES 2001b). School nurses are in a position to recognise the potential impact mental ill-health can have on pupils' development and can act as strong advocates for the promotion of positive child mental health.

School nurses may also provide 'drop in' sessions for students to access school nursing advice and host parent support groups to parents with school age children and conduct selective reception health interviews with new pupil entrants and parents, respond to individual requests for support via negotiated referral systems. They may also work with other professionals and agencies to devise and implement anti-bullying strategies, facilitate friendship clubs and young person's clinics and respond to issues of emotional well-being.

School nurses may act as the liaison point between pupils and local adolescent mental health services, the family and school staff. They may also enhance the effectiveness of their interventions by joining forces with other health professionals to promote a 'total' school-wide approach to mental health surveillance. School nurses also work with educational psychologists, clinical psychologists, educational social workers, special educational needs coordinators, counsellors, social workers, learning mentors and other support staff to plan and implement strategies to respond to mental health challenges.

The challenges for school nurses and other health professionals contributing to mental health promotion within the school setting are to eliminate stigma and discrimination, to reduce fragmentation of services and work towards achieving a comprehensive wider community model that includes partnership, prevention, early identification and intervention services.

The need for marketing

Adopting a marketing perspective to promote the role of the school nurse is a strategy for survival (Edwards 1992). Polnay (1998), ten years ago, noted there had been a 'conspicuous lack of marketing surrounding school health, with many people, parents, children, teachers, health purchasers and providers being devoid of informed knowledge about the service' (p. 98).

The Chief Nursing Officer's review on choosing health (DH 2004b) highlighted the need to increase the size of the school nursing workforce and recommended that every cluster or group of primary schools and their related secondary school should have a full time, whole year, qualified school nurse responding to the needs of local populations. Alongside this promotional policy, changes in health education in schools have meant that the role of the school nurse, in both primary and secondary schools, has become more wide ranging and far better known. School nurses were further advertised within the document *Looking for a School Nurse?* (DfES/DH 2006a), aimed at head teachers, which set out the advantages and some of the practical considerations of having a school nurse either onsite, or assigned to a school or cluster of schools. Teachers are perhaps school nurses' closest allies and many appreciate the importance of establishing health promoting partnership strategies. With local trusts seeking to match services to their local communities, school nurses need to be working with pupils and their parents in locally based practice groupings.

Conclusion

The past ten years have witnessed public health becoming established as a core component of school nursing. This is evidenced further in the *School Nurse: Practice Development Resource Pack* (DfES/DH 2006b) which emphasises the importance of inter-professional work at its most demanding.

With the development of children's trusts and the provision of statutory guidance on inter-agency working, and cooperation to improve the well-being of children and young people, school nurses need to work hard to build links with education and social care teams. In so doing their aim must be to develop their role to bridge agencies and to become expert clinicians, leaders and managers in the new public health arena. School nurses are ideally placed to help make the UK the best place for children and young people to grow up. If they are to achieve this aim they must continue to raise

their profiles within PCTs, local authorities and children's trusts and demonstrate the effectiveness of their contribution to the transaction of the government's reformed health care agenda.

References

Bagnall, P. & Dilloway, M. (1996a) *In Search of a Blueprint: A Survey of School Health Services.* Department of Health and Queen's Nursing Institute, London.

Bagnall, P. & Dilloway, M. (1996b) *In a Different Light: School Nurses and Their Role in Meeting the Health Needs of School Age Children.* Department of Health and Queen's Nursing Institute, London.

Ball, J. & Pike, G. (2005) *School Nurses Results From a Census Survey of RCN School Nurses in 2005.* Royal College of Nursing, London.

Baptiste, L. & Drennan, V. (1999) Communication between school nurses and primary care teams. *British Journal of Community Nursing,* **4**, 13–18.

BBC (2006) Anger at school nurse's workload. Available at http://news.bbc.co.uk/1/hi/england/cornwall/6091524.stm (accessed 25 May 2008).

Blair, M., Stewart-Brown, S., Waterson, T. & Crowther, R. (2003) *Child Public Health.* Oxford University Press, Oxford.

Burns, J. (1978) *Leadership.* Harper and Row, New York.

Clark, J., Buttegeig, M., Bodycombe-James, M., Eaton, N., Kelly, A., Merrell, J., Palmer-Thomas, J., Parke, S. & Symonds, A. (2000) *A Review of Health Visiting and School Services in Wales.* University of Wales, Swansea.

Community Practitioners' and Health Visitors' Association (1998a) *The Cambridge Experiment.* Community Practitioners' and Health Visitors' Association, London.

Community Practitioners' and Health Visitors' Association (1998b) *The Principles of School Nursing: Foundations for Good Practice.* Community Practitioners' and Health Visitors' Association, London.

Cotton, L., Brazier, J., Hall, D., Lindsay, G., Marsh, P., Polnay, L. & Williams, T. (2000) School nursing: costs and potential benefits. *Journal of Advanced Nursing,* **31**, 1063–1071.

Council for the Education and Training of Health Visitors (1977) *An Investigation into the Principles of Health Visiting.* Council for the Education and Training of Health Visitors, London.

Cowley, S. & Houston, A. (1999) *Health Visiting and School Nursing: The Croydon Story.* King's College/Croydon Community Health Council, London.

Crown copyright (2005) *Statutory Instrument 2005* (no. 2038). The Education (School Inspection) (England). Available at www.opsi.gov.uk/si/si2005/20052038.htm (accessed 21 May 2008).

DeBell, D. (2000) Translating school nursing research into practice. An assessment of change in the management and delivery of school nursing. Report to the Department of Health.

DeBell, D. & Jackson, P. (2000) School nursing within the public health agenda: a strategy for practice. CPHVA/Queen's Institute/RCN, London.

Debell, D. & Tomkins, A.S. (2006) Discovering the future of school nursing. The evidence base. Community Practitioners' and Health Visitors' Association, London.

Department for Children, Schools and Families (2007) *The Children's Plan: Building Brighter Futures*. The Stationery Office, London.

Department for Children, Schools and Families (2008) *Children's Trusts Statutory Guidance on Interagency Cooperation to Improve Well-Being of Children, Young People and their Families*. The Stationery Office, London.

Department for Education and Employment (1997) *Excellence in Schools*. Department for Education and Employment, Nottingham.

Department for Education and Employment (1999) *National Healthy School Standards*. Department for Education and Employment, Nottingham.

Department for Education and Skills (2001a) *The Special Educational Needs and Disability Act*. Available at www.dfes.gov.uk (accessed 28 November 2008).

Department for Education and Skills (2001b) *Guidance: Promoting Children's Mental Health within Early Years and School Settings*. Department for Education and Employment 0121/200, Nottingham.

Department for Education and Skills (2002a) *Extended Schools: Providing Opportunities and Services for all*. Department for Education and Skills, Nottingham.

Department for Education and Skills (2002b) *Special Educational Needs Codes of Practice*. Department for Education and Skills, Nottingham.

Department for Education and Skills (2003) *Every Child Matters*. Department for Education and Skills, Nottingham.

Department for Education and Skills (2004) *Health Living Blueprint for Schools*. DfES, Nottingham.

Department for Education and Skills/Department of Health (2006a) *Looking for a School Nurse?* DfES, Nottingham.

Department for Education and Skills/Department of Health (2006b) *School Nurse: Practice Development Resource Pack*. The Stationery Office, London.

Department of Health (1999a) *Making a Difference: Strengthening the Nursing, Midwifery and Health Visiting Contribution to Health and Health Care*. Department of Health, London.

Department of Health (1999b) *Saving Lives: Our Healthier Nation*. Department of Health, London.

Department of Health (1999c) *The School Fruit Scheme. Healthy Schools*. London.

Department of Health (2000a) *National Service Framework for Coronary Heart Disease: Modern Standards and Service Models*. Department of Health, London.

Department of Health (2000b) *National Diet and Nutrition Survey: Young People Aged 4–18 years*. Volume 1: Report of the Diet and Nutrition Survey. Department of Health, London.

Department of Health (2000c) *The NHS Plan: A Plan for Investment. A Plan for Reform*. The Stationery Office, London.

Department of Health (2002) *Extended Schools: Providing Opportunities and Services for All*. Department for Education and Skills, Nottingham.

Department of Health (2003) *Getting the Right Start: The National Services Framework for Children, Young People and Maternity Services – Emerging Findings*. Department of Health, London.

Department of Health (2004a) *Practice Based Commissioning: Promoting Clinical Engagement*. Department of Health, London.

Department of Health (2004b) *Chief Nursing Officer's Bulletin*. Available at: www.dh.gov.uk/en/Publicationsandstatistics/Bulletins/Chiefnursingofficerbulletin/Browsable/DH_4098626 (accessed 21 May 2008).

Department of Health (2008) *What is Practice Based Commissioning?* Available at: www.dh.gov.uk/en/Managingyourorganisation/Commissioning/Practice-basedcommissioning/DH_4138698 (accessed 25 May 2008).

Department of Health/Department for Education and Skills (2004) *National Service Framework for Children, Young People and Maternity Services: Disabled Children and Young People and those with Complex Health Needs*. Department of Health, London.

Education Reform Act (1988) Available at: www.opsi.gov.uk/acts/acts1988/ukpga_19880040_en_1 (accessed 21 May 2008).

Edwards, J. (1992) Market in practice. *Health Visitor*, **65**, 352–353.

European Network of Health Promoting Schools (2001). World Health Organization, Geneva.

Graham, A., Moor, L., Sharpe, D. & Diamond, I. (2002) Improving teenagers' knowledge of emergency contraception: cluster randomised controlled trial of a teacher led intervention. *British Medical Journal*, **324**, 1179–1185.

Graham, H. & Power, C. (2004) Effects of childhood socioeconomic circumstances on persistent smoking. *American Journal of Public Health*, **94**, 279–285.

Hall, D.M.B. & Elliman, D. (2003) *Health for All Children*, 4th edition. Oxford University Press, Oxford.

House of Commons (2004) *Health Committee Obesity*. The Stationery Office, London. Available at www.parliament.the-stationery-office.co.uk/pa/cm200304/cmselect/cmhealth/23/23.pdf (accessed xxx).

House of Commons (2006) *Education and Skills – Third Report*. Available at www.publications.parliament.uk/pa/cm200506/cmselect/cmeduski/478/47802.htm (accessed 21 May 2008).

Kuss, T., Proulx-Girouard, L., Lovitt, S., Katz, C.B. & Kennelly, P. (1997) A public health nursing model. *Public Health Nursing*, **14**, 81–91.

Madge, N. & Franklin, A. (2003) *Change, Challenge and School Nursing*. National Children's Bureau, London.

Meltzer, H., Gatward, R., Goodman, R. & Ford, T. (2000) *Mental Health of Children and Adolescents in Britain*. A survey carried out in 1999 by the social survey division of the ONS. The Stationery Office, London.

Meltzer, H., Gatward, R., & Corbin, T. (2003) *The Mental Health of Young People Looked After by Local Authorities in England*. The Stationery Office, London.

Mental Health Foundation (2006) *Truth Hurts: Report of the National Inquiry into Self-Harm Among Young People*. Mental Health Foundation, London.

NHS Institute for Innovation and Improvement (2006) *NHS Leadership Qualities Framework*. Available at: www.NHSLeadershipQualities.nhs.uk (accessed 26 May 2008).

National Statistics (2004) *Child Population*. Available at www.statistics.gov.uk/children/ (accessed 25 May 2008).

Nursing and Midwifery Council (2004) *Standards of Proficiency for Specialist Community Public Health Nurses*. Nursing and Midwifery Council, London.

Nursing and Midwifery Council (2007) *Statistical Analysis of the Register 1 April 2006 to 31 March 2007*. Nursing and Midwifery Council, London.

Office for National Statistics (2004a) *The Health of Young People*. Available at www.statistics.gov.uk/.children (accessed xxx).

Ofsted (2005) *Personal, Social and Health Education in Secondary Schools*. Ofsted, London.

Osborne, N. (2000) Children's voices: evaluation of school drop-in health clinic. *Community Practitioner*, **73**, 516–518.

Polnay, L. (1998) A school health service for children: a commentary. *Children and Society*, **12**, 98–100.

Ramrakha, S., Caspi, A., Dickinson, N., Moffit, T.E. & Paul, C. (2000) Psychiatric disorders and risky sex in young adulthood: a cross sectional study in a birth cohort. *British Medical Journal*, **321**, 263–266.

Richardson-Todd, B. (2002) GPs: Do they know what school nurses do? *Primary Health Care*, **12**, 38–41.

Rosener, J. (1990) Ways women lead. *Harvard Business Review*, **Nov–Dec**, 119–125.

Royal College of Nursing (2005) *Analysis of the Nursing Workforce*. Royal College of Nursing, London.

Social Exclusion Unit (1999) *Teenage Pregnancy*. Social Exclusion Unit, London.

Social Exclusion Unit Report (2004) *Mental Health and Social Exclusion*. Office of the Deputy Prime Minister, Yorkshire.

Thurtle, V. (1996) Why nurses choose to enter school nursing. *Health Visitor*, **69**, 231–233.

Thurtle, V. & Wright, J. (2008) *Promoting the Health of School Age Children*. Quay Books, London.

Townsend, P., Davidson, N. & Whitehead, W. (1992) *Inequalities in Health*. Penguin, London.

United Kingdom Central Council for Nursing, Midwifery and Health Visiting (1994) *The Future of Professional Practice, The Council's Standards for Education and Practice Following Registration*. United Kingdom Central Council for Nursing, Midwifery and Health Visiting, London.

UNicef Innocenti Research Centre (2007) *Child Poverty in Perspective: An Overview of Child Well-Being in Rich Countries*. Innocenti Research Centre, Florence.

World Health Organization (2001) The World Health Report. Available at: www.who.int/whr2001/2001/archives/1998/exsum98e.htm (accessed xxx).

Young Minds. Available at: www.youngminds.org.uk/ym-newsroom/media-resources/fast-facts/?searchterm=statistics (accessed 26 May 2008).

Chapter 12 **Occupational Health Nursing**

Anne Harriss

Introduction

Occupational health nurses (OHNs) provide specialised nursing care in a specific public health care setting – the workplace. The National Health Service (NHS) does provide occupational health for its staff but many OHNs practise in settings outside the NHS. The International Labour Organisation (ILO) and the World Health Organization (WHO) are two international institutions that regularly comment on both health and health and safety at work. They have defined the aims and objectives of an occupational health (OH) service. One of the ILO's recommendations, Recommendation 112, highlights that the aim of an OH service is to protect workers against health hazards arising out of their work, or their working environment, and adapting work processes so that optimum physical and mental health of the worker can be achieved (ILO 1959). The WHO (1973) takes a similar stance and also comments on the identification and control of all 'chemical, physical, mechanical, biological and psychosocial agents that are known to be or expected to be very hazardous'.

Occupational health nurses as specialist practitioners

This chapter provides an overview of the role of the OHN as a specialist practitioner. In order to give the reader an understanding of contemporary OH nursing practice, a historical perspective which outlines the influencing factors and domains of OHN practice is explored. Lewis & Thornbory (2006) comment that 'Occupational health nurses are probably the biggest group of occupational health professional in the UK' (p. 81). OHNs practise within a public health

framework and have the potential to make a significant contribution to the health of the working population. As Marmot (2005) highlights, inequalities in health arise as a result of the complex interplay between employment, socioeconomic status, housing and education. It is not an easy task for nurses who practise in other settings to be able to influence these factors but proactive OHNs do have the opportunity to engage with a workforce that may consist of a 'crunchy social mix' of people of differing ages, cultures, ethnicity and social backgrounds. This engagement can lead to health improvements as not only are OHNs well placed to offer impartial general health advice to employees they can also assist employers prevent, or at least reduce, the incidence of workplace accidents and work-related ill-health, thus meeting the aims proposed by the ILO and WHO.

Occupational health nursing is a distinct specialty within the family of public health nursing. OH nursing practice is multi-faceted; it involves the utilisation of a unique blend of specialised nursing skills including:

- Undertaking health needs assessments for their specific client group – people at work
- Devising strategies which reduce work-related ill-health and accidental injury
- Working collaboratively with other practitioners and management to identify and address health needs

A specialist OHN as a nurse who holds a role-preparation qualification in occupational health nursing conferring registration with the Nursing and Midwifery Council (NMC) as a Specialist Community Public Health Nurse (SCPHN). The scope of practice and competencies of an

OHN is further described in the Royal College of Nursing document *Competencies: an Integrated Career and Competency Framework for Occupational Health Nursing* (Royal College of Nursing 2005). This document highlights the range of skills of a competent OHN; these include those of risk assessment, health surveillance and health promotion and health protection. It underlines the importance of the role of the OHN in attendance management and the development of strategies that facilitate a successful return to work following an accident or serious illness.

The NMC sets, and the RCN describes, standards for practice. Unfortunately, there is currently no mandatory requirement for nurses employed to provide care in the workplace to hold a specialist qualification in OH nursing. Many employers do not provide an OH service for their staff. Of those that do, many do not require the nurses they employ to hold a qualification in the specialty. Indeed there is now a move to employ technicians to support specialist OHNs. Such technicians undertake a task-driven role. Universities are now offering programmes that prepare technicians for this role, which is dependent on the needs of the employing organisation. It commonly includes participation in statutory health surveillance programmes. Such programmes may incorporate audiometry for workers who are exposed to noise in the workplace or spirometry for those exposed to respiratory sensitisers. Technicians have their place but do not operate at the strategic level of the OHN specialist. They may hold a nursing or health qualification but there is no requirement to do so. However, the author proposes that holding an appropriate qualification is essential in this very specialist area of nursing practice that encompasses independent functioning, autonomous decision-making, and employee health management (Rogers 1994, p. 34). It is the role of the OHN specialist practitioner that will be explored in this chapter.

The model of OH service provision is influenced by a multitude of factors including the current state of the economy, legal requirements and the hazards to which employees could be exposed (Smedley *et al.* 2007). OHNs practise nursing in a unique way. Working with specific populations in the workplace, they perform an important public health function. Although their role is diverse and complex, it is primarily concerned with promoting general health status and preventing work-related ill-health and accidents. Experienced OHNs play an important part in organisational health policy development, risk and health assessment. They are thus in a prime position to contribute to attendance management and rehabilitative interventions assisting those with chronic health issues to remain in productive and paid employment. These interventions will be explored later in this chapter.

An effective OH service adds value to the organisation that employs it; there are clearly benefits to both employee and employer by improving the quality of working life as well as having a positive impact on business productivity. Employer commitment to employee health improvements not only contributes to the long-term health status of the community but also benefits the organisation through an improvement in worker retention, a reduction in sickness absence and accident rates, and an increase in productivity. As the Health and Safety Executive (1995) has long asserted 'good health means good business'. Organisations providing an OH service do so because it adds value. OHNs recognise that well-designed work processes should do employees no harm, indeed there are benefits, as Manos & Silcox (2007, p.17) comment: 'good work is good medicine'.

It can be argued that there is a paradoxical relationship between work and health; work is usually a financial necessity and often socially rewarding but it must be acknowledged that under some circumstances it may result in significant adverse health effects. Some work areas such as construction sites have obvious dangers including working in a hazardous environment, perhaps in adverse climatic conditions, using dangerous machinery and possible exposure to harmful chemicals. It is important to note that the construction industry employs a predominantly itinerant workforce. Although many construction industry workers are highly skilled, others are semi- or unskilled employees; a large proportion of these people speak English as a second or subsequent language and a number may speak no English at all. The combination of these factors results in an increased risk of accidents. Indeed construction sites are probably the most dangerous work areas in the UK today.

The Health and Safety Executive recognises the dangers associated with construction work and notes that in the period 1999–2004 almost 300 people died following workplace accidents. These accidents resulted from falls during work carried out at heights; incidents involving the movement of vehicles and machinery and accidents occurring during the lifting of heavy loads. Despite their strategy to target health and safety in the construction industry the Health and Safety Executive (2007) reported that there were still 77 fatal injuries among construction workers in the year 2006–7, a 28% increase on the previous year. Construction workers are more likely to be involved in serious accidents than people employed in less dangerous work areas and their work is also associated with a range of occupational illnesses. Working with noisy, vibrating tools can result in them developing occupational deafness and circulatory disorders such as hand arm vibration syndrome. (Health and Safety Executive 2005) Their exposure to materials such as oils and cement predisposes them to developing occupational dermatitis and chemical burns. There are now a growing number of OHNs who choose to work in the construction industry as a result of the diversity of the hazards associated with such employment.

Other occupations also have illnesses associated with them, for example, work-related upper limb disorders are associated with repetitive tasks such as poorly designed work involving extensive keyboard use. Occupational asthma is a work-related condition associated with a number of work processes including exposure to flour in food production; exposure to isocyanates in the paint spraying of motor vehicles; and exposure to dander and body fluids from working with animals. Noise-induced hearing loss is not confined to the construction industry and is also associated with a number of occupations including factory work and among professional musicians. Unsurprisingly a number of high-profile rock musicians are reputed to have developed noise-induced hearing loss. These performers are particularly at risk due to both their ongoing exposure to noise and their probable reluctance to wearing hearing protection.

Members of other performing arts such as actors, singers and dancers are also predisposed to developing occupation-related conditions. Dancers are prone to joint and other musculoskeletal injuries while singers and actors may develop problems with their voice. There is a small group of OHNs working specifically in this highly specialised field of OH practice. Their client group is interesting and unusual as it includes every age range from children (including babies) to older age actors.

An appreciation of the effect of work on health is not new. Indeed more than 300 years ago, Ramazzini, a professor of medicine at Padua, Italy, acknowledged that work impacts on health. Ramazzini is widely considered to be the father of occupational medicine and his practice involved looking after the health needs of artisans and labourers. He stressed the importance of asking patients this question 'What is your occupation?'. This question is often forgotten by many medical (and nursing) practitioners of today but is not forgotten by nurses working in occupational health as they appreciate the possible adverse effects of work on health and health on work performance.

Historical perspective

OH nursing has a long history in the UK. The first nurse to work in the industrial setting is reputed to be Phillipa Flowerday, who was employed in the late nineteenth century in Coleman's mustard factory in Norwich. Her role was innovative at that time and encompassed a public health dimension as she offered a treatment service in the factory during the morning then spent the rest of her working day working with sick employees and their families in their own homes. Contemporary OHN practice has evolved from such a treatment-based approach to one that is both evidence-based and proactive and has a preventive focus.

OH services of the twenty-first century are directly involved in employee health management and they work towards reducing employee exposure to health risks and preventing illnesses associated with occupation. This is congruent with the ILO/WHO's (1973) stated aim of occupational health as being:

> 'the promotion and maintenance of the highest degree of physical, mental and social well-being of workers in all occupations by preventing departures from health, controlling risks and the adaptation of work to people, and people to their jobs'.

In order to accomplish this aim OHNs must have an understanding of the factors impacting on the health of workers and be innovative in their approach to the client care offered by them to all strata within the organisation. They have an understanding of how organisations function and an appreciation of the social influences on health status. The Acheson report (Department of Health [DH] 1998) indicates that poverty continues to exert a negative effect on health with the gap between the social classes widening. OHNs are able to work with employees at all levels and within all social groups. Consequently, they contribute to the improvement of the health of all strata of the workforce and can focus on particularly vulnerable groups. One such group are people, often low-paid unskilled workers, employed to operate hazardous processes. These people are already disadvantaged and such exposure to workplace hazards has the potential to further contribute to the health divide between the social classes.

Provision of occupational health services in the UK

Unfortunately, there is currently no legal requirement in the UK for employers to provide an OH service for their employees. Large organisations, or those with exposure to workplace hazards such as dangerous chemicals, often choose to provide one. The provision of such a service is not mandatory and is therefore an option for businesses rather than an obligation. The decision whether to provide an OH service is usually a financial one. A consequence of the provision of OH services not being obligatory is that OH provision in the UK is patchy; in short there is no 'national occupational health service'. The government's strategy to promote the health and well-being of working age people: *Health, Work and Wellbeing – Caring for Our Future* (HM Government 2005) could make this a reality. Central to this strategy was the appointment of a National Director for Occupational Health, Dame Carol Black (Manos & Silcox 2007) and initiatives to help and encourage people to return to the workplace after a period of sickness absence (O'Reilly & Gee 2007). A proactive OH service is well placed to develop high-quality return to work recovery programmes. O'Reilly (2007, p. 16) comments that 'Rehabilitation is a key part of the OH contribution to cutting long-term absence rates'. Important elements of this initiative include promoting health and assisting people with chronic health problems to stay in work and out of a benefit trap, thus reducing both the financial burden on society and the social exclusion of those living with chronic health deficits.

Whether a national OH service will indeed become a reality in the foreseeable future is yet to be confirmed. It has been suggested that OH as a specialty has been slow to progress owing to its exclusion from the NHS at its inception in 1948. This omission was probably due to financial reasons resulting from concerns regarding the cost of developing a new national health service. The government's stance that employers are responsible for OH provision has resulted in this inconsistent approach and, until recently, there was little collaborative working evident between the NHS and the workplace. NHS Plus, which is discussed later in this chapter, is helping to bridge this gap. Dame Carol Black's review of the health of Britain's working population, *Working for a Healthier Tomorrow* for the Department of Work and Pensions indicates that detachment of OH from mainstream health care undermines holistic patient care (Department of Work and Pensions 2008a).

The changing nature of UK workplaces

The nature of UK workplaces is changing and the role of the OHN is developing to meet the challenges these changes present. Their role can be as diverse as the workplaces in which they are employed. There is now a decline in the number of large manufacturing industries in the UK and work is increasingly undertaken within a multi-cultural context. Non-discriminatory governmental policy has resulted in employers being required to make arrangements to facilitate the employment of people with a range of physical and mental disabilities. Employers must also offer equality of opportunity for both men and women; women of all ages now form a much larger proportion of the workforce, particularly so in what had previously been occupations dominated by male workers. This raises particular health and safety issues in respect of those who are pregnant or those who have recently returned to work following maternity leave. Pregnant women and new and nursing mothers are at risk from some work processes including exposure to some chemicals or the moving and handling of heavy or cumbersome loads.

The rapid growth of information technology has had a significant influence on work practices. This development has led to a growth of 'call centres' in which people are employed to undertake work that depends on the use of both telephones and computers. On the face of it this would appear to be a safe place of work. However, on closer inspection there are a number of health problems associated with work of this nature. One of the most significant is voice strain; it is arguable that there is also the potential for some degree of damage to the ear with possible hearing loss associated with loud noise from a poorly adjusted volume control on telephone headsets (Maltby 2005). Other health problems are not specific to workers in call centres but are common to other occupations requiring work with computers such as work-related upper limb disorders. Working in a call centre is generally more stressful than other occupations. Careful work planning and equipment design can alleviate some of this stress and an OHN can advise on such issues.

OHN practice requires an appreciation of the bio-psychosocial sciences recognising that employment is an integral part of adult life and health should not be harmed as a result of it. The ability to participate productively in workplace activities can, and should, contribute to ongoing physical and psychological well-being. However, not all work is free from risk. Workers of lower social status experience more injuries and work-related ill-health than those from the middle classes. The financial circumstances of those living in socially deprived areas, single parents or those without skills or qualifications may be forced into hazardous, low-paid occupations. Cognisance of this situation enables OHNs to focus workplace health promotion activities on this group of workers – people who may not access such information from other sources.

Semi-skilled and unskilled workers frequently undertake tasks on poorly designed production lines pre-disposing them to musculo-skeletal disorders such as work-related upper limb disorders and back pain. An example of a successful initiative put in place by one company is the protection of people working on a poultry processing production line. Their work tasks had hitherto included lifting plucked, semi-processed turkeys from a production conveyor belt located behind them and at waist height. The birds were then lifted onto a hook positioned in front of, and at the shoulder height, of the operatives. Many of these workers subsequently developed a range of work-related musculo-skeletal disorders including neck, shoulder and back pain. Both the design of the equipment with which they worked and their work tasks pre-disposed them to such pain due to the resulting repetitive twisting actions of the trunk, lifting a load (the turkeys) away from the body and re-positioning and anchoring it at shoulder height. The high-risk operations they were required to undertake included twisting, reaching and handling a heavy load held at a distance from the body. The OH service took a pro-active involvement in the redesign of both the work process and work equipment. Risk assessment proformas were developed in order to identify any future problems associated with the process. The OHNs were able to refer clients with musculo-skeletal problems into a fast track, in-house, physiotherapy service. These initiatives resulted in a dramatic reduction in musculo-skeletal disorders with reduced costs relating to labour relations and turnover, sickness absence and possible future litigation. These employees were fortunate to have access to such a proactive OH service that was funded by their employer. This was possible due to the size and financial turnover of their company. Employees in many other workplaces in similar factories are not so fortunate.

Changing work patterns

It must be acknowledged that the world of work is rapidly changing with fewer large industries and a higher proportion of small- and medium-sized business enterprises. Even in large organisations, employment does not always take place in a conventional workplace. Paton (2004) comments that more than a million people are estimated to regularly work from home. Such working has been facilitated by developments in information technology. Paton goes on to discuss the benefits and challenges of using the home as a workplace. Reduced travel costs with fewer distractions are appealing, however, isolation, the potential for longer working hours and higher levels of stress may result in workers employed in this way experiencing more emotional difficulties than their colleagues employed in a conventional office environment. Home working brings challenges to the OHNs who provide a service for people who work in this way.

Employers have a duty of care under legislation including the Health and Safety at Work etc. Act 1974. They must ensure the health, safety and welfare of their staff no matter where they work. It is also in the employer's financial interest to reduce absences resulting from work-related ill-health. OHNs are suitably positioned and experienced to work collaboratively with workers, their representatives, management and other health and health and safety practitioners to improve worker health. Changing work

patterns, work requirements and improved control strategies have resulted in a reduction of health deficits linked to exposure to hazardous chemicals. However, there has been an increase in work-related upper limb disorders associated with the use of computers. Likewise, workplace stress seems to be a topical subject of much debate. Work should not lead to mental ill-health. There is poorer mental health among those who are unemployed than among those in employment (Smedley *et al.* 2007).

Workplace practices

The role of the OHN requires cognisance of the organisational, sociological and psychological factors that affect workplace practices impacting on worker health status. They advise and work with management, employees and their representatives towards ensuring a safe and a health-promoting workplace. OHNs are well placed to influence the health of the community as the workplace provides a captive audience for interventions, which further promote health among a group of well adults who are often otherwise difficult to access. As the DH states, the workplace offers potential for improving the health status of the population because of:

- 'Access to a large number of people many of whom are at risk for adverse health effects
- A potentially low level of attrition as the population is relatively stable
- Cohesion of the working community which can offer benefits such as positive peer pressure and peer support
- Established channels of communication which can be used to publicise programmes, encourage participation, provide feedback and assist in the process of change'

(DH 2003)

Some OH services offer a very limited service with an emphasis on pre-employment screening and attendance management – sadly, this is a lost opportunity and reflects a service which has not moved forward. Such limited services were highlighted more than a decade and a half ago

(Pickvance 1993). By contrast other services have a much more proactive and holistic approach more closely aligned to a broader public health agenda. Such proactive services provide very much a preventive role integrating the skills of risk and health assessment. Many OHNs are highly experienced in formulating return to work recovery programmes for employees who have been absent from work as the result of accidents or following serious ill-health.

The discussion so far has indicated that OHNs are specialist practitioners, aware of the effect of work on health and health on work, who work with both individuals and groups to improve health. Their advice to all concerned aims to minimise any adverse effects of work on health and assist in reducing accidents (Harriss 2004). Most OHNs undertake health and risk management to achieve this aim whereas experienced and more senior OHNs operate at a more strategic level, contributing to policy formation and professional leadership in the organisations in which they work.

The domains of occupational health nursing practice

OHNs face challenges and practice in a way that differs from that undertaken by nurses employed in other community or hospital settings. Although their practice has a different emphasis, OHNs bring with them the values and beliefs developed as a result of having initially qualified as general or mental health nurses. Much, but not all, of what OHNs undertake as part of their practice would be unrecognisable to many other nurses as 'nursing skills' and their role will now be explored. The role of the OHN incorporates a number of domains including professional, managerial, environmental and educational spheres. How these are applied depends on the OHN's area of practice and the needs of their employing organisation, but there are certain commonalities.

The professional domain

The professional domain is very broad and encompasses the 'nitty-gritty' of practice as nurses in the workplace setting. They must be able to work within the requirements of both legislation and the NMC professional code of conduct. This is often challenging as many of the people with whom OHNs work, including managers and human resources professionals, do not fully appreciate the implications of their professional code of conduct particularly in relation to client confidentiality.

OHNs have the potential to undertake an important role in research and epidemiology – identifying work-related health issues. They use their nursing skills in the assessment of health in a range of activities including pre-employment health assessments to ensure that prospective employees are fit to take on the requirements of their proposed job. They are involved in providing ongoing health surveillance for workers exposed to workplace hazards such as work involving exposure to a vast array of hazardous chemicals including iso-cyanates, chrome, lead and solvents. Chemicals used in the workplace can have numerous patho-physiological effects of which the OHN should be aware. They have the potential to impact on a number of organs and body systems including organs such as the skin, liver, kidneys and the respiratory, reproductive, haematopoietic and central nervous systems. Health surveillance provides an opportunity to identify early changes linked to such exposure in order to identify people at risk.

The focus on promoting health, reducing the number of people on incapacity benefit and effective vocational rehabilitation is central to Dame Carol Black's review of the health of Britain's working population (Department of Work and Pensions 2008a). Her report emphasises the importance of vocational rehabilitation and multi-disciplinary working. The report highlights the links between health and employment and their effects on productivity. The promotion of health and well-being benefits all as it raises employability, and reduces worklessness. These in turn assist in achieving greater social justice, promoting economic growth and reducing poverty benefiting the individual and the community alike. In November 2008 the government responded to Black's review supporting her recommendations. Of particular

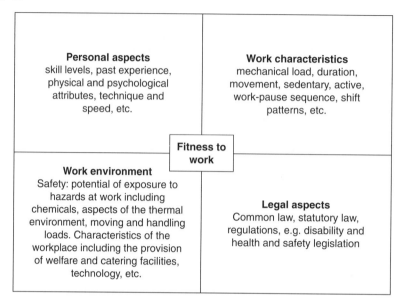

Figure 12.1 The fitness to work framework of assessment (source: Murugiah *et al.* 2002. Reproduced with permission).

note is a move to piloting a 'Fit for Work service' and replacing the existing approach to medical certification for absence from work with an electronic 'fit note' (Department for Work and Pensions 2008b).

OHNs are well placed to take a strategic role in this strategy. Over the past two decades they have increasingly been undertaking a role in attendance management. The costs of sickness absence is a significant drain on the profitability of many organisations and is consistently estimated to cost the UK economy more than £11 billion each year in direct costs of sick pay. OHNs' knowledge of health and work requirements means that they can make a valuable contribution to an attendance management strategy (Harriss 2001). However, it is essential that they clarify their role to ensure that there is no conflict between maintaining an impartial role as employee advocate and acting as an adviser to management. Part of their contribution to attendance management strategies put in place by organisations is the undertaking of health assessments for employees following periods of repeated short-term or one episode of long-term

absence prior to their return to work. This offers an ideal opportunity to identify whether a health problem is caused, or exacerbated, by job requirements. The OHN can then devise recovery programmes facilitating a successful and productive return to work, a benefit to all concerned.

It is appropriate that the OHN is asked for an opinion on the health of employees with a tendency to repeated short-term absences as well as those who have had a long-term absence, whether or not these are work related. An automatic OH review is advisable following a period of long-term sickness absence of, perhaps, three weeks' duration, or following a reportable workplace accident as this offers the opportunity to decide whether the person is now fit enough to carry out the full requirements of their job or whether a phased return to work programme should be negotiated with both the client and their manager.

A competent assessment of a worker's fitness to return to work involves consideration of the extent of fitness or any degree of impairment and current health status in the light of their job demands. A skilled and competent assessment requires consideration of aspects of the individual, their job and the hazards to which they may be exposed at work, each considered in the light of a range of legal requirements. These requirements are incorporated into the Murugiah *et al.* health assessment model: fitness to work (Figure 12.1). This model, developed by three practising OHN educators, is designed specifically for use in the OH setting and assists in the decision-making process regarding whether a worker who had previously experienced a significant health deficit is fit to return to work. Their return to work may, in the short term, be on restricted duties (Murugiah *et al.* 2002).

There are occasions when a return to work following serious illness or injury would be difficult without modifications being made to the work-process and/or the equipment used at work. The Disability Discrimination Act 1995 requires employers to make such reasonable adjustments for people who are disabled, as defined by the Act. In order to do so they need access to competent and professional advice. The specialist OHN is well placed to do this as they have knowledge of health and illness, the requirements of the worker's job coupled with an understanding of both employment and health and safety legislation. They are able to integrate clinical and problem-solving skills with other expertise such as the skills of risk assessment, problem-solving and multi-disciplinary team working.

In order to facilitate a successful return to work programme, it may be necessary for the OHN to make effective links with a range of practitioners including medical practitioners and those who work in the allied health professions such as occupational therapists, physiotherapists and disability advisers. This facilitates them giving the best possible advice to both worker and manager. Although an employee may be fit to undertake work of some type, a multitude of factors, not least continuing health problems, may preclude them from returning to their previous post. Unfortunately under such circumstances redeployment may be the only option. Occasionally even redeployment is not possible owing to the nature, severity or circumstances

of their health status and the person chooses to retire from work on the grounds of ill-health seeing this as a positive step. The OHN can give valuable advice and support at this time.

Senior OHNs manage and lead multi-disciplinary teams, a role previously only assigned to a physician. The managerial domain of OHN practice incorporates policy development. The range of health-related policies an organisation may need to formulate is very broad and reflects the type of work they undertake. Some of these include those covering home working, work with computers, moving and handling of loads, food hygiene, waste management, and working with chemical and microbiological hazards. OHNs also contribute to the formulation of policies focused on human resources including attendance management policies and strategies as already discussed.

Increasingly many OH services outsource their services; this is particularly the case since the advent of NHS Plus, which has facilitated services initially set up for NHS establishments offering their services to businesses leading to valuable income generation. This process must be well managed if it is to be successful. There are commonalities with managing any OH service as both require significant leadership and business acumen. Outsourcing involves the setting and negotiation of service level agreements, effective budgeting and procurement of human and other resources. The final part of the process is the effective management of both these contracts and the staff required to service them.

The environmental domain

The environmental domain is perhaps the aspect that is least recognisable to a 'generalist' as 'nursing care'. This can be the most challenging owing to the range of skills required in order to perform it with any degree of competence. An in-depth understanding of health and safety and employment legislation is therefore required. Particularly pertinent is an appreciation of the requirements of the myriad of regulations covering both health and safety and disability, much of which results from the UK being part of the European Union. In 1992 six regulations under the Health and Safety at Work Act 1974 became law. These regulations are generally known as the 'six-pack'. A recurring theme is the need for both risk and health assessments. All employers are required to undertake a general risk assessment, supplemented with health surveillance, for people exposed to hazards that have an identifiable adverse effect on their health such as exposure to respiratory or skin sensitising agents. In addition to the need for a general risk assessment, further risk assessments are included within the 'six-pack' for workers who use computers or who manually handle loads or patients. OHNs are considered competent to undertake, or teach others to undertake, such risk assessments. They are able to contribute to the evaluation of control measures such as local exhaust ventilation extracting chemicals in work areas such as laboratories or car spraying booths.

Many people work in industries that are intrinsically noisy. OHNs who practice in such industries are well placed to undertake a risk assessment to identify if employees are at risk, measure noise levels, comment on current exposure and suggest ways of reducing exposure by putting in place engineering or other controls. They are also able to comment on the suitability of personal protective equipment such as ear defenders including in-ear devices and ear muffs. They can interpret legislation covering noise in the workplace and decide which employees could be at risk of developing noise induced hearing loss. Under such circumstances they undertake audiometry in order to detect its very early signs enabling protective strategies to be instigated as a matter of urgency.

The educational domain of practice

The educational domain interlinks with the environmental domain previously discussed. It involves the OHN in teaching managers and workers on a range of issues as part of workplace health promotion. This is complementary to, but often different from, the health promotion interventions undertaken by nurses outside the OH setting. An example of such an activity is raising awareness of workplace hazards with managers and 'shop floor' staff and being involved in developing strategies and policies to prevent exposure. This may, for example, involve developing and presenting a health education package teaching people who work with hazardous chemicals how they can protect themselves from exposure. This may include highlighting safe and unsafe working practices during the storage, use and disposal of hazardous material, protective mechanisms including local exhaust ventilation and finally advising on the suitability of personal protective equipment. This is a health promotion activity but not as most nurses would recognise it.

Public health strategies

OHNs can influence the health of the community, and as such they are public health nurses, and it is appropriate that those who hold a qualification in occupational health nursing are eligible to register as SCPHNs. Having discussed the domains of their practice the contribution they are able to make to the government's public health strategy will now be briefly explored. The end of the twentieth and start of the twenty-first century has seen the publication of a number of public health documents including *Saving Lives: Our Healthier Nation* (DH 1999); *Revitalising Health and Safety* (Department of the Environment, Transport and the Regions 2000); and the Occupational Health Advisory Committee report on improving access to occupational health support (Health and Safety Commission 2000). These publications acknowledge the extent and costs of work-related ill-health and recognise the potential for the workplace to become a platform to achieve the government's overall aim of reducing accidents and improving the health of the population. They have influenced the practice of OHNs by engaging them in public health agendas and are essential if they are to meet the aims of the ILO and WHO already highlighted earlier in this chapter. The DH in association with the RCN and Association of Occupational Health Nurse Practitioners has underlined the contribution of OHNs to public health in the document *Taking a Public Health Approach in the Workplace* (DH 2003). This guide states: 'Occupational health nurses are a key part of the public health workforce. Changing health needs, increasing public expectations and new Government policies make this role more important than ever before.' It acknowledges the contribution that OHNs may make in reducing health inequalities and improving physical and mental health of the community through workplace interventions. Thornbory (2004) refers to the Health and Safety Commission's strategy for improving health and safety in Great Britain to 2010 and beyond whereby 'occupational health is acknowledged as a rising challenge now that "causes of safety failure" have been brought under some sort of control' (Health and Safety Commission 2004).

Specialist community public health nursing – part 3 of the Register maintained by the Nursing and Midwifery Council

So what will the future hold for OH nursing? The year 2004 saw the NMC open a new three-part register incorporating the 15-part register previously maintained by the United Kingdom Central Council for Nursing, Midwifery and Health Visiting. Incorporated within the register is one part specifically for SCPHNs. There is no direct access for those not already registered with the NMC. Health visitors along with those school and OH nurses holding appropriate qualifications are eligible to registration on this part of the register. The NMC has demonstrated its commitment to the public health agenda by supporting a new qualification for qualified nurses leading to additional registration on this part of the register. The NMC had debated whether the SPCHN qualification should be of a generic nature covering all aspects of specialist community public health nursing. This concept was rejected as it was quite rightly decided that it would be very difficult to ensure that graduates from such a programme would be 'fit for practise' across the whole field of public health nursing.

Validating a qualification that leads to registration on a separate part of the nursing register is a significant move. Previously qualifications in OH nursing were recordable, but in contrast to the position with health visitors, such a qualification did not lead to registration of the holders on a special part of the register. The establishment of a part of the register for public health nurses, which includes OHNs, recognises their contribution to the public health agenda. In the view of many practitioners a registerable qualification for OHNs is essential to ensure public protection. There may be implications for nurses who are practising in the OH setting without such a specialist practitioner qualification.

Conclusion

This chapter has presented to the reader an overview of the aim of OH services and the role of the OHN as a specialist practitioner within them. The context of their practice and historical perspective has been explored with particular reference to their contribution to public health initiatives. The OHN can directly influence the health, health and safety, and productivity of the workforce. They therefore make a contribution to promoting the health of the nation as a whole. It is an excellent career choice for nurses who enjoy a high degree of autonomy working with a predominantly well population.

References

Department of the Environment, Transport and the Regions (2000) *Revitalising Health and Safety: Strategy Statement*. The Stationery Office, London.

Department of Health (1998) *Report of the Independent Inquiry into the Inequalities in Health*. Department of Health, London.

Department of Health (1999) *Saving Lives: Our Healthier Nation*. Department of Health, London.

Department of Health (2003) *Taking a Public Health Approach in the Workplace*. Department of Health, London.

Department for Work and Pensions (2008a) *Working for a Healthier Tomorrow*. The Stationery Office, London.

Harriss, A. (2001) Attending to sickness absence. The experience of OH nursing degree students. *Occupational Health Review*, **92**, 24–27.

Harriss, A. (2004) Erring on the side of danger. *Occupational Health*, **56**, 24–27.

Health and Safety Commission (2000) *Occupational Health Advisory Committee: Report and Recommendation on Improving Access to Occupational Health Support*.

Health and Safety Commission (2004) *A Strategy for Workplace Health and Safety in Great Britain to 2010 and Beyond*. The Stationery Office, London.

Health and Safety Executive (1995) *Good Health is Good Business: An Introduction to Managing Health risks at Work*. Health and Safety Executive, London.

Health and Safety Executive (2005) *Hand-Arm Vibration the Control of Vibration at Work Regulations*. HSE Books, Norwich.

Health and Safety Executive (2007) *Occupational Health Standards in the Construction Industry*. Prepared by the Health and Safety Laboratory, RR-584, London.

HM Government (2005) *Health, Work and Wellbeing – Caring for Our Future*. Department of Work and Pensions, London.

International Labour Organisation (1959) *International Labour Organisation Occupational Services Recommendation, no. 112*. International Labour Organisation, Geneva.

Lewis, J. & Thornbory, G. (2006) *Employment Law and Occupational Health: A Practical Handbook*. Blackwell Publishing, Oxford.

Maltby, M. (2005) *Occupational Audiometry*. Butterworth-Heinemann, Oxford.

Manos, J. & Silcox, S. (2007) Health, work and wellbeing: the occupational contribution. *Occupational Health Review*, **May/June**, 17–18.

Marmot, M. (2005) *Status Syndrome*. Bloomsbury Publishing, London.

Murugiah, S., Thornbory, G. & Harriss, A. (2002) Assessment of fitness. *Occupational Health*, **54**, 26–29.

O'Reilly, J. & Gee, J. (2007) Helping Hands. *Occupational Health*, **59**, 16–17.

O'Reilly, S. (2007) Healing Partnership. *Occupational Health*, **59**, 18–19.

Paton, N. (2004) Putting OH centre stage. *Occupational Health*, **56**, 10–11.

Pickvance, S. (1993) In: *Health and Work Critical Perspectives* (eds Daykin & Doyal). Macmillan Press Ltd, London.

Rogers, B. (1994) *Occupational Health Nursing Concepts and Practice*. W.B. Saunders, London.

Royal College of Nursing (2005) *Competencies: An Integrated Career and Competency Framework for Occupational Health Nursing*. Royal College of Nursing, London.

Smedley, J. Dick, F. & Sadhra, S. (eds) (2007) *Oxford Handbook of Occupational Health*. Oxford Medical Publications, Oxford.

Thornbory, G. (2004) In with the new. *Occupational Health*, **56**, 20–21.

World Health Organization (1973) *Environmental and Health Monitoring in Occupational Health*. Report of a WHO expert committee. Technical report series 535. World Health Organization, Geneva.

Chapter 13 Community Mental Health Nursing

Derek McLaughlin and Ann Long

Introduction

The role of the community mental health nurse (CMHN) is continuing to evolve. CMHNs practise a wide variety of therapies ranging from behavioural psychotherapy, family interventions and grief counselling to psychodynamic psychotherapy, relaxation and visualisation. Further, CMHNs are increasingly engaged in innovative ways of working, such as non-medical prescribing, and extended roles arising from recent changes in mental health legislation (Jones & Jones 2008a). Their *raison d'être* is to represent people with mental health needs and to provide high-quality therapeutic care founded on a code of professional practice (Nursing and Midwifery Council [NMC] 2008). Being accountable to that code gives CMHNs licence to enhance and own a personal practice methodology which is unique to each individual nurse's style and personhood.

Five defining characteristics underpin the professional practice of community mental health nursing:

- A guiding paradigm
- Therapeutic presence
- The therapeutic encounter
- The *National Service Framework*
- The principles of community mental health nursing

These essential aspects are not displayed in order of priority. They are operationalised continuously and simultaneously. It is their dynamic combination in practice that illustrates the distinctive nature of community mental health nursing.

A guiding paradigm

The axioms underpinning community mental health nursing are to respect, value and facilitate the self-propelling and self-generating growth unique within each individual (Rogers 1990). For CMHNs the adoption of a person-valuing paradigm serves as a means of utilising systematically the powerful healing forces both within and between individuals, families, groups and nations. This notion is supported in the Chief Nursing Officer's *Review of Mental Health Nursing* (Department of Health [DH] 2006a). A person-valuing paradigm necessitates the use of a co-participative, person-centred perspective of a nurse *being* with and for the individual who is in need of mental health care as advocated by Long (1997a).

Being as a therapeutic experience

At an individual level, *being with* and *caring for* the person is both a valuable and therapeutic experience (Benner 1984; Leininger 1978; Long 1997a; Travelbee 1971; Watson 1985). It emphasises the role of the nurse as caring for the person with an illness. The person-valuing paradigm demands that CMHNs work alongside people as they endeavour to make meaning out of their journey in life (Casey & Long 2003). CMHNs work by listening, exploration, clarification and interpretation rather than by observing and explaining illnesses and behaviours. The person-valuing paradigm suggested here has its foundations in, and was developed from, a synthesis of Parse's (1992) theory of human becoming, Rogers' (1980) human science perspective of a unitary human being and existential phenomenology (Heidegger 1987; Merleau-Ponty 1974; Satre 1969).

Therapeutic ambience

CMHNs create a therapeutic ambience marked by a high degree of emotional nourishment and containment for feelings (conscious and unconscious), acceptance, genuine concern for, and openness to sharing. The person-valuing paradigm implies, paradoxically, that mental health and well-being are embroiled in the process of 'becoming' (Rogers 1990). Mental health and well-being are embedded into each individual's chosen way of living, their cherished ideals; and into the way in which he or she works to become an autonomous person (Mills 1986). At the *same time*, it means believing oneself to be part of and concerned for the general community and a wider universe of people (Long 1997a). Mental health is profoundly featured in each person's own lived experience (Heidegger 1992) of both valuing and living in their internal and external world; and this can be made known to the nurse only by their personal description. Herein lies the complexity, quality and richness of the process of community mental health nursing.

Mental health providers, at all levels, benefit from recognising that everyone in distress is an individual and has different needs, preferences and ways of coping. Thus, clients need to be included in the decision-making processes involved in the planning, delivery and evaluation of care (National Service Framework, 1999a; DH 2006a; Mental Capacity Act 2005; Mental Health Foundation 2000; Mental Health Act 2007).

Becoming a mirror image for the person

Clients need to see that their descriptions of lived experiences and personal histories of distress are reflected and validated in the eyes of non-judgemental nurses who demonstrate empathy with, mutuality, genuineness and concern for them. The healing journey begins from within the essence of the person/client's own perception of their needs. Moreover, as catalysts for healing and change, nurses must rely on the client for the direction, pace and movement of the healing process (Long 1999; Rogers 1961).

Providing a new focus of care: shifting the power base

Shifting to a new person-valuing paradigm as a guide to practice means more than adding to or replacing wide and unacceptable variations

in provision (DH 1999a, 2006a). It presents a formula for helping to raise standards, tackle inequalities and meet the special needs of women, men and different ethnic groups (DH 1999a, 2006a). A person-valuing paradigm, because of its integral, unifying, community and global aspects, is an ideal foundation on which to build the practice methodology of community mental health nursing (DH 2006a).

Self-monitoring

In view of these humanistic, esoteric, and essential health-giving and life-nurturing dimensions, CMHNs must come to believe that they, too, possess essential life-affirming and health-giving inner strengths and resources including the human quality to care (Brykczynska 1999; Heidegger 1992). Therefore, CMHNs need to be awarded protected opportunities to become self-reflective and self-receptive practitioners (Schon 1983). According to Schon, the two processes of reflection-on-action and reflection-in-action form the core professional artistry of the reflective practitioner. However, while reflective practice is concerned with improving practice and developing additional competence, *effective* reflective practice is defined by a broader model than Schon's essentially rational one; that is predicated upon an understanding of self, society and moral purposes. This goal may be achieved through attending structured, sensitive, clinical supervision (Cutcliffe 2001).

Therapeutic presence

Community mental health nursing in its uniqueness attributes precedence to the interpersonal, dynamic process of enabling individuals, families and nations to restore equilibrium between their internal and external worlds (Long & Chambers 1993). Through the therapeutic use of self, the nurse embraces the concept of self to influence all therapeutic approaches to care (O'Brien 2001). Implicit in this concept is the belief that a nurse's therapeutic presence has a complex role to play in the promotion of healing and in the recovery process. The unique attributes of the CMHN, coupled with the salience of what he or she says, feels, thinks and believes, when accepted and introjected, can lead to clients internalising a positive experience of self. *Being with* and *for* clients is the quintessential health-giving way in which CMHNs can meet the psychotherapeutic needs of clients (Slevin 1999).

A central tenet of the nurse–client relationship is therapeutic communication. It is a two-way process. Communication embraces the notions of giving and receiving, opening up, reflecting and responding. Working within a therapeutic encounter, communication also involves *empathic being* and having an ability to invite, 'stay with', contain and interpret a client's painful thoughts and emotions, thus help the person to work through distressing experiences. Unexamined life histories, coupled with unexplored and unresolved conflicts and feelings of their own, may render nurses unable to stay with and contain clients' painful thoughts and feelings. When this happens, a nurse's presence is no longer that of a catalyst for healing and recovery rather she or he becomes instead atherapeutic. Therefore, CMHNs require an understanding and awareness of their own *therapeutic presence* in order that they may be able to stay with and contain their clients' innermost thoughts, feelings and emotions. Otherwise, they may find it impossible to integrate their therapeutic presence into the nurse–client relationship. Rogers (1990) narrated: 'Recently I find that when I am closest to my inner intuitive self whatever I do seems to be full of healing, simply my presence is releasing and helpful.'

The therapeutic encounter

The essence of the therapeutic relationship is referred to by Buber (1937, 1987), as the *inter-human*. The inter-human is not owned by either the nurse or the client, it exists between them. Community mental health nursing is, therefore, located within the inter-human. The central tenet in Buber's philosophy is that to be human is to relate (Buber 1988; Buber & Rogers 1965; Slevin 1999). In community mental health nursing, then, the nurse–client relationship *takes centre stage* as a therapeutic channel for healing and growth and as such it is an end in itself. Each therapeutic encounter is, therefore, a lived experienced for both the nurse and the client on the basis of co-partnership.

In co-participation with clients, specific goals and plans are designed and implemented (DH 1999a, 2006a; Mental Health Act 2007). The promotion of such decision-making and decision-taking contributes greatly to empowerment and to the holistic healing process (DH 1999a, 2006a; Long 1999; Mental Health Foundation 2000).

The *National Service Framework*

The *National Service Framework* for mental health was designed to drive quality by setting national standards and defining service models for promoting mental health and treating mental illness. It emphasises the need to ensure that programmes of care can be delivered locally. In addition, it established milestones and a specific group of high-level performance indicators against which progress within agreed time-scales can be measured. To ensure this framework remains up to date, a national group has been set up to oversee both implementation and future development. The standards have been set out in seven areas:

- Standard one: mental health promotion
- Standards two and three: primary care and access to services
- Standards four and five: effective services for people with severe mental illness
- Standard six: caring about carers
- Standard seven: preventing suicide

The standards are realistic, challenging and measurable, and are based on the best available evidence. Interestingly, all of these standards had already been interwoven within the principles of community mental health nursing, which were designed prior to the framework and, even more motivating, they are raised again in the Chief Nursing Officer's *Review of Mental Health Nursing* (DH 2006a). They are now integrated into the following discussion.

The principles of community mental health nursing

In its uniqueness, community mental health nursing recognises the diversity and breadth of the role of CMHNs, who provide a proactive outreach service that embraces a professional responsibility to seek out, challenge and influence public policy related to mental health. Government, public health and health promotion agencies have been asked to support and promote positive images of people living with mental health problems (DH 2006a; Mental Health Foundation 2000). Hence, the overall objective of CMHNs is to work alongside clients, their carers and communities to maximise overall mental health potential.

In this section the standards and service models prioritised in the *National Service Framework* (DH 1999a), the major statutes in the Mental Capacity Act (2005), The Chief Nursing Officer's key issues for mental health nursing (DH 2006a); and the strategic directives in the Mental Health Act (2007) are incorporated into five principles of community mental health nursing. They are:

- The search for recognised and unrecognised mental health needs
- The prevention of a disequilibrium in mental health
- The facilitation of mental-health-enhancing activities
- Therapeutic approaches to mental health care
- Influences on policies affecting mental health.

These principles draw on the notion that principles state a relationship between two or more facts that may be used to explain, guide and predict action.

The first principle: the search for recognised and unrecognised needs

The search for and identification of recognised and unrecognised mental health needs is integral to the concept of a facilitative and empowering partnership with clients and communities. In order to practise this principle, CMHNs are required to research, analyse and audit detailed health and social profiles of the specific recognised and unrecognised needs they identify within the population they serve. A systematic health and social-needs-based model

is suggested here, which is based on four key factors:

- Health and social needs profiling
- Prioritising mental health care
- Primary care and access to services
- Specification of mental health targets and the identification of measurable mental health outcomes

Health and social needs profiling

Mental health cannot be divorced from the socio-economic and cultural context in which it is experienced (Long 1997b; DH 1999a, 2005; Mental Health Act 2007). However, 'There are people who are not receiving care according to the NICE Guidelines, which would never be tolerated for any physical condition' (Lord Layard, cited in Hodson & Browne 2008). In his presentation to government, Lord Layard widened the concept of material deprivation to include psychic deprivation. This was seen as an important change in the government's mindset about an increase in improving access to psychological therapies (IAPT).

Health and social profiling is one way of endeavouring to redress this situation as it is a specific attempt to identify the level and distribution of poverty and poverty-related health and social needs (current and potential) in a defined population (Blackburn 1992; World Health Organization [WHO] 2001). A health and social profile is essentially a contextualising profile. It assigns identified health information about recognised and unrecognised mental health needs into a social context. It offers CMHNs an overview of poverty and an awareness of how people's experience of poverty shapes their lives and affects their mental health.

Further, a health and social profile acts as a baseline and information source for prioritising, planning, implementing and evaluating practice (DH 1999a; Rowe *et al.* 1997). In addition, it generates objective and comparable information and data that can be used by practitioners and addresses a major deficit in the information base that exists regarding mental illness in the communities and GP practices within which CMHNs work (DH 1999a). At a wider level, the development and updating of community mental health and social profiles provides evidence for the evaluation of the effectiveness of mental health services by using approaches that are tailor-made to meeting clients' needs and aspirations rather than simply recording the activities and skills of each individual practitioner (DH 1999a, 2006a).

Prioritising

Practitioners will require the support of managers skilled in their area of professional practice if they are to draw up priorities and develop their work to the highest standard and effectively and efficiently deliver community mental health nursing care. Standards two and three of the *National Service Framework* (DH 1999a) indicate that primary care and access to services are fundamental to the effective delivery of mental health services. This seems justifiable as mental health indicators range on a continuum from suicide, severe depression and phobia through to the whole range of identity, sexual, marital and human relationship problems, for which it is both humane and realistic to offer high-quality nursing care (DH 2006a; Long & Chambers 1993; WHO 2001).

Primary care and access to services

A primary-care-led National Health Service (NHS) is a fundamental health service priority that is built on the proposition that primary care professionals are best placed to assess, plan, deliver and evaluate services that are based as near to service users as possible (DH 1999a, 2006a; NHS Management Executive [NHSME] 1996). Further strengthening of clinical effectiveness initiatives and extending the role of primary health care through primary care trusts that emphasise health care quality and prevent social exclusion are currently features of the government's evolving health service strategies (Office of Deputy Prime Minister [ODPM] 2004). Such features include reductions in the number of people admitted to psychiatric hospitals and in the onset of mental illnesses together with

support for carers and cost-effectiveness (Mental Health Act 2007).

Clearly, services must be developed to ensure that all members of the community are helped to overcome social exclusion and have equal access to health services (DH 1999a, 2006a; ODPM 2004). The vast majority of CMHNs work as part of multi-disciplinary teams. This requires competencies in communication and an understanding of others' perspectives as well as mutual respect (DH 2006a). It is essential that the guidance provided by all team members is transparent and consistent. In terms of first-level guidance, members of the primary care teams work with other agencies and the voluntary sector organisations, for example, the Samaritans and Saneline, to ensure that access is available 24 hours daily. Whatever the point of contact the principles of the new NHS Direct (DH 1998b) and the Mental Health Act (2007) should apply. However, it must be acknowledged that not all members of the primary care team are educated and trained in contemporary evidence-based interventions. Consequently, CMHNs often act as consultants to other team members on mental health issues (DH 2006a). The importance of conducting on-going accurate needs assessment is stressed.

Specification of targets and the identification of measureable outcomes

The ways in which mental health services are commissioned need further development to ensure that resources and priorities reflect a planned approach and an overall strategy for promoting mental health, preventing mental ill-health and ensuring the therapeutic care of people who are mentally ill and their carers (DH 1999a; National Institute for Clinical Excellence [NICE] 2003). Indeed, CMHNs should develop their leadership skills and use the commissioning process to improve, change and expand services to meet the needs and preferences of users, carers and communities (DH 2006a). Moreover, mental health outcomes/objectives must be identified and evaluated yearly to measure how effectively the objectives have been met. Contracts can be informed by the *needs profile*, which will need annual updating (Rowe *et al.* 1997).

The second principle: the prevention of disequilibrium in mental health

This principle reflects standard one, mental health promotion, of the *National Service Framework* (DH 1999a) and paragraph 21 of the *Chief Nursing Officer's Review of Mental Health Nursing* (DH 2006a). The Caplan (1961) model of primary, secondary and tertiary prevention is used here as a practical guide to focus on this principle. Primary preventative measures are carried out by CMHNs through designing mental health promotion programmes and health education packages, for example, the promotion and maintenance of healthy relationships (Duck 1992; Kelley *et al.* 1988); pre-conceptual mental health care; promoting healthy bonding (Bee 2001; Sluckin & Sluckin 1992); facilitating emotional health and well-being; healthy, non-shaming and non-punitive communication patterns (Dwindell & Middleton-Moz 1986); human sexuality and education for love (Higgins *et al.* 2006); and death, dying and letting go as natural experiences in living (Leader 2008; Tugendhat 2005). CMHNs are in a key position to initiate, develop, implement and research such health promoting and life-enriching programmes. Such mental health activities challenge nurses to redirect their focus and promote positive mental health at a wider level as recommended by the WHO (2005). However, mental health promotion research has been hindered by the deficit of reliable and validated psychometrically tested instruments to use in empirical studies. Further work is needed in this area.

Secondary prevention

Secondary preventative measures are conducted by CMHNs who provide a diversity of health promoting strengths and strategies to individuals, families, groups and communities to enable them cope with identified disequilibrium in mental health. Some examples of such health-giving activities are anxiety and stress management (Kabat-Zinn 2006); dealing with rational fear (Beck 1979); resolving anger, resentment and shame (Bradshaw 1992); screening and identifying 'at-risk' indicators for self-destructive and self-abusive behaviours (Beck *et al.* 1979; Santa Mina *et al.* 2006; Spandler & Warner 2007) and planning screening programmes for the early identification and remediation of chemical addictive behaviours (Bryant-Jefferies 2001; DH 2002; Shinebourne & Adams 2007) and sexual addictive behaviours (Carnes 2005). Examples of service models and of good practice include the provision of 24-hour crisis response teams, assertive outreach teams, one-stop clinics, the CALM programme (Campaign Against Living Miserably), local mental health helplines and self-harm intervention services (cited in the *National Health Framework*, DH 1999a, pp. 34–39). Activating and implementing these programmes requires an advanced level of planning, educative, therapeutic and management skills.

Tertiary prevention

Tertiary prevention embraces standards four and five, effective services for people with severe mental illnesses, of the National Service Framework (DH 1999a). Tertiary prevention involves planning current mental health care and preventing further deterioration in people who endure chronic mental ill-health. To be successful in carrying out this role, CMHNs must be competent in advanced skills, which include monitoring clients and carers' satisfaction. In addition, they must be competent to assess, monitor and evaluate the therapeutic modalities provided including their own health care skills.

The evidence-based (or evidence-informed) paradigm was introduced in the 1980s and this has grown in dominance since that time. While this process has clearly contributed much to the provision of clear evidence regarding what works and for whom, there is always unease where one paradigm is dominant. Accordingly, in recent years a complementary paradigm has emerged, namely practice-based evidence. It is important to view these two paradigms as complementary and not as being in competition with each other as the knowledge base in any discipline is considerably stronger when one paradigm informs the other. A core principle of a practice-based approach is that evidence must indeed be practice-based and practice is the core driver of the process – driven by practitioners and managers' desires to provide a quality service to their patients. At this level, it is crucial for practitioners to take ownership of the research activity, as they strive to innovate and generate solutions to local service delivery issues. Practice-based evidence can be gathered and evaluated through the use of, for example, a robust research tool such as the Clinical Outcomes Routine Evaluation assessment form (CORE-OM) (Evans *et al.* 2002).

Using CORE as an approach to practice-based evidence

We believe that there is merit in considering the use of the CORE-OM approach and the CORE system within the context of the developing paradigm of practice-based evidence. The CORE-OM approach was devised so that it could be adopted widely by both practitioners and researchers. It is a short and *free* outcome measure that is used widely in the UK. The complementarity of the client and practitioner individually completing forms both pre- and post-therapy means that it has been possible to collapse a series of forms into a coherent system called the CORE System. This is used for profiling the delivery of the psychological therapies. Further, the CORE-OM instrument covers the subject of 'risk assessment' and has a benchmark that specifically focuses on service safety (National Service Framework, standard seven [DH 1999a]). To this end, performance indicators explore levels of agreement between patient and practitioner risk assessment as recorded on the CORE-OM form and the practitioner assessment form, respectively, before concluding with a discussion on the clinical and managerial implications of discrepancies.

CORE-OM comprises 34 items condensed into four domains. These are:

- W – which refers to subjective well-being
- P – which refers to problems/symptoms
- F – which refers to functioning
- R – which refers to risk assessment

The purpose of CORE is to provide a free, user-friendly, pan-theoretical outcome measurement tool that is sensitive to both high-intensity and low-intensity ranges of distress and which utilises positive attributes as well as pathological symptoms, and can be used in both research and practice settings (Evans *et al.* 2002).

Further, the fourth principle embraces the notion that CMHNs are proficient in assessing, monitoring and evaluating the uses, benefits and positive and negative side effects of drugs and other chemicals used in psychiatry and in nurse prescribing (DH 2006a; Jones & Jones 2008a,b), as well as in the field of addictions (Shinebourne & Adams 2007) and sexual health education for people with a mental illness (Higgins *et al.* 2006). For further information on service models and examples of good practice please see the Chief Nursing Officer's review (DH 2006a) and the *National Service Framework* (DH 1999a, p. 52).

The third principle: the facilitation of mental-health-enhancing activities

Long & Chambers (1993) defined mental health as a process of equilibrium both within and between the inner and the outer self the social environment and the natural world in which people live. They state that:

'Within individuals it is manifest by self awareness; self acceptance; and the ability to cope with changing life circumstances… Positive mental health leads to a true value of all people as unique individuals and, therefore, the awareness of the existence of one humanity in an evolving world.'

Feely *et al.* (2007a,b) support and advance this definition in their theory of connectivity to include the spiritual dimension of health as recommended in the *Chief Nursing Officer's Review of Mental Health Nursing* (DH 2006a). The facilitation of mental-health-enhancing activities is promoted by designing health- and self-awareness programmes. Such educative experiences are designed and implemented in ways that empower people to come to *believe in* themselves as unique individuals and to help understand and accept both self and others hence improving relationships; increasing their understanding of life's meaning and purpose; and realising their creative potential (DH 2006a; National Institute for Mental Health in England [NIMHE] 2003). One of the key findings in the Strategies for Living report (Mental Health Foundation 2000) demonstrated that the total sample group interviewed with mental distress (n = 71) highlighted the need for professionals to acquire 'people-valuing' strategies. People-valuing strategies were categorised into: on-going survival strategies; crisis or life-saving strategies; medication; physical exercise; religious and spiritual beliefs; and money and other activities, such as hobbies, receiving information and the need for creative expression.

At community level, to protect the individual's autonomy within defined limits, society imposes norms of behaviour on its members. In the most permissive range, compliance brings personal acceptance and the enhancement of social-esteem as well as social status and material rewards. Alternatively, it is difficult, if not impossible, for others to sustain and maintain mental health and retain their dignity in a climate where: poverty and unemployment are paramount; there is gross inequality and social injustice; the young, the homeless, and those who are socially disadvantaged, including those who belong to minority groups, are undervalued and deprived of equitable opportunities and equal civil liberties for personal, social, educative and futuristic self-growth and development (DH 1999a, 2006a; Long 1997b).

The fourth principle: therapeutic approaches to mental health care

The role of the CMHN has undergone significant re-clarification as community mental health care services have continued to expand and develop. The *Chief Nursing Officer's Review* (DH 2006a, p. 12) aims to identify how mental health nursing can provide effective, truly holistic care, helping meet the needs of those with mental health problems as whole individuals as opposed to simply tackling their illness.

There is a developing trend that CMHNs should become specialised. However, Barker *et al.* (1998) indicated that specialisation did little to improve the quality of community health care nursing. These authors contended that the needs of certain clients would be overlooked if particular clients and their needs did not match the appropriate specialty. In the present era, CMHNs care for a wide variety of clients in the community. Hence, it is argued here that all CMHNs are specialist practitioners in that they are concerned with the totality of mental health care at individual, family, community, society and global levels. It is imperative, therefore, that they have a solid, eclectic and integrated theoretical grounding on a wide range of contemporary psychotherapeutic approaches to mental health care. Meanwhile, in order to function holistically, they need to remain purists in community mental health care nursing. The extent of the clients' needs for specialist mental health nursing intervention, however, requires further research.

Community mental health nurses: using therapeutic modalities to facilitate change

Examination of the differing approaches to care demonstrates that CMHNs are continuing to advance new, culturally sensitive approaches to nursing and a new epistemology of change for clients, carers and communities. As their role has evolved a number of level of change have been witnessed:

- Change at *level one*: refers to a change in a specific behaviour such as smoking, which can be brought about by the provision of a behaviour modification technique.
- Change at *level two*: refers to a change in a set of behaviours that are controlled by a belief or a construct regarding how to operate in the world. Change is brought about for anxiety and depression through insight and this can be achieved by the use of cognitive therapy (Beck *et al.* 1985; NICE 2006a, 2006b; Sanders & Wills 2005) or rational emotive therapy (Ellis 1984) or the 'gentle art of reframing' (Watzlawick 1974).
- Change at *level three*: refers to a change in a set of beliefs that are held within a

worldview or paradigm. An example of such a change might take place when individuals meet a crisis of identity. Their sense of the meaning and purpose of life and their previous identities become confused and lost. Most 'depth' therapies, such as psychoanalytic, psychodynamic and mindfulness (Williams *et al.* 2007) operate at this level.

- Change at *level four*: refers to a change in a set of paradigms or world views. Level four is related to not being identified in any world view but rather being truly oneself. Work at this level does not involve therapy as such but spiritual discipline such as meditation or yoga.
- Change at *family/carer level*: research has demonstrated that people experiencing severe psychotic symptoms are very sensitive to their environments (Gournay 1995a,b). Since families provide the essential psychosocial environment for patients, working with families is a necessary part of caring for people with severe and enduring mental ill-health. The evidence of the efficacy of practical family interventions in schizophrenia is well documented (Kelly & Newstead 2004; Leff 1998) and was the focus of a systematic review by the Cochrane Collaboration (Mari & Steiner 1996).

One significant attempt to enhance community mental health nursing skills in the area of psychosocial interventions was the development of the Thorn course, which began in 1992. The programme provides education and training for mental health professionals on evidence-based psychosocial interventions and family work. Since this time, policy service provision and needs have changed. Brooker *et al.* (2002) argued that Thorn courses are highly relevant to the implementation of the *National Service Framework*. O'Carroll *et al.* (2004) claim that the Thorn course reflects current policy and demonstrates how policy can be translated into practice. However, there is a deficit in evidence that user and carer involvement in the provision of psychosocial interventions has moved beyond rhetoric (Brooker & Brabban 2004).

Further, CMHNs continue to lack opportunities and support to implement the psychosocial skills acquired in training (Couldwell & Stickley 2007; Rolls & Davis 2002). It is important that all stakeholders contribute to the advancement of the Thorn course in order to integrate service and training provision.

Change at European and global levels

Mental health and social inclusion have been chosen as key priorities for care at the WHO Collaborating Centre for Research and Training for Nursing Development in Primary Health Care (WHO Collaborating Centre for Research and Training for Nursing Development in Primary Health Care 1999) and in the *Chief Nursing Officer's Review of Mental Health Nursing* (DH 2006a).

The WHO highlighted six priority areas to advance and strengthen cross-national cooperation, invigorate new activity and redefine priorities in the field of mental health care. This European innovation provides a dais for listening to the voice of users of mental health services and recognising their expertise and also to nurses together with all those involved in mental health care. All have a role in shaping and influencing the care and service delivery of the future. Priorities are:

- Enhancement of the value and visibility of mental health
- Development of mental health indicators
- Promotion of mental health of children and young people
- Promotion of mental health in old age
- Working life, employment policy and promotion of mental health

Examination of these levels and styles of change, in combination with Long's (1998) work on the stages of healing, demonstrates that some people might wish to change only their behaviours. Others might wish to change a particular belief without wishing to change their world view. Appreciating the different levels of change enables CMHNs to assess both at what level clients want to change and at what level they want to remain the same. Therapeutic approaches to care are enhanced when they are matched accordingly.

Listening to the voice of users and their carers

This section embraces standard six of the *National Service Framework* (DH 1999a). People who are ill, and their carers, have a right to expect considerate and competent care. This principle was reinforced in the Chief Nursing Officer's review (DH 2006a, p. 19), which states that: 'The assessment of the needs of carers and subsequent support for carers remains, in many instances, poor'. Newbronner & Hare (2002) concluded that mental health workers saw their role as primarily about treating people with a mental health problem and viewed supporting and involving carers as 'extra work'. Support for carers' needs to be integrated into local mental health services and may best be achieved by 'changing attitudes, systems and practices' (DH 2006a, p. 19). It is acknowledged that carers play a vital role in helping to look after service users, particularly those with severe mental illness (DH 1999s).

All too often mental health service users and their carers have been the subject of research – providing details of their lives – to be used by others. Some published studies that are worth reading are, for example, one study on service users and carers' experiences of a psychosis service in Lancaster (McKenzie 2006) and another on consumer predication in mental health services in Australia (Lamer & Happell 2003). Two excellent scholarship papers on the topic, by Rush (2004) and Stickley (2006), are also recommended. Further, pressure groups and consumer organisations add an important dimension to the debate.

The fifth principle: influencing policies affecting mental health

Mental health is political. It cannot be divorced from the decisions made by local councils or from policies created and legislated at government level. As such, CMHNs should be politically aware and assume positive action roles on behalf of their clients. This could be achieved through the creation and utilisation of local networks with the aim of influencing the political agenda and promoting positive images of people with mental health problems and advancing provision of care for the mental health population.

The legislative framework and policy context

Two new acts have impacted on the work of CMHNs. They are the Mental Capacity Act (2005) and the Mental Health Act (2007).

Mental Capacity Act 2005

Mental Capacity Act (2005) was introduced into England and Wales in 2007. The Act defines mental capacity as an individual's ability to understand the information provided and the skills to retain the information long enough to be able to make an informed and rational decision. This includes the capacity to weigh the information provided and the skill to communicate the resultant informed decision. If some or all of these skills are missing, some form of incapacity may be deemed to exist. The Act stipulates that all individuals must be given total assistance to support them in making their own decisions. All of us make unwise decisions at times and this can be true for our clients. The Act instructs that when clients make an unwise decision this does not mean that they lack capacity to make decisions. When a person is lacking in mental capacity to make decisions, however, any decision made or action chosen by a professional must be in the best interests of the person. It is important to note that using the term 'in the best interests of the person' is insufficient without justification for this deduction.

The Act specifies that a detailed assessment must be carried out to investigate if the person has the capacity to make a particular decision at a specific point in time. Moreover, assessments conducted must be the least restrictive to the person in relation to their human rights and freedom. The Act demands that having a particular mental health diagnosis is not a good enough reason to deem an individual to be incapable of making their own decisions. Similarly unjustifiable assumptions about people's behaviours, age, or appearance cannot inform decisions regarding lack of mental capacity.

The Act protects all people's right to document, in writing, their wishes about issues that might occur in the future if their capacity were affected. Carers can be consulted on their notions of the person's 'best interests'. The Act helps protect professionals providing care for individuals who lack capacity. It covers issues relating to the use, or threat, of restraint, which can only be used when it is necessary to prevent harm to people who lack capacity: and is in proportion to the risk posed. The Act does not cover deprivation of liberty within the terms of the European Convention on Human Rights. The Mental Capacity Act (2005) includes the following provisions:

- *Lasting Power of Attorney* (LPA): meaning that individuals can appoint a solicitor to act on their behalf if they should lose capacity in the future.
- *Court of Protection*: comprising the inauguration of a new Court of Protection that holds jurisdiction relating to the complete Act. This Court will constitute orders relating to individuals who lack the capacity to make health and well-being decisions.
- *Court Appointed Deputies*: these are appointed to replace the present system of receivership in the existing Court of Protection.
- *Independent Mental Capacity Advocates* (IMCAs): these are appointed for people who lack capacity and do not have anyone to represent their wishes. IMCAs will only become involved when issues about serious treatment or, a change in accommodation, has been raised.
- *Advanced Decisions*: before individuals lose their capacity, they can make advanced decisions regarding their acceptance or refusal of treatments-to-be.
- *Criminal Offence*: if professionals ill-treat or neglect any individual who lacks capacity they face a jail sentence of up to five years.
- *Research*: people without capacity will only be involved in research when the study aims to improve the condition that has caused the lack of capacity, or the care of people who lack capacity.

The Mental Health Act, 2007

The new Mental Health Act (2007) covers the following provisions:

- Definition of mental disorder
- Criteria for detention
- The right to advocacy
- Mental health review tribunal (MHRT)
- Professional roles
- Nearest relative
- Supervised community treatment

Definition of mental disorder

The new Act simplifies the definition and includes all disorders and disabilities of mind, which include promiscuity and other immoral conduct and also sexual deviancy. In keeping with the old Mental Health Act (1983) dependence on alcohol and drugs is excluded from the definition.

Criteria for detention

A major and far reaching aspect of this Act relates to detention with the introduction of the appropriate treatment test. Professionals involved in deliberating on an individual's need for detention must:

- First, carry out a holistic assessment of the person prior to detention, which includes identifying risks posed to self and other
- Second, categorise the proposed treatment regimen
- Third, assess if this treatment is culturally appropriate and available, as well as the distance from home and how this treatment might affect potential contact with family and friends
- Fourth, demonstrate that detention has a clinical purpose
- Fifth, validate clear anti-discriminatory and anti-oppressive practices.

These five strands make up the appropriate treatment test.

The Act advances the previous legislation on detention, which relied heavily on the provision of diagnosis. It broadens the term medical treatment to include nursing care, habilitation and rehabilitation, hence ensuring that assessed holistic needs are met. The Act abolishes the 'treat-ability test' from the 1983 Act. Evidence demonstrates that some people in need of mental health care were denied this and often ended up in the Criminal Justice system by default. The Mental Health Act decrees when it should take precedence over the Mental Capacity Act, which does not possess the legislative power to deprive individuals of their liberty. Overall, the Act is resolute that the least restrictive approach to care should be provided for people with disorders or disabilities of mind.

The right to advocacy

The Act takes endorses Human Rights legislation and relates it to people who are detained. This, in itself, is a paradox because detention without offence is possibly one of the most oppressive of actions a government can execute. However, the Act maintains that individuals who are detained have the right to access independent advocacy from the point they are detained. The possession of rights enhances the dignity of the rights held and so exemplifies the idea of respect for persons. CMHNs are required to protect and defend the rights of their clients to ensure that their strengths and needs and not just their diagnoses are recognised. Barnes *et al.* (2002) and Carver & Morrison (2005) call for a national independent specialist advocacy service. It is imperative that the individual's autonomy is respected at all times. If their ability to make decisions about their health is significantly impaired, the Mental Capacity Act (2005) will be invoked.

Mental health review tribunal

The legislation guarantees that people should have automatic access to the MHRT. For example, those who are in supervised community treatment and have not asked for an appraisal will be reviewed after six months, thus sanctioning the rights of the person and also assuring that 'best possible' care is provided.

Professional roles

The role of approved social worker (ASW) has been replaced with that of approved mental health professional (AMHP) and the role of responsible medical officer (RMO) has been changed to clinical supervisor, which is known as approved clinician (AC). These roles are open to all professionals and include a commitment to 'Expand the skill-base of professionals who are responsible for patients' treatment without their consent.' CMHNs are of course included in these new role definitions.

Nearest relative

The key changes here relate to the policy where, when reasonable grounds exist, a county court can take over this position. The Act permits civil partners to be considered as nearest relatives. Nearest relatives will also be involved in the process of supervised community treatment. Nearest relatives, and indeed recipients of the Act, can ask for and will receive a full assessment of all their needs proactively, prior to a crisis arising.

Supervised community treatment

This Act summons supervised community treatment. The government aims to ensure that people with serious mental health problems will continue their treatment following discharge from hospital into the community. Supervised community treatment will be invoked after individuals have been assessed as suitable for admission and treatment and both the AC and AMHP must be agreement with the decision. Moreover, supervised community treatment is only sanctioned when individuals are held on Section 3 of the Act or are detained under Part III without restriction. Supervised community treatment will not be approved for people who have never admitted to hospital. A full free care package must be put in place before individuals are discharged.

The goals of supervised community treatment are to: allow people to live comfortable and safely in the community; prevent readmission; reduce stigma and exclusion; and also avert disruption to their lives. Supervised community treatment is only considered when there is a risk to self or others and if there has been failure to comply with prescribed treatment. While receiving supervised community treatment, individuals must stay in contact with their named professionals. Professionals can decide to return individuals to hospital if their mental state deteriorates. However, clear criteria must be established on recall to hospital. For example, the AC is obliged to obtain a second opinion from an AMPH in order to re-detain a person and trust management must refer cases to the MHRT if a person has been detained in hospital for more than 72 hours. Further, if individuals refuse treatment in the community they cannot be forced to receive it, therefore, they are recalled to hospital for this essential clinical treatment. Supervised community treatments are reviewed at six months following discharge and from that point on annually and these reports are entrusted to the trust management. A number of safeguards in the Act protect individuals' rights. Examples are the nearest relatives' rights and the right to access a second opinion doctor (SOAD) for those who have medication as part of their supervised community treatment.

Managed care

The concept of *managed care* is a variant of the terms care management and case management (Cochrane 2001). Managed care has been established largely against a backdrop of the dialogue on best practice versus best value. Essentially, it involves designing planned programmes that specify what will be provided, the range of interventions, the diagnostic tests and the protocols to be followed in providing the services. Care provision, therefore, is determined by guidelines that are broad in that they state the general range of provision and some guidelines on delivery. In addition, managed care involves the formation of *integrated care pathways*, which state the activities that will take place at each stage in the course of the care provided to users.

Designing integrated care pathway involves cooperation and collaboration among health and social services providers to meet the holistic needs of people with mental health problems and their carers. This includes all those people who will be, or have been, discharged from mental hospitals and other institutions (Mental

Health Act 2007). Further, as primary care trusts were implemented against a background of growing public and media concern, greater emphasis is currently placed on ensuring the provision of effective support systems and continuing holistic, psychotherapeutic care for people with serious and enduring mental illness. The most prominent response to the reporting of high-profile incidents where risk has been poorly managed has been the call for greater powers to ensure compliance with medication in the community setting.

Overall, nurses and other mental health professionals, could design strategies to meet the current government's five challenges set out in the *National Framework for Mental Health* (DH 1999a). They are:

- Tackling the causes of inequalities
- Ensuring fast and easy access to a range of therapeutic interventions
- Keeping patients fully informed at all stages of their illness and the recovery process
- Involving patients in their own care by working in partnership with them and planning their care with them
- Designing actions to improve both the clinical performance and the productivity of the NHS
- Promoting flexibility in education and training and also in working practices and removing fudged professional boundaries to ensure that the NHS has the right skills, organised in the right way, to deliver modern, flexible and patient-centred services

Ultimately, mental health care means supporting individuals and communities to make choices, to explore and test out their options and to learn from their experiences in life. It does not ignore the need to protect individuals and others from potential harm, but it strives for a better balance between professional enforcement and patient choice, which needs to take place in a therapeutic and nurturing environment.

Risk assessment

Clearly, the benefits to be achieved by real community care and concomitant increased normalisation for people who are mentally ill and their carers far outreach the deficits. This may be especially true for our future generations. However, there are real concerns about the dangers that a minority of people with serious mental illness may pose to the community. These concerns have been focused on a small, but tragic, number of high-profile incidents of violence and suicide, prompting an internal review by the government on the care of vulnerable people with mental health problems who might slip through the net of services (Mental Capacity Act 2005). There is an urgent need to review current practice and to define ways which help identify and protect individuals 'at risk', and also safeguard the community. The implementation of the managed care approach, involving the concept of a 'named' key worker, requires mental health nurses to offer more formal specifications of their risk assessment methods, including the criteria underpinning clinical judgements. *Assessing and Managing Risk* is a training package that could be used nationally to establish some systematic multi-disciplinary approaches to this complex issue (Morgan 1999).

Risk management falls into three distinct categories: before, during and after an incident or event. Prevention is the key as neither practitioners nor patients wish to be on the giving or receiving end of serious harm. Assessing risk at first contact with the mental health services assumes special place in this regard. Evidence demonstrates that a modified version of the Sainsbury risk-assessment tool fits well as an inial risk assessment tool together with an overall assessment system (Stein 2005). The content of the care plan will also help to prevent risk. Risk assessment can be carried out through the channel of continuous assessment and reassessment of holistic needs together with an open policy on information sharing and exploration of the thoughts and feelings of patients and carers and an openness to mutual learning. Risk management should be an implicit or explicit goal for interventions. The most appropriate activity for risk minimisation is initiating and maintaining a safe and therapeutic relationship with the services that can be achieved for example through

assertive outreach (Allen 1998; Morgan 1999). The provision of evidence-based psychosocial interventions together with collaborative approaches to medication management further enhances risk minimisation. Paradoxically, risk taking is also an important part of risk assessment and management. Positive risk-taking means supporting patients to make and take decisions about their lives, to explore and test out their choices and to learn from the experience of 'failure' as this is what living is about. This suggests that CMHNs take positive risks in the carrying out of their role.

Homeless and 'rootless' people

Little attention has been given to the bulk of individuals who are mentally ill and have no home and generally few relatives (Bean & Mounser 1993). Further, the issue of discharge from hospitals to the streets and shelters has been seldom explored in the literature, but is all too commonly experienced by individuals experiencing mental disorders (Forchuk *et al.* 2006). Nevertheless, it is fair to say that some progress has been made in this area. CMHNs have a key role in working alongside people who are homeless and motivating them to experiment with ideas and learn social and life skills. They may even encourage people who are homeless to share their real experience of what it means to be a homeless person in a wealthy society (Dewdney *et al.* 1994; Long 1997b).

Prevention of suicide

Suicidal ideations produce features of both a private depression and a public failure where there is a need to come to terms with the split between sentimental and unrealistic ideals and the reality and pain of living. Hence, the act of suicide can be defined as a shortcut to dying (Long *et al.* 1998).

Standard seven of the *National Service Framework* (DH 1999a) relates to preventing suicide. Statistics on suicide are a real cause for concern. In 2000 approximately one million people died from suicide: a 'global' mortality rate of 16 per 100000, or one death every 40 seconds. Suicide is among the three leading causes of death among those aged 15–44 years

(WHO 2007). Internationally, epidemiological trends show that there has been a rapid increase in suicide rates in many countries, including America (10.4/100 000 in 2000; 11.0/100 000 in 2004); Japan (24.1/100 000 in 2000; 27.0/100 000 in 2005); and Taiwan (11.14/100, 00 in 2000; 19.3/100 000 in 2006) (WHO 2007). Alternatively, there has been a slow decrease in suicide rates in a few Western countries, including the UK (7.5/100 000 in 1999; 7.0/100.000 in 2004), Germany (13.5/100 000 in 2000; 13.0/100 000 in 2004) and Australia (12.5/100 000 in 2000; 10.8/100 000 in 2003) (WHO 2007). In the UK, the male/female ratio for completing suicide is approximately three males to one female (WHO 2007). Further, in the UK in 2006, the most common methods of suicide used were hanging, firearms and poisoning by gases (University of Oxford Centre for Suicide Research 2007).

The *National Suicide Prevention Strategy for England* (DH 2002) documents six key goals as part of a programme of activity to reduce suicide:

- Reducing risk in key high-risk groups
- Promoting mental well-being in the wider population (see the third principle above)
- Reducing the availability and lethality of suicide methods
- Improving the reports on suicidal behaviour in the media (see the fifth principle above)
- Promoting research on suicide and suicide preventions
- Improving the monitoring of progress towards *Saving Lives: Our Healthier Nation* target for reducing suicide.

The national strategy for England, as for other countries, demonstrates a commitment to enhancing and advancing health care professionals' skills in the assessment of suicidal behaviour (DH 2002, 2006b; Ministry of Health 2001).

Suicide is an avoidable form of mortality. Hawton *et al.* (2000) provide explicit direction on commonly identified motives, whereby the person may express the wish:

- To die
- To escape from unbearable anguish

- To escape from a situation
- To show desperation to others
- To change the behaviour of others
- To get back at other people/make them feel guilty
- To get help

Anderson *et al.* (2003) provide evidence demonstrating that nurses and doctors are aware of such motives, particularly when unsatisfactory personal relationships are present. Riesch *et al.* (2008) present results from a rigorous study that identified factors providing a foundation from which nurses can assess actual or potential suicide risk among later elementary school-aged youth who are encountered in schools, community settings and the variety of settings in which nurses practice. There remains much that CMHNs might do to reduce the risk of suicide, especially through the development of more cohesive, functional and realistic forms of assessment of suicide risk. The Nurses' Global Assessment of Suicide Risk (NGASR) risk assessment instrument (Cutcliffe & Barker 2004) provides CMHNs with a template for assessment that can be used as one aspect of a more thorough, ethical risk assessment process.

Suicide prevention must be targeted at individual, family, community and global levels. An example of an impressive suicide prevention strategy is designed by Murray & Wright (2006) for young people, which includes a youth suicide risk assessment and intervention model. The model integrates a range of theories to establish a comprehensive risk assessment and diagnosis and a reparative intervention.

A multi-agency approach is required in the sphere of suicidology and in the provision of care for bereaved families and friends (Sun & Long 2008). Practitioners need time to reflect on the impact that issues relating to suicide has on them both personally and professionally. This will include reflecting on their spiritual, ethical, moral and philosophical perspectives on suicide and developing an awareness of how these perspectives facilitate or hinder their therapeutic contract with clients (Fox & Cooper 1998; Reeves & Mintz 2001). CMHNs work with a range of non-statutory organisations such as Re-think, Survivors of Bereavement by Suicide, Mindout and the Samaritans. Connecting with people in a variety of ways is the reality of suicide prevention work.

Therapist–client matching and multicultural community mental health care

The important challenge of meeting the needs of an increasingly diverse society remains controversial. Nonetheless, the *special needs* of people who belong to ethnic groups and women who are mentally ill must be identified and met under the principle of influence.

Since many people who are mentally ill are female and from ethnic minorities and many CMHNs remain both white and male, it is imperative that CMHNs receive multi-cultural education and training. CMHNs working with different ethnic groups should be encouraged to examine their own values in relation to the needs of clients. Multi-cultural approaches require the avoidance of stereotyping and the encouragement of clients to explore their full potential, while realistically acknowledging social barriers to their aspirations. In one study of African and African Caribbean users' perceptions of inpatient services, the participants' accounts revolved mainly around a sense of loss of control as well as experiencing overt and covert racism (Secker & Harding 2002). Appropriate local responses to national priorities could help cut a swathe through the barriers confronted by ethic minority mental heath service users in a cross-cultural context (Pierre 2002).

Delivering Race Equality (DRE) in Mental Health Care (DH 2005) is a five year action plan for achieving equality and tackling discrimination in mental health services in England. The aims of DRE include:

- Reducing fear of mental health services among black and minority ethnic communities (BME) and service users
- A reduction of the disproportionate rates of compulsory detention of BME service users
- Reducing violent incidents that are secondary to inadequate treatment of mental illness

There are many challenges facing CMHNs in delivering race equality (DH 2006a).

A voice for women

Similar to the above discussion, there is a need to critique and recast assumptions about the mental health of women in a way which elevates women's experiences. Women frequently find their views being undervalued or discounted. CMHNs provide a voice for women who are mentally ill. They can also be instrumental in highlighting the real concerns of women's issues. CMHNs aim to provide gender-sensitive mental health care. There is also a need to acknowledge and address the link between violence and abuse, most notably childhood sexual abuse and women's mental ill-health (DH 2006a). The multifactorial dimensions of mental health services for women were explored in the mental health nursing review (DH 1994).

A platform for children

The mental health care of infants (Young Minds 2006), children and young people is fundamental to enable them to reach their full potential. Marshall & Parvis (2004) write comprehensively on Human Rights and the quality of life for children. Their book is invaluable for CMHNs who work with families as it depicts both information and evidence of salutary good practice.

In safeguarding children (DH 2006a), the effectiveness with which children's needs are assessed is the key to the efficacy of subsequent interventions and ultimately to their health, growth and development (Department of Education and Skills [DfES] 2003). The duty to protect children from the emotional challenge of mental illness demands knowledge, understanding, guidance and multi-disciplinary working. Determining who is in need and what those needs are and providing services to safeguard and care for children requires urgent attention. All professionals must strive to ensure that children are honoured and grow up in circumstances consistent with the provision of nurturing, safe and effective care. However, there is a deficit of research into the care of children with mental health needs and in the care of children who are living with parents who have a mental illness (Aldridge 2006; Knutsson-Medin *et al.* 2007; Polkki *et al.* 2004).

Conclusion

Community mental health nursing services should be organised in a way that will help to accomplish the vision expressed about 'mental health for all' in the *National Service Framework for Mental Health* (DH 1999), The Chief Nursing's Officer's Review (DH 2006a) and throughout this chapter. CMHNs search for recognised and unrecognised mental health needs at individual, family and community levels. They take cognisance of the primacy of mental health promotion and prevention and they provide proactive and responsive services, which are delivered as close as possible to where clients live. They provide therapeutic care to clients throughout the lifespan. This eclectic and integrative model of working enables the creative potential of professional practice to be fulfilled. It is essential that the unique expertise of CMHNs and their unique and dynamic combination of therapeutic skills and psychotherapeutic approaches to care are used to maximum effect for individuals, families and communities. The views and perceptions of service users, their advocates and their families/carers remain paramount.

The key features addressed in this chapter emphasise the *empowerment* of clients, families, carers and communities and also of all practitioners who work in the field of mental health care. The fundamental principles of mental health for all, universal services for all and openness and availability for all remain unchanged. Finally, partnership between government, local authorities, the voluntary and statutory services and community groups, both at national and local levels, is vital to improve the nation's mental health.

References

Allen, D. (1998) *Mental Health and Nursing*. Sage, London.

Aldridge, J. (2006) Experiences of children living with and caring for parents with a mental illness. *Child Abuse Review*, **15**, 79–88.

Allen, D. (1998) *Mental Health and Nursing*. Sage, London.

Anderson, M., Standen, P. & Noon, J. (2003) Nurses and doctors' perceptions of young people who engage in suicidal behaviour: a contemporary grounded theory study analysis. *International Journal of Nursing Studies*, **40**, 587–597.

Barker, P.J., Keady, J., Croom, S., Stevenson, C., Adams, T. & Reynolds, B. (1998) The concept of serious mental illness: modern myths and grim realities. *Journal of Psychiatric and Mental Health Nursing*, **5**, 247–254.

Barnes, D., Brandon, T. & Webb, T. (2002) *Independent Specialist Advocacy in England and Wales: Recommendations for Good Practice*. University of Durham, Durham.

Bean, P. & Mounser, P. (1993) *Discharged From Mental Hospital*. Macmillan Press, London.

Beck, A.T. (1979) *Cognitive Therapy and Emotional Disorders*. New American Library, New York.

Beck, A.T., Kovacs, M. & Weissman, A. (1979) Assessment of Suicidal Intention. The Scale for Suicidal Ideation. *Journal of Consulting and Clinical Psychology*, **47**, 34352.

Beck, A.T., Emery, G. & Greenburg R.L. (1985) *Cognitive Therapy of Depression*. Guilford, New York.

Bee, H. (2001) *The Developing Child*. Harper Collins College Publishers, New York.

Benner, P. (1984) *From Novice to Expert*. Addison-Wesley, Reading, Massachusetts.

Blackburn, C. (1992) *Poverty Profiling*. Health Visitors Association, London.

Bradshaw, J. (1992) *Healing the Shame That Binds You*. Health Communications, Florida.

Brooker, C. & Brabban, A. (2004) Measured success: a scoping review of evaluated psychosocial interventions training for work with people with serious mental health problems. NIMHE/Trent Workforce Development Confederation.

Brooker, C., Gournay, K.O., Halloran, P., Bailey, D. & Saul, C. (2002) Mapping training to support the implementation of the National Service Framework. *Journal of Mental Health*, **11**, 103–116.

Bryant-Jefferies, R. (2001) Counselling the person beyond the alcohol problem. Jessica Kingsley, London.

Brykczynska, G. (1999) *Caring: The Compassion and Wisdom and Nursing*. Arnols, London.

Buber, M. (1937) *I and Thou*. T & T Clark, Edinburgh.

Buber, M. (1987) I *and Thou*. Translated by Walter Kaufmann. Scribners, New York.

Buber, M. (1988) *Knowledge of Man: Selected Essays*. Atlantic Highlands, Humanities Press, New York.

Buber, M. & Rogers, C. (1965) Transcriptions of dialogue held 18 April 1965. Ann Arbor, Michigan. Unpublished manuscript.

Caplan, G. (1961) *An Approach to Community Mental Health*. Tavistock Publications, London.

Carnes, P. (2005) *Facing the Shadow*. Gentle Path Press, Arizona.

Carver, N. & Morrison, J. (2005) Advocacy in practice: the experiences of independent advocates on UK mental health wards. *Journal of Psychiatric and Mental Health Nursing*, **12**, 75–84.

Casey, B. & Long, A. (2003) Meanings of madness: a literature review. *Journal of Psychiatric and Mental Health Nursing*, **10**, 89–99.

Couldwell, A. & Stickley, T. (2007) The Thorn Course: rhetoric and reality. *Journal of Psychiatric and Mental Health Nursing*, **14**, 625–634.

Cutcliffe, J. (2001) *Clinical Supervision: Advancing Clinical Practice or the Nursing Novelty of the 1990s?* Routledge, London.

Cutcliffe, J. & Barker, P. (2004) The Nurses' Global Assessment of Suicide Risk (NGASR): developing a tool for clinical practice. *Journal of Psychiatric and Mental Health Nursing*, **11**, 393–400.

Department for Education and Skills (2003) *Every Child Matters*. Department for Education and Skills, London.

Department of Health (1994) *Working in Partnership. A Collaborative Approach to Care*. Report of the Mental Health Nursing Review Team. HMSO, London.

Department of Health (1998a) *Information for Health: An Information Strategy for the Modern NHS*. HSC (98) 168. Department of Health, London.

Department of Health (1998b) *A First Class Service: Quality in the New NHS Health Services, Circular 1998/113*. Department of Health, London.

Department of Health (1999a) *National Service Framework for Mental Health: Modern Standards and Service Models*. Department of Health, London.

Department of Health (1999) *Saving Lives: Our Healthier Nation*. HMSO, London.

Department of Health (2002) *National Suicide Prevention Strategy for England*. HMSO, London.

Department of Health (2005) *Delivering Race Equality in Mental Health Care. An Action Plan for Reform Inside and Outside Services and the Government's Response to the Independent Inquiry into the Death of David Bennett*. London, Department of Health.

Department of Health (2006a) *From Values to Action: The Chief Nursing Officer's Review of Mental Health Nursing*. HMSO, London.

Department of Health (2006b) *National Suicide Prevention Strategy for England: Annual Report on Progress 2005*. HMSO, London.

Dewdney, A., Gray, C., Minnion, A. & the residents of Rufford Street Hostel (1994) *Down But Not Out*. Trentham Books, Stoke-on-Trent.

Duck, S. (1992) *Human Relationships*. Sage Publications, London.

Dwindell, L. & Middleton-Moz, J. (1986) *After the Tears*. Health Communications, Pompano Beach, Florida.

Ellis, A. (1984) Rational emotive therapy. In: *Current Psychotherapies* (ed. R. Corsini). Peacock, Itasca, IL.

Evans, C., Connell, J., Barkham, M., Margison, F., Mellor-Clark, J., McGrath, G. & Audin, K. (2002) Towards a standardised brief outcome measure: Psychometric measures and utility of the CORE-OM. *British Journal of Psychiatry*, **180**, 51–60.

Feely, M., Sines, D.T. & Long, A. (2007a) Naming of depression: nursing, social and personal descriptors. *Journal of Psychiatric and Mental Health Nursing*, **14**, 21–32.

Feely, M., Sines, D.T. & Long, A. (2007b) Early life experiences and their impact on our understanding of depression. *Journal of Psychiatric and Mental Health Nursing*, **14**, 393–402.

Forchuk, C., Russell, G., Kingston-MacClure, S., Turner, K. & Dill, S. (2006) From psychiatric ward to the streets and shelters. *Journal of Psychiatric and Mental Health Nursing*, **13**, 301–308.

Fox, R. & Cooper, M. (1998) The effects of suicide on the private practitioner. A professional and personal perspective. *Clinical Social Work Journal*, **26**, 143–157.

Gournay, K. (1995a) Mental health nurses working purposefully with people with serious and enduring mental illness: an international perspective. *International Journal of Nursing Studies*, **32**, 341–352.

Gournay, K. (1995b) Future directions in community psychiatric nursing research. In: *Stress and Coping in Mental Health Nursing* (eds J. Carson, L. Fagin & S. Ritter). Chapman and Hall, London.

Hawton, K., Fagg, J. & Simkin, S. (2000) Deliberate self harm in adolescents in Oxford, 1985–1995. *Journal of Adolescence*, **23**, 47–55.

Heidegger, M. (1987) *On Being and Acting: From Principles to Anarchy*. Translated by R. Shurrnann. Indiana University Press, Bloomington.

Heidegger, M. (1992) *The Concept of Time From the 1924 German Edition* (translated by W. McNeil). Blackwell Publishers, Oxford.

Higgins, A., Barker, P. & Begley, C.M. (2006) Sexual health education for people with a mental health problems: what can we learn from the literature? *Journal of Psychiatric and Mental Health Nursing*, **13**, 687–697.

Hodson, P. & Browne, S. (2008) Bringing up IAPT. *Therapy Today*, **19**, 4–7.

Jones, A. & Jones, M. (2008a) Mental health nurse prescribing: issues in the UK. *Journal of Psychiatric and Mental Health Nursing*, **12**, 743–749.

Jones, A. & Jones, M. (2008b) Choice as an intervention to promote wellbeing: the role of the nurse prescriber. *Journal of Psychiatric and Mental Health Nursing*, **15**, 75–81.

Kabat-Zinn, J. (2006) Full catastrophe living. The program of stress reduction. Clinic at the University of Massachusetts Medical Center. Delta, New York.

Kelley, H.H., Berscheid, E., Christensen, A., Harvey, J.H. & Houston, T.L. (1988) *Close Relationships*. W.H. Freeman, New York.

Kelly, M., Newstead, L. (2004) Family Interventions in Routine Practice: it is possible. *Journal of Psychiatric and Mental Health Nursing*, **11**, 64–72.

Knutsson-Medin, L., Edlund, B. & Ramklint, M. (2007) Experiences in a group of grown up children of mentally ill parents. *Journal of Psychiatric and mental Health Nursing*, **14**, 744–752.

Lamer, J. & Happell, B. (2003) Consumer participation in mental health services: looking from a consumer perspective. *Journal of Psychiatric and Mental Health Nursing*, **10**, 385–392.

Leader, D. (2008) *The New Black: Melancholia and Depression*. Hamish Hamilton, London.

Leff, J. (1998) Needs of the families of people with schizophrenia. *Advances in Psychiatric Treatment*, **4**, 277–284.

Leininger, M. (1978) *Transcultural Nursing*. Wiley, New York.

Long, A. (1997a) Nursing: a spiritual perspective. *International Journal of Nursing Ethics*, **4**, 496–510.

Long, A. (1997b) Avoiding abuse amongst vulnerable groups in the community: people with a mental illness. In: *Achieving Quality in Community Health Care Nursing* (ed. C. Mason). Macmillan, London.

Long, A. (1998) The healing process, the road to recovery and positive mental health. *Journal of Psychiatric and Mental health Nursing*, **5**, 1–9.

Long, A. (1999) *Interaction for Practice in Community Nursing*. Macmillan, London.

Long, A. & Chambers, M. (1993) Mental health in action. *Senior Nurse*, **13**, 79.

Long, A., Long, A. & Smyth, A. (1998) Suicide: a statement of suffering. *International Journal of Nursing Ethics*, **1**, 3–15.

Mari, J.J. & Steiner, D. (1996) Family interventions for people with schizophrenia (Cochrane Review). In: *The Cochrane Library*, Issue 1. Oxford: Update Software.

Marshall, K. & Parvis, P. (2004) *Honouring Children*. St Andrews Press, Edinburgh.

McKenzie, L.H. (2006) service users and carers' experiences of a psychosis service. *Journal of Psychiatric and Mental Health Nursing*, **13**, 636–640.

Mental Capacity Act 2005. HMSO, London

Mental Health Act 2007. HMSO, London.

Mental Health Foundation (2000) *Strategies for Living*. Mental Health Foundation, London.

Merleau-Ponty, M. (1974) *Phenomenology of Perception*. Humanities Press. New York.

Mills, J.S. (1986) *On Liberty*. Penguin, London.

Ministry of Health (2001) *District Health Board Toolkit: Suicide Prevention: To Reduce the Rate of Suicides and Suicide Attempts*. Ministry of Health: Wellington, NZ.

Morgan, S. (1999) *Assessing and Managing Risk*. Pavilion: London.

Murray, B.L. & Wright, K. (2006) Integration of a suicide risk assessment and intervention approach: a perspective on youth. *Journal of Psychiatric and Mental health Nursing*, **13**, 157–164.

National Institute for Health and Clinical Excellence (2006a) *Depression and Anxiety – Computerised Cognitive Behavioural Therapy (CCBT)*. Technology appraisal TA97. NICE, London. Available at: www.nice.org.uk/TA97 (accessed 28 November 2008).

National Institute for Health and Clinical Excellence (2006b) *Computerised Depression and Anxiety – Cognitive Behaviour Therapy – Panic and Phobia*. Available at www.nice.org.uk (accessed 28 November 2008).

Newbronner, E., Hare, P. (2002) *Services to Support Carers of People with Mental Health Problems. Consultation Report for the National Co-ordinating Centre for NHS Service Delivery and Organisation RnD*. Department of Health, London.

NHS Management Executive (1992). *Guidance on the Extension of the Hospital and Community Health Services Elements of GP Fundholding Scheme from 1 April 1993EL* 48 (92). NHS Management Executive, London.

NHS Management Executive (1994) *Introduction of Supervision Registers for Mentally Ill People*. HSG (94). NHS Management Executive, Leeds.

NHS Management Executive (1996) *Annual Report 1995/96*. Department of Health, London.

NIMHE/Mental Health Foundation (2003) *Inspiring Hope: Recognising the Importance of Spirituality in a Whole Person Approach to Mental Health*. Available at: www.mentalhealth.org.uk/html/content/spirituality_project.pdf (accessed 2 December 2008).

Nursing and Midwifery Council (2008) *Code of Professional Practice*. Nursing and Midwifery Council, London.

O'Brien, A.J. (2001) The therapeutic relationship: historical development and contemporary significance. *Journal of Psychiatric Nursing*, **8**, 129–137.

O'Carroll, M., Rayner, L. & Young, N. (2004) Education and training in psychosocial interventions. *Journal of Psychiatric and Mental Health Nursing*, **11**, 602–607.

Office of the Deputy Prime Minister (2004) *Mental Health and Social Exclusion. Social Exclusion Unit Report*. Office of the Deputy Prime Minister, London.

Parse, R.R. (1992) Human becoming: Parse's theory of nursing. *Nursing Science Quarterly*, **5**, 35–45.

Polkki, P., Ervast, S.A. & Huppoonen, M. (2004) Coping and resilience of children of a mentally ill parent. *Society of Work Health Care*, **39**, 151–611.

Pierre, S.A. (2002) Legal, social, cultural and political developments in mental health care in the UK: the Liverpool black mental health service users' perspective. *Journal of Psychiatric and Mental Health Nursing*, **9**, 103–111.

Riesch, S.K., Jacobson, G., Sawdey, L., Anderson, J. & Henriques, J. (2008) Suicide ideation among later elementary school-aged youth. *Journal of Psychiatric and Mental Health Nursing*, **15**, 263–277.

Rogers, C.R. (1961) *On Becoming a Person*. Houghton-Mifflin.

Rogers, C.R. (1990) *Client Centred Therapy*. Constable, London.

Rogers, M. (1980) Nursing: a science of unitary man. In: *Conceptual Model for Nursing Practice*, 2nd edition (eds A. Reihl & C. Ray). Appleton-Centur, Crofts, New York.

Rolls, L. & Davis, L. (2002) Improving serious mental health illness through inter-professional education. *Journal of Psychiatric and Mental Health Nursing*, **9**, 317–324.

Rowe, A., Mitchinson, S., Morgan, M. & Carey, L. (1997) *Health Profiling; All You Need to Know*. Liverpool John Moores University/Premier Health NHS Trust, Liverpool.

Roy, S. (1990) *Nursing in the Community*. Report of a working group, North West Thames Regional Health Authority, Sheila Roy (Chair). HMSO, London.

Rush, B. (2004) Mental health user involvement in England: lessons from history. *Journal of Psychiatric and Mental Health Nursing*, **11**, 313–318.

Sanders, D. & Wills, F. (2005) *Cognitive Therapy*. Sage, London.

Santa Mina, E.E., Gallop, R., Links, P., Heslegrave, R., Pringle, D., Wekerle, C. & Grewal, P. (2006) The self-injury questionnaire: evaluation of the psychometric properties in a clinical population. *Journal of Psychiatric and Mental Health Nursing*, **13**, 220–227.

Satre, J.P. (1969) *Being and Nothingnesss*. Routledge, London.

Schon, D.A. (1983) *The Reflective Practitioner: How Professionals Think in Action*. Basic Books, New York.

Secker, J. & Harding, C. (2002) African and African Caribbean users' perceptions of inpatient services. *Journal of Psychiatric and Mental Health Nursing*, **9**, 161–167.

Shinebourne, P. & Adams, M. (2007) Therapists' understanding and experience of working with clients with problems of addiction: a pilot study using Q methodology. *Counselling and Psychotherapy Research*, **7**, 211–219.

Slevin, O. (1999) The nurse-0patient relationship. In: *Interaction for Practice in Community Nursing* (ed. A. Long). Macmillan, London.

Sluckin, W. & Sluckin, A. (1992) *Maternal Bonding*. Blackwell, Oxford.

Spandler, H. & Warner, S. (2007) *Beyond Fear and Control. Working With Young People Who Self-Harm*. PCCS Books, London.

Stein, W. (2005) Modified Sainsbury tool: an initial risk assessment too for primary care mental health and learning disability services. *Journal of Psychiatric and Mental Health Nursing*, **12**, 620–633.

Stickley, T. (2006) Should service user involvement be consigned to history? A critical realist perspective. *Journal of Psychiatric and Mental Health Nursing*, **13**, 570–577.

Sun, F.K. & Long, A. (2008) Family care of Taiwanese patients who had attempted suicide: a grounded theory study. *Journal of Advanced Nursing*, **62**, 53–61.

Travelbee, J. (1971) *Interpersonal Aspects of Nursing*, 2nd edition. F.A. Davis, Philadelphia.

Tugendhat, J. (2005) *Living with Grief and Loss*. Sheldon, London.

University of Oxford Centre for Suicide Research (2007) *Methods Used for Suicide*. Available at http://cebmh.warne.ox.ac.uk/csr/resmethods.html (accessed 11 August 2007).

Watson, J. (1985) *Nursing: Human Science and Human Care*. Appleton-Century-Crofts, New York.

Watzlawick, P. (1974) *Change: The Principle of Problem Formation and Problem Resolution*. W.W. Norton, New York.

Williams, M., Teasdale, J., Segal, Z. & Kabat-Zin, J. (2007) *The Mindful Way Through Depression: Freeing Yourself from Chronic Unhappiness*. Guilford Press, New York.

World Health Organization (2001) *Community Health Needs Assessment: An Introductory Guide for the Family Health Nurse in Europe*. World Health Organization, Copenhagen.

World Health Organization Collaborating Centre for Research and Training for Nursing Development in Primary Health Care (1999) *Initiatives in European Mental Health*. WHO Collaborating Centre for Research and Training for Nursing Development in Primary Health Care, University of Manchester.

World Health Organization Europe (2005) *Mental Health: Facing the Challenges, Building Solutions*. Report from the WHO Ministerial Conference. WHO, Copenhagen.

Young Minds (2006) *Mental Health in Infancy*. Available at www.youngminds.org.uk (accessed 28 November 2008).

Chapter 14 **Community Nursing Learning Disability**

Owen Barr

Introduction

This chapter commences with an introduction to the definition of learning disabilities, an overview of the number of people with learning disabilities and their overall health status. This is followed by a review of the changing service principles within services for people with learning disabilities that have arisen as a result of the series of policy reviews that have been published since 2000. Following this the growing evidence on the role of CNLDs and their families is presented. The key challenges presented in providing an effective community nursing services for people with learning disabilities are then explored before considering the future direction for community nursing in services for people with learning disabilities.

People with learning disabilities

The term 'learning disability' is used within the UK in the context of service planning and provision. The definitions used in the current reviews in England, Scotland and Northern Ireland (Department of Health [DH] 2001; Department of Health, Social Services and Public Safety [DHSSPS] 2005; Scottish Executive [SE] 2000) consider learning disabilities to have three components, namely:

- A significantly reduced ability to understand new or complex information, to learn new skills (impaired intelligence)
- A reduced ability to cope independently (impaired social functioning)
- Having started before adulthood (before the age of 18), with a lasting effect on development

Some clarification was provided within *Valuing People* (DH 2001) that 'the presence of a low intelligence quotient, for example an IQ below 70, is not, of itself, a sufficient reason for deciding whether an individual should be provided with additional health and social care support' (p. 15). The guidance went on to state that in determining the level of need, an assessment of social functioning and communication skills should also be undertaken. Furthermore it was clarified that the definition of learning disability, is not the same as the term 'learning difficulty', which has been defined more broadly within the corresponding legislation relating to education.

The position of adults with autistic spectrum disorders in relation to the definition of learning disabilities is not always clear. Within the definition used in *Valuing People*, it was further stated that the definition covers adults with autism who also have learning disabilities, but not those with a higher level autistic spectrum disorder who may be of average or even above average intelligence – such as some people with Asperger's syndrome (p. 22). The review undertaken in Northern Ireland does not include this caveat and a separate stream of work has been undertaken. In contrast, within the policy review undertaken in Scotland (SE 2000) it was stated that the definition of learning disabilities was taken to include people with autistic spectrum disorders, for the purposes of that review (p.116).

The above definitions provide an overview of the criteria that may be applied by service planners and providers in determining who has learning disabilities, and it is accepted that the term may be viewed from differing perspectives and the detail of the interpretation of the nature of learning disabilities alters to some degree depending on the perspective it is being viewed. However, it is generally agreed that if services for people with learning disabilities are to be effective they must be holistic in nature. The need for an effectively co-orientated inter-disciplinary and inter-agency approach to working with people with learning disabilities is recognised as central to making a holistic approach to service a reality (DH 2007).

The number of people who have learning disabilities

The numbers of people in the UK who are considered to have learning disabilities are estimates based on reported prevalence rates and have been revised within major policy reviews or as a result of census findings. The currently quoted figures in planning services were developed from the policy reviews undertaken in over the past decade. These reported prevalence rates have been reported differently across different countries within the UK. Within England, a prevalence rate of as 3–4 people per 1000 of the population for people with severe and profound learning disabilities and 20–25 people per 1000 of the population has been used to estimate the numbers of people with mild and moderate learning disabilities. On the basis of these figures it has been estimated there are about 210 000 people with profound and severe learning disabilities in England, of which approximately 65 000 are children and young people, and 120 000 are adults of working age and 25 000 are older people. In using the prevalence rate of 25 people per 1000 for people with mild and moderate learning disabilities it was estimated there was 1.2 million people with this condition in England (DH 2001). A figure of 120 000 has been given for the estimated number of people with learning disabilities in Scotland, using a prevalence rate of 3–4 per 1000 for profound and severe learning disabilities and 20 people in every 1000 for people with mild/moderate learning disabilities. Increasingly, it was further estimated that only about a quarter of people with learning disabilities had regular contact with local authorities

or the health service in Scotland. A survey to calculate the prevalence of people with learning disabilities in Northern Ireland reported the overall prevalence rate for all levels of learning disability as 9.7 persons per 1000 people in the population. In 2003, this calculated to a population of 16 366 people with learning disabilities in Northern Ireland (McConkey *et al.* 2003).

The number of people with learning disabilities across the UK has been increasingly since the 1960s with an estimated annual rate of increase of 1.2%. The life expectancy of people with learning disabilities has increased considerably in the past 50 years with many people living into their sixties, and although still lower, it is now approaching that of other members of the general population (Cooke 1997). At the other end of the age continuum, children with learning disabilities who may have died as children now more frequently live into adulthood due to advances in and increased accessibility to treatment. At times these children and young adults may have complex health needs, which can lead to an increased need for physical care and support, such as specialist seating equipment, intensive physiotherapy, the availability of suction equipment and enteral feeding.

Given the increasing success in children with profound and severe learning disabilities surviving into adulthood and the increasing life expectancy of adults people with learning disabilities it is expected that the number of people with learning disabilities will continue to rise year on year over the next 10–15 years. It has been projected that the rate of increase will be approximately 1% per year, this will primarily be seen among younger people with profound and severe learning disabilities and the growth in the number of older people with learning disabilities (DH 2001; SE 2000).

The majority of people with learning disabilities continue to live in community-based settings with almost all people under 20 years of age living in their family home, as do about three- quarters of adults with learning disabilities (McConkey *et al.* 2003). Increasingly, people with learning disabilities who move out of their family home seek accommodation in residential accommodation in the local community and a growing number are successfully living within supported living settings (Simons & Watson 1999). However, many adults with learning disabilities are living with older parents or other family carers who are often reluctant to see their son or daughter move into residential accommodation. It has been reported that in Scotland, that a quarter of people with learning disabilities live with a family carer over 65 years of age. Furthermore, 20% of people with learning disabilities have two carers aged 70 or over, and 11% have one carer aged 70 or over (SE 2000).

Changing service principles – but what progress?

The past ten years has seen the unprecedented level of revision in the policies that define how services for people with learning disabilities should be delivered. Policy reviews were published in Scotland under the title of *Same as You?* in 2000, and in England the first major review of learning disability policy in 30 years entitled *Valuing People* was published in 2001. A new framework was presented in Wales during 2002 under the title of *Fulfilling the Promises* (Welsh Office [WO] 2001) and the most recent review in Northern Ireland has been published under the title of *Equal Lives* (DHSSPS 2005). Across these policy reviews, there is a consistent emphasis on the rights of people with learning disabilities to be included as valued citizens in the countries they live in the principles identified to guide future services. The policy reviews within Scotland, England, Wales and Northern Ireland have presented their future vision as a series of service principles (Boxes 14.1 and 14.2).

Box 14.1   Principles identified in policy reviews in the Scotland, England and Northern Ireland since 2000

Scotland: *Same As You?* (SE 2000)

- People with learning disabilities should be valued. They should be asked to and encouraged to contribute to the community they live in. They should not be picked on or treated differently from others.
- People with learning disabilities are individual people.
- People with learning disabilities should be asked about the services they need and be involved in making choices about what they want.
- People with learning disabilities should be helped and supported to do everything they are able to.
- People with learning disabilities should be able to use the same local services as everyone else, wherever possible.
- People with learning disabilities should benefit from specialist social, health and educational services.
- People with learning disabilities should have services which take account of their age, abilities and other needs.

England: *Valuing People* (DH 2001)

- *Legal and civil rights*: The government is committed to enforceable civil rights for disabled people in order to eradicate discrimination in society. All services should treat people with learning disabilities as individuals with respect for their dignity, and challenge discrimination on all grounds including disability. People with learning disabilities will also receive the full protection of the law when necessary.
- *Independence*: The starting presumption should be one of independence, rather than dependence, with public services providing the support needed to maximise this. Independence in this context does not mean doing everything unaided.

Box 14.1   (Continued)

- *Choice*: This includes people with severe and profound disabilities who, with the right help and support, can make important choices and express preferences about their day-to-day lives.
- *Inclusion*: Inclusion means enabling people with learning disabilities to do those ordinary things, make use of mainstream services and be fully included in the local community.

These principles were revised by the DH (England) in 2007.

- Personalisation – so that people have real choice and control over their lives and services
- What people do during the day (and evenings and weekends) – helping people to be properly included in their communities, with a particular focus on paid work
- Better health – ensuring that the NHS provides full and equal access to good quality health care
- Access to housing – housing that people want and need with a particular emphasis on home ownership and tenancies
- Making sure that change happens and the policy is delivered – including making partnership boards more effective

Northern Ireland: *Equal Lives* (DHSSPS 2005)

- *Citizenship*: People with learning disabilities are individuals first and foremost and each has a right to be treated as an equal citizen

- *Social Inclusion*: People with a learning disability are valued citizens and must be enabled to use mainstream services and be fully included in the life of the community

- *Empowerment*: People with a learning disability must be enabled to actively participate in decisions affecting their lives

- *Working Together*: Conditions must be created where people with a learning disability, families and organisations work well together in order to meet the needs and aspirations of people with a learning disability.

- *Individual Support*: People with a learning disability will be supported in ways that take account of their individual needs and help them to be as independent as possible

---

Box 14.2   Principles that underpin the vision of future services for people with learning disabilities in Wales (WO 2001)

- Provide comprehensive and integrated services to achieve social inclusion
- Be person-centred
- Improve empowerment and independence
- Ensure effortless and effective movements between services and organisations at different times of life
- Be holistic in approach and delivery taking fully into account an individual's preferences, hopes and lifestyle.
- Ensure that a range of appropriate advocacy services is available for people who wish to use them
- Be accessible – in terms of both service users and their carers and families having full information
- Have fully developed collaborative partnerships to deliver flexible services
- Services should be developed on evidence of their effectiveness and transparency about their costs
- Be delivered by a competent, well-informed, well-trained and effectively supported and supervised workforce
- The early completion of the National Assembly's resettlement programmes to enable all people with learning disabilities to return to live in the community

A report published four years after *Valuing People*, which presented the findings of a review of information from government departments and service providers, concluded that after considering the responses received that there had been progress towards the implementation of the *Valuing People* policy including:

- People are being listened to more
- Person-centred planning, done properly, makes a difference in people's lives
- The *Supporting People* programme has helped many more people live independently
- Direct payments are helping to change people's lives
- Organisations are working together better at a local level (Valuing People Support Team [VPST] 2005, p. 6).

However, it was also noted that change was not universal and in particular more work was needed to support people in ethnic minority communities. In responding to the report the DH (2007, pp.16,17) noted that:

- There has been good progress in many areas but disappointing change in others
- Getting some mainstream services to be properly inclusive of people with learning disabilities has been difficult
- Too many people and organisations have failed to deliver on the policy promises
- Where change has happened, some people now feel it is getting difficult to move on to the next stage of change

To put things another way in the language of the original evaluation

'Big change is only happening where people wanted it to happen and were willing to listen to why people with learning disabilities must be seen and treated as equal citizens. In some other places, little has changed. Put bluntly, too many people in public services see *Valuing People* as being "optional" – something they can get away with not doing.'

(VPST 2005, p. 6)

The report concluded that the major challenge to be overcome was to 'make sure that everyone takes the lives of people with learning disabilities a lot more seriously' (VPST 2005, p. 7).

Time to reflect?

Further evidence of the limited process made was repeatedly highlighted during 2006 and 2007. During that time several independent investigative reports have been published which highlighted the poor quality of care which had components of institutional abuse and promoting dependency in some services within newer models of services, including dispersed community housing, respite care, services for people who presented challenges to services and day activities (Healthcare Commission/Commission for Social Care Inspection 2006, Healthcare Commission 2007a,b.) These reports have further criticised the governance arrangements in place and the attention given to assessing, planning, implementing and evaluating care within services; one has challenged and criticised the actions of the body responsible for undertaking regulation and quality of services as not being effective (Regulation and Quality Improvement Authority 2007).

These reports should be a reality check for people working in services for people with learning disabilities and impress on them the need for attention to person-centred care that focuses on the individual and does not become complacent about how much 'new' services have improved from the previous long-stay hospital services. There continues to be a need for nurses in community services to pay attention to all stages of the nursing process from assessment through to the evaluation of care, taking seriously their advocacy role in supporting people with learning disabilities and their professional accountability for actions and omissions as nurses. The implications of failing to do so are clearly visible within reports issued in 2006 and 2007, which bear unsettling similarities to the reports that criticised the long-stay hospitals in the 1960s and 1970s, such as Ely and Normansfield. The recent reports have clearly demonstrated that the removal of large hospitals and congregated living settings has not removed the risk of institutionalisation, as this not require a large hospital, if the essential ingredients of depersonalisation, 'block treatment', and failure to recognise the value of each person as a citizen are present in any service, including community teams that do not have residential services.

Moving forward

Despite the limitations highlighted in the previous reports referred to, much as been learnt about what characterises a 'good service'. The Healthcare Commission noted that it can be difficult to work in services for people with learning disabilities, and that in their review of 154 services (of which six were found to have safety concerns requiring immediate actions) that succeeded in providing a quality service as reported by people with learning disabilities had the following characteristics (HCC 2007b, p. 5):

- Placed people with learning disabilities at the centre of care, particularly in relation to planning for their care and helping them to make choices
- Provided care in an attractive environment
- Had clear arrangements for safeguarding
- Provided access to independent advocacy services
- Were open to internal and external scrutiny, with the organisations' leaders playing an important role in this
- Had good practices in place for the training of staff.

In response to the review of progress to date in implementing *Valuing People*, revised priorities for the implementation of *Valuing People* over the next three years was published in December 2007 for a three-month consultation period (see Table one for a summary of these priorities).

A central theme running across all policy reviews within the UK, including the most recent reports noted above is the need to make the inclusion of people with learning disabilities as equal citizens in society a reality. Inclusion emphasises the rights to people with learning disabilities as citizens of their respective countries and as citizens their entitlement to the same

services as all other citizens. Inclusion challenges the need for people with learning disabilities to meet extra conditions/criteria to use community facilities, make decisions about their lives or to receive the same services as other members of the local population. In delivering an inclusive service, people with learning disabilities 'must be seen as valued citizens and must be fully included in the life of the community (e.g. education, employment and leisure, integration in living accommodation and the use of services and facilities not least in the field of health and personal social services)' (DHSSPS 2005).

The respect of citizenship means that community nurses will have to further develop their knowledge and skills in the establishment of anti-discriminatory practice. This is a legal requirement, rather than an 'optional extra' (VPST 2005). Over the past few years there have been implications from major changes in legislation such as the implementation of the Disability Discrimination Act 1995 which covered access to areas such as goods, services and employment, together with the acceptance of the European Convention on Human Rights into UK law in 1997 and the corresponding Human Rights and capacity-based legislation. This requires a considerable shift in emphasis in which the onus is on professionals, members of the public and local communities to make reasonable adjustments to accommodate people with learning disabilities, instead of the previous emphasis on people with learning disabilities having to 'fit in' to existing structures. Failure to make reasonable adjustments may be challenged as unlawful discrimination. The implementation of legislation such as the Disability Discrimination Act and the Human Rights Act are being used to further support to move towards development of inclusive services.

Another particular focus in policy reviews has been the need to deliver services in a person-centred manner and the need to promote choice for people with learning disabilities. The development of clearer policies in relation to consent to examination, treatment and care, as well as legislation covering capacity in Scotland and England further reinforce the need to clear steps to be taken to include people with learning disabilities in all decisions that affect them to the degree to which this is possible, with each decision being treated separately, in so far as someone may be able to make a decision about day activities, but not surgery, and this should be accommodated. The starting point is the expectation that people will be involved, with the onus on services to make this a possibility, and only when efforts taken and reasonable adjustments have been made that have not been successful, should a best interests pathway be followed and the decision taking by others. Attention will also need to be given to the criteria for informed consent in order to ensure that the procedures involved in providing information to people with learning disabilities and including them in overall decision-making process is consistent with these guidelines. This is consistent with the expectations of citizenship, inclusion and a holistic model to services. A particular challenge in making active involvement in decision-making a reality is access to information for people with learning disabilities. While considerable progress has been made in increasing the amount of accessible information available, the lack of information, particularly about health care and health services continues to be highlighted as a gap in services. Overcoming this will require a focus on the provision of information in a manner accessible to a person's individual abilities and needs.

The health of people with learning disabilities

The need to improve the health of people with learning disabilities continues to be identified as a major challenge to future services (DRC 2006; Healthcare Commission 2007b; Mencap 2007). There is a body of evidence that has accumulated since the mid-1990s which now conclusively shows that people with learning disabilities have a wide range of unmet health needs. Community nurses for people with learning disabilities have been identified as potentially having a significant role in promoting and maintaining the health of people with learning disabilities (DH 2001). However, in the past few years further evidence has emerged about the

concerns over the access to health care for people with learning disabilities, in particular the risk of diagnostic overshadowing with potentially fatal consequences, due to the lack of coordinated services between primary care, acute secondary care and learning disability services (DRC 2006; Mencap 2007). It is worrying that CNLDs as collaborating partners with primary care and secondary care services, or advocates for people with learning disabilities and their families are largely noticeable by their absence, rather than presence in these reports.

In order to benefit from increased longevity, people with learning disabilities need to be able to maintain a high level of overall health. Physical and mental health is crucial if people are to have a satisfactory quality of life and be able to avail of the developing opportunities for valued social inclusion. However, although the available evidence clearly shows an increasing life expectancy of people with learning disabilities, associated with this is the growing prevalence of physical and mental ill-health. As for other members of the general population, the physical and mental health of people with learning disabilities is influenced by broad factors such as their living and working conditions, their behaviour and way of life, and aspects within their wider environment including the degree of disadvantage or social exclusion they experience (DHSSPS 2002). The influence of several of these factors may be stronger in the lives of people with learning disabilities, for instance, these may be a greater impact from disadvantage and social exclusion arising from higher rates of poverty, unemployment and low educational achievement (Emerson *et al.* 2001; Northway 2001). Limited opportunities for involvement in local community activities arising from a number of factors including lack of awareness of these opportunities, dependence on others for transport (often older carers) and the costs involved can result in people with learning disabilities leading a more sedentary lifestyle. Furthermore, poor nutrition and the long-term use of a large number of medications (polypharmacy) have been identified as particular risk factors among people with learning disabilities (Beange 2002).

In addition to the above factors, the health of people with learning disabilities may be further compromised by co-morbidity in which the presence of particular syndromes or conditions associated with their learning disabilities may increase their likelihood of having physical health problems (e.g. Down's syndrome, epilepsy, associated physical disabilities). The situation for people with learning disabilities may be future compounded by barriers in access to health care facilities and a resultant delay in the detection of their health needs and instigation of effective treatment (DRC 2006; ECNI 2007; Mencap 2007).

Physical health

It is clear that the pattern of morbidity and mortality among people with learning disabilities is altering to become similar to that of the general population, with the increasing longevity of people with learning disabilities considered to be a major contributing factor to these reported changes. There has been an increase in deaths arising from cardiovascular disease, such as stroke and cancers but, at the same time, there has been a reduction in the number of deaths from infections (Hatton *et al.* 2003).

Much debate has taken place in respect of whether the health of people with learning disabilities is comparatively less healthy than that of the general population. Two main strategies have been used to answer this question; the first approach has involved the inclusion of control or comparison groups within research projects investigating the health of people with learning disabilities. In the main these studies have focused on hearing and visual impairments, conditions of the nervous system, skin disorders and obesity. These conditions are more 'visible' and data obtained from observation and measurement can usually be collected to support the presence of these conditions without the need for most intrusive investigations that other conditions may need to confirm their presence. In undertaking a review of comparative studies on the health problems of people with learning disabilities, Jansen *et al.* (2004) located eight studies that they considered robust and included control groups, undertaken since 1995. The evidence

from these studies indicates that people with learning disabilities have increased prevalence rates for epilepsy, diseases of the skin, sensory loss and increased risk of fractures.

A second approach for conditions that require more intrusive investigation or have a lower frequency of occurrence has been the comparison between the reported rates of particular conditions and illness among people with learning disabilities and the national prevalence rates for that condition. The most comprehensive review in this area has been undertaken in relation to cancer among people with learning disabilities. The authors concluded that although the overall prevalence rates of cancer among people with learning disabilities are similar to that of the general population there is evidence of an increased prevalence of particular types of cancer among people with learning disabilities (Hogg *et al.* 2000). Cancers of the stomach and oesophagus, as well as testicular cancer have been reported at rates higher than those present in the general population. Conversely people with learning disabilities appear to have lower rates for lung, breast, urinary tract and prostate cancers (Cooke 1997; Duff *et al.* 2001; Patja *et al.* 2001). Irrespective of whether to overall rates for the above conditions are higher among people with learning disabilities, there is growing evidence of unmet health needs among people with learning disabilities in a number of areas (Table 14.1).

Mental health

A review of available studies found reported prevalence rates of mental health problems (excluding challenging behaviour) among adults with learning disabilities range from 25% to 40% (Emerson *et al.* 2001). This compares with rates of 15–25% for adults without learning disabilities. A recently published population-based study reported prevalence rates of mental health problems among children with learning disabilities as 39% compared with a rate of 8.1% for children who did not have learning disabilities (Emerson 2003).

A consistent finding across studies investigating the mental health of people with learning

Table 14.1 Overview of the findings of health screening projects in the UK and internationally (Cassidy *et al.* 2002; Hatton *et al.* 2003; Horwitz *et al.* 2000; Hunt *et al.* 2001; Turner & Moss 1996)

Area of health screen	Examples of conditions detected
Optical/visual impairments	Reduced vision, need for prescription glasses, cataracts, eye infections
Ear, nose and throat	Hearing loss, ear wax
Dermatology	Eczema, psoriasis, dry skin
Mobility problems	Arthritis, obesity, foot problems
Dental health	Problems with teeth, gums and mouth ulcers
Sexual health	Menstrual problems, testicular and breast anomalies
Cardiovascular	Obesity, hypertension
Endocrine	Diabetes, thyroid problems
Gastrointestinal	Pain and discomfort, reflux problems, peptic ulcers, constipation
Continence problems	Reduced continence, urinary tract infections, pain and discomfort

disabilities is that a wide range of mental health problems, similar to that found among the general population, can be present. In addition, on occasions the presentation of the mental health problems among people with learning disabilities may be atypical due to their level of verbal and cognitive abilities. Furthermore, some mental health problems may be over-prevalent among people with learning disabilities, including affective disorders, phobic states and dementia (Hassiotis *et al.* 2003). In children similar rates have been reported for depressive disorders, eating disorders and psychosis, with higher rates reported for conduct disorders, anxiety disorders, hyperkinesis, and pervasive developmental disorders (Emerson 2003). While any attempt to provide definitive prevalence rates of mental illness among people with learning disabilities comes up against a number of difficulties it is clear that children and adults with learning disabilities do develop mental health problems and at a higher rate that members of the general population (Foundation for People with Learning Disabilities [FPLD] 2002; Fraser & Kerr 2003).

Action to promote and maintain the health of people with learning disabilities is likely to become an increasing area of work for community nurses, both in relation to the direct care they provide and the need for more effective collaboration with staff in mainstream primary, care, acute general hospitals and mental

health services. Research on the role of community nurses demonstrates that they have already taken steps to improve the health status of people with learning disabilities, among a range of other roles they fulfil in present services. However, despite this process many mental health services available to other members of the general public continue to present barriers for people with learning disabilities wishing to access services and do not seem to have made the process towards inclusive services that has been achieved within primary care and secondary acute services (DHSSPS 2005; FPLD 2002).

What community nurses for people with learning disabilities do – the emerging evidence base

The first research papers on the role of the CNLD appeared in the late 1980s (Mackay 1989), with several others published since that time. The findings from these studies show that CNLDs report that they have a reasonably consistent range of reasons for visiting people with learning disabilities. These include support in responding to the presence of challenging behaviour, mental health problems, physical disability, epilepsy, and sensory disability (Jenkins & Johnson 1991; Mackay 1989). More recently the degree of community nurse support for issues relating to physical care needs, issues associated with people with learning disabilities growing older, and sexuality appear to becoming more prevalent (Parahoo & Barr 1996). It is also noted that although the majority of people with learning disabilities visited by community nurses are adults, community nurses are also actively involved with people with learning disabilities across a wide age range from young children through to people with learning disabilities who are over 60 years of age.

Mobbs *et al.* (2002) used postal questionnaires, this time to managers of community learning disabilities services across 170 National Health Service (NHS) trusts in England and obtained responses from 136 NHS trusts (81%). This study showed that 99% of NHS trusts responding employed one or more CNLD. However, it is clear from the information provided on clinical grades which range from A to I that this survey sought information on all nurses working in community learning disability services. It was reported that 44% of NHS trusts employed support staff at B grade, while staff at clinical grades D, E, F, G, and H were employed by 12%, 57%, 30%, 97% and 43% of NHS trusts, respectively, but no information was provided on the numbers of staff employed at each grade or grade mixture within individual services. Mobbs *et al.* (2002) outlined the increasing range of specific posts within community nursing services for people with learning disabilities and reported the presence of dedicated clinical posts in the following percentage of NHS trusts surveyed: challenging behaviour (27%), child health (25%), epilepsy (20%) and forensic (18%). However, despite these developments, this study also reported that CNLDs were not employed to work with children less than 5 years of age, or between 6 and 19 years of age in 27% and 21% of NHS trusts, respectively. They also reported that 18% of NHS trusts provided an out-of-hours or on call service.

The top ten areas of clinical practice as identified by the managers on the basis of the time they felt allocated by nurses were:

- Assessment
- Advice and support
- Health monitoring (on-going)

- Nursing care
- Counselling
- Health promotion
- Clinical procedures
- Health screening (assessment)
- Crisis intervention
- Client reviews

While this study provides an overview from the perspective of managers, it does not provide information on the composition of services or the function of nurses within individual services. The authors also acknowledge that the views of managers may not reflect the views of individual community nurses in practice settings. It is also appears that all nurses working with community services for people with learning disabilities have been considered as a homogeneous group, despite the range of specific posts identified, which will impact on the activities the individual nurses will undertake.

In a qualitative study into the role of CNLDs, Boarder (2001) interviewed 20 experienced CNLDs (more than five years experience as a CNLD in Wales about the key aims and features of their role. Participants reported caseloads of between 15 and 35 clients, three working with children and 17 with adults. In the analysis of the interview data a number of main themes were identified pertaining to the role of community nurses. Participants highlighted the increasing health focus on the community nurses and the continuing development of dedicated clinical posts, such has those reported by Mobbs *et al.* (2002).

They reported an emphasis on place interdisciplinary teamwork, and a wide range of tasks undertaken by community nurses was identified. These highlighted the role of community nurses in working with people with learning disabilities in relation to health maintenance and responding to specific physical and mental health difficulties they may experience. Community nurses also had key roles in respect of assessment, advocacy, assisting to maintain people with learning disabilities in a range of community settings, supporting people who present with behaviours that challenge skills development and personal relationships. Unfortunately the findings of this study may be confounded by the fact that two nurses were not registered learning disability nurses and four nurses (20% of sample), although working in the community, did not work as part of community learning disability nursing teams, but rather in two residential settings, one in a challenging behaviour service and one within a case management team (Boarder 2002).

The views that other professionals within community learning disability teams had of CNLDs was explored by Mansell & Harris (1998). They used postal questionnaires to collect information from a range of 96 professionals (including 32 nurses) working in community learning disability teams in south Wales and achieved a response rate of 83%. Respondents identified the top five skills of nurses to be:

- Client-based interventions
- Coordination and planning of care
- Training
- Care management
- Health promotion

The authors reported that the majority of respondents (74 of the 96) indicated that if the registered nurse for people with a learning disability was not a team member, another professional could not undertake their role.

Powell *et al.* (2004) reported similar support for the role undertaken by community learning disability nurses working within community-based residential services. In a questionnaire-based survey of 40 staff, the top five areas reported as part of the role of community nurses were consultancy, assessment, treatment, training and promoting access to services, care planning and health promotion. The need to improve communication with other services and take further action to promote the health of people with learning disabilities were identified as two areas that the services provided by community nurses could be further improved upon. Overall, the respondents rated the community nursing service as effective and valued the broad and varied role that community nurses undertook.

These developments in the role of community nurses are further evidenced in published papers on individual service developments that provide detail of similar developments (Barr *et al.* 1999; Cassidy *et al.* 2002; Hunt *et al.* 2001; Martin 2003; Meehan *et al.* 1995). Overall, emerging research knowledge about the role of CNLDs demonstrates a continued wide-ranging role and also notes an increasing focus on health-orientated practice, accompanied by an increasing number of people appointed into dedicated clinical posts. These studies also provide a growing body of evidence as to the value attached to the role of community nurses by other heath and social care professionals, in particular the importance attached to the comprehensive knowledge and package of skills community nurses have, to work with people with learning disabilities across a wide range of tasks (Mansell & Harris 1998; Stewart & Todd 2001).

While the above research findings do show considerable progress in the development of the role of CNLDs, there also identify four challenges that need to be considered in developing future services were also reported. First, the emphasis on trying to justify the role of the CNLD by reducing it into tasks undertaken, risks missing the key value of a CNLD, which should be evaluated on the basis on the totality of their role performance and productivity. Individually, each of the discrete skills can be found in other professionals in the community and among other carers, but it is the combination of knowledge, skills and expertise that is the contribution of CNLDs to the services. Second, there appears to have been a reduction in the number of community nurses who work with children with learning disabilities, as it has been reported that up to quarter of CNLDs in England do not work with children under 5 years of age and one-fifth do not work with children under the age of 16 years old (Mobbs *et al.* 2002). Third, there continues to be a lack of recognition and understanding by staff in mainstream services as to the role of the CNLDs and the need for greater role clarity within learning disability services. Finally, there is a need to keep under review the impact that the development of dedicated clinical posts and care management/coordination types of post have, as distinct from engaging in direct caseload work with individuals, on the access to these services for people with learning disabilities and fragmentation of services, and the effect this has on the role of the domiciliary CNLD.

The future role of community nursing services for people with learning disabilities

A review of the structure of nurse education within the UK tends to arise about once every decade and within this the question is asked as to whether learning disability nursing is required as a separate branch of nursing. Once again in this decade, during 2006 the Nursing and Midwifery Council launched a consultation of the future of pre-registration nursing and although not yet complete, it is likely that it will find that, as did previous reviews in the past 30 years, learning disability nursing is a required pathway with pre-registration nursing within the UK. Building on the reports discussed earlier in this chapter, the direction of the future role of CNLD services appears clearly to be within a more health-orientated framework than was previously the situation and developments within this area have been noted across the UK. The future CNLD role will be different in a number of ways from the previous role, namely:

- More work with people with complex physical and mental health needs
- A greater role in facilitating access to primary, secondary and tertiary care services
- A refocusing on the role and contribution of the 'nursing' component of the CNLD role and an increased 'throughput' in CNLD caseloads with more effective admission and discharge procedures

Existing services in many areas continue to be characterised by either perceived 'medical' or 'social' models of care. At times these models are unfortunately portrayed has having irreconcilable differences and that the medical model is less acceptable in developing services for people with learning disabilities. However, as Thomas & Woods (2003) have highlighted, both models have their strengths and limitations and it is important that a medical model is not mistaken as representing all health care provision. Evidence has clearly shown a high level of unmet health need among people with learning disabilities and action must be taken to address this (DRC 2006; Mencap 2007). Future services will be required to become more holistic and accommodate a broader 'health' perspective. Health is holistic in nature as it encompasses physical, psychological and social aspects as well as primary, secondary and tertiary aspects. The emphasis should be on comprehensive holistic assessment of an individual's abilities and needs while giving due recognition to their social circumstances (Valuing People Support Team 2005). A holistic model of health such as that proposed by Seedhouse (1986) who defined health as 'the set of conditions which fulfil or enable a person to work to fulfil his or her realistic chosen and biological potentials' (p. 61), is consistent with services principles identified as guiding future services for people with learning disabilities and is in keeping with the need for increase inter-disciplinary and inter-agency collaboration.

The assessment of health requires inter-disciplinary collaboration in the completion of comprehensive assessments. The key rationale for a comprehensive assessment is the bringing together the thoughts of the main people involved. Each professional inputs into the assessment either with a specific assessment instrument or as part of the process of joint assessments with other people. Nursing assessments can provide important information, on which future decisions will be based, and it is essential that nursing assessments are grounded in nursing models. Community nurses must be careful to match the assessment instrument/strategy they choose to the individual needs of the person with learning disabilities. Following the completion of a nursing assessment, nurses will be able to contribute to a comprehensive assessment. Failure to complete a 'nursing' assessment and instead relying only on limited information obtained in some broader-ranging but more superficial assessments considerably weakens the nursing contribution to a comprehensive assessment (Barr & Devine 2006).

As more people with learning disabilities have their health needs met within primary care and other mainstream services, CNLDs will increasingly become a secondary specialist service working with people with more complex needs than can be meet within mainstream services alone. This will involve the continued need for frequent visits to people with learning disabilities and their families together with close liaison with other support services that are being provided. Community nurses will need to develop closer links with services such as community children's services, staff in dedicated clinical posts such as behaviour support, epilepsy services, mental health and child and adolescent psychiatry services, primary care, acute hospitals and at times palliative care services. Collaborative working in which some joint visits, as well as the exchange of knowledge and skills, will need to be further developed to move beyond the separateness of some of these services, which now often work in comparative isolation from each other with differing priorities, aims and objectives. While this does not necessarily require community nurses to be physically based within primary and acute care services, at the very least it requires the development of more formal links between nurses and other professionals in learning disability and primary care services. For instance, CNLDs could attend local community nurse meetings within their trust and forge links with nursing colleagues or be nominally attached to general practices and develop effective liaison with local acute general hospitals. Actively promoting these links will increase the opportunities for CNLDs to make positive contributions in collaboration with other community nursing services to the lives of people with learning disabilities and their families. In relation to adults with learning disabilities, such links will assist in overcoming barriers to accessing primary and acute care services for the increasing number of people with learning disabilities who need to access such services. In contrast, the continued 'isolation' of community nurses within separate learning disability and social work networks will do little to inform other nursing colleagues of their role and possible contributions.

While it is important that more people become aware of the possible contribution of CNLD services, the admission to the people to caseloads should be more effectively managed and prioritised (Barr & Devine 2006; Caffery & Todd 2002). Only on the completion of a nursing assessment and consideration by the CNLD of the contribution they can make in relation to specific nursing objectives should an individual be admitted to a CNLD caseload. This is not to argue against the need for person-centred planning approaches, and it is strongly believed that nursing assessments should contribute to person-centred planning discussions. However, it is not acceptable professionally that nurses should become involved in nursing care that is not based on a nursing assessment. Nor is it acceptable to deliver nursing care to people and not record this intervention, for instance in case of the nurses who have direct involvement with people not on their nursing caseload. While it is recognised that nurses may be asked for advice and support it is recommended that a note (not necessarily a complete file) be kept of this interaction. Such changes as outlined above are likely to require a revision of nursing assessments to ensure these reflect current approaches to nursing assessment and are suitable to CNLD services. More specific nursing assessment and determination of nursing needs will also go some way to removing the vagueness and uncertainties around the role of the CNLD (Boarder 2001).

When a nursing assessment identifies no nursing need (defined as a need identified within a structured nursing assessment undertaken by a registered nurse), this should be communicated to the referring professional and alternative services can then be sought by them. It should not fall to the CNLD to fill the gap in existing services by responding to non-nursing needs; rather this should be identified as an unmet need and dealt with by the person making the referral through local arrangements for responding to such needs. A more focused approach to nursing assessment will contribute to smoother admission processes and to more effective discharge procedures. It follows that if an individual is admitted to a nursing caseload with specific identified objectives then once these objectives are achieved the person could be potentially discharged. However, in order for this to happen there is a need for comprehensive discharge policies that clearly provide procedures to staff, as evidence exists that without such policies that address staff concerns they will not discharge clients (Caffery & Todd 2002; Walker *et al.* 2003). CNLDs should start this process by reviewing the nursing needs of all people they have infrequent contact with (less than once a month) and determine what the current nursing needs are that justify retaining these people on a CNLD caseload. If the need identified is primarily one of monitoring health (physical or mental), steps should be taken to work collaboratively with primary care services towards a situation when they undertake this monitoring as they would for other members the community with ongoing health needs.

Conclusion

The role of CNLDs has altered considerably in the past few years and is becoming increasingly health focused. Community nurses continue to work with people who have a wide range of abilities and needs, however there are some indications that a particular emphasis on their future role will be with people who have increasingly complex physical and mental health needs. CNLDs must remain cognisant of the core values within policy reviews, the limitations of services highlighted within recent independent reviews (Healthcare Commission/ Commission for Social Care Inspection 2006; Healthcare Commission 2007a,b) and take seriously their role to support people with learning

disabilities and their families through the provision of high-quality, person focused and coordinated services.

The continued development of CNLD services requires the commitment of community nurses, their immediate managers and those managers within the services responsible for agreeing service structures and policies. Services planners need to consider how the comprehensive package of skills that a CNLD brings to community services can be most effectively used within services that seek to take forward services for people with learning disabilities in line with revised principles that should underpin future services. Equally there is also a need for CNLDs to recognise that although the role they have performed for many years has been valued, it also will need to evolve further if it is to continue to be of value to people with learning disabilities and their families.

References

Barr, O., Devine, M. (2006) Care planning in community learning disability nursing. In: *Care Planning and Delivery in Intellectual Disability Nursing* (ed. B. Gates). Blackwell Science, London, 212–238.

Barr, O., Gilgunn, J., Kane, T. & Moore, G. (1999) Health screening for people with learning disabilities by a community nursing service in Northern Ireland. *Journal of Advanced Nursing*, **29**, 1482–1491.

Beange, H. (2002) Epidemiological issues. In: *Physical Health of Adults with Intellectual Disabilities* (eds V.P. Prasher & M. Janicki). Blackwell Publishing/ IASSID, London.

Boarder, J. (2001) *Perceptions of Experienced Community Learning Disability Nurses of their Roles and ways of Working: An Exploratory Study.* Report for Welsh National Board Training Research Fellowship.

Boarder, J.H. (2002) The perceptions of experienced community learning disability nurses of their roles and ways of working: an exploratory study. *Journal of Learning Disabilities*, **6**, 281–296.

Caffery, A. & Todd, M. (2002) Community learning disability teams: the need for objective methods of prioritisation and discharge planning. *Health Services Management Research*, **15**, 223–231.

Cassidy, G., Martin, D.M., Martin G.H.B. & Roy, A. (2002) Health checks for people with learning disabilities: community learning disability teams working with general practitioners and primary care teams. *Journal of Learning Disabilities*, **6**, 123–136.

Cooke, L.B. (1997) Cancer and learning disability. *Journal of Intellectual Disability Research*, **41**, 312–316.

Department of Health (2001) *Valuing People. A New Strategy for Learning Disability for 21st century.* Department of Health, London.

Department of Health (2007) *Valuing People Now. From Progress to Transformation.* Department of Health, London.

Department of Health, Social Services and Public Safety (2002) *Investing in Health.* Department of Health, Social Services and Public Safety, Belfast.

Department of Health, Social Services and Public Safety (2005) *Equal Lives: Report of Learning Disability Committee.* Department of Health, Social Services and Public Safety, Belfast.

Duff, M., Hoghton, M., Scheepers, M., Cooper, M. & Baddeley, P. (2001) Helicobacter pylori: has the filler escaped from the institution? A possible cause of increased stomach cancer in a population with intellectual disability. *Journal of Intellectual Disability Research*, **45**, 219–225.

Emerson, E. (2003) Prevalence of psychiatric disorders in children and adolescents with and without intellectual disability. *Journal of Intellectual Disability Research*, **47**, 51–58.

Emerson, E., Hatton, C., Felce, D. & Murphy, G. (2001) *The Fundamental Facts.* Foundation for People with Learning Disabilities, London.

Foundation for People with Learning Disabilities (2002) *Count Us. In: The Report of the Committee of Inquiry into Meeting the Mental Health Needs of Young People with Learning Disabilities.* Foundation for People with Learning Disabilities, London.

Fraser, W. & Kerr, M. (eds) (2003) *Seminars in the Psychiatry of Learning Disabilities*, 2nd edition. Gaskell Press, London.

Hassiotis, A., Tyrer, P. & Oliver, P. (2003) Psychiatric assertive outreach and learning disability services. *Advances in Psychiatric Treatment*, **9**, 368–373.

Hatton, C., Elliot, J. & Emerson, E. (2003) Key highlights of research evidence on the health of people with learning disabilities. Personal Social Services Research, University of Kent, Canterbury.

Healthcare Commission (2007a) *Investigation into the Service for People with Learning Disabilities Provided by Sutton and Merton Primary Care Trust.* Healthcare Commission, London.

Healthcare Commission (2007b) *A Life Like No Other: A National Audit of Specialist Inpatient Healthcare Services for People with Learning Difficulties in England.* Healthcare Commission, London.

Healthcare Commission/Commission for Social Care Inspection (2006) *Joint Investigation into the Provision of Services for People with Learning Disabilities at Cornwall Partnership NHS Trust.* Healthcare Commission, London.

Hogg, J., Northfield, J. & Turnbull, J. (2000) *Cancer and People with Learning Disabilities.* British Institute of Learning Disabilities, Kidderminster.

Horwitz, S., Kerler, B.D., Owens, P. & Zigler, E. (2000) *The Health Status and needs of Individuals with Mental Retardation.* Yale University, Connecticut.

Hunt, C., Wakefield, S., Hunt, G. (2001) Community nurse learning disabilities – a case study of the use of an evidence-based health screening tool to identify and meet health needs of people with learning disabilities. *Journal of Learning Disabilities*, **5**, 9–18.

Jansen, D., Krol, B., Groothof, J. & Post, D. (2004) People with intellectual disabilities and their health problems: a review of comparative studies. *Journal of Intellectual Disability Research*, **48**, 93–102.

Jenkins, J. & Johnson, B. (1991) Community nursing learning disability survey. In: *The Community Mental Handicap Nurse-Specialist Practitioner in the 1990's* (ed. P. Kelly, pp. 39–54). Mental Handicap Nurses Association, Penarth.

Mackay, T. (1989) A community nursing service analysis. *Nursing Standard*, **4**, 32–35.

Mansell, I. & Harris, P. (1998) Role of the registered nurse learning disability within community support teams for people with learning disabilities. *Journal of Learning Disabilities for Nursing, Health and Social Care*, **2**, 190–195.

Martin, G. (2003) Annual health reviews for patients with severe learning disabilities: five years of a combined GP/CLDN Clinic. *Journal of Learning Disabilities*, **7**, 9–22.

McConkey, R., Spollen, M. & Jamison, J. (2003) *Administrative Prevalence of Learning Disability in Northern Ireland. A Report to the Department of Health, Social Services and Public Safety.* DHSSPS, Belfast.

Meehan, S., Moore, G. & Barr, O. (1995) Specialist services for people with learning disabilities. *Nursing Times*, **91**, 33–35.

Mencap (2007) *Death by Indifference.* Mencap, London.

Mobbs, C., Hadley, S., Wittering, R. & Bailey, N.M. (2002) An exploration of the role of the community nurse, learning disability, in England. *British Journal of Learning Disabilities*, **30**, 13–18.

Northway, R. (2001) Poverty as a practice issue for learning disability nurses. *British Journal of Nursing*, **10**, 1186–1192.

Parahoo, K. & Barr, O. (1996) Community mental handicap nursing services in Northern Ireland: a profile of clients and selected working practices. *Journal of Clinical Nursing*, **5**, 211–228.

Patja, K., Eero, P. & Iivanainen, M. (2001) Cancer incidence among people with intellectual disabilities. *Journal of Intellectual Disability Research*, **45**, 300–307.

Powell, H., Murray, G. & McKenize, K. (2004) Staff perceptions of community learning disability nurses' role. *Nursing Times*, **100**, 40–42.

Regulation and Quality Improvement Authority (2007) *Annual Report – 2006–2007*. The Stationery Office, Belfast.

Scottish Executive (2000) *The Same As You? A Review of the Services for People with Learning Disabilities*. Scottish Executive, Edinburgh.

Seedhouse, D. (1986) *Health: Foundations for Achievement*. Wiley, Bristol.

Stewart, D. & Todd, M. (2001) Role and contribution of nurses for people with learning disabilities: a local study in a county of the Oxford-Anglia region. *British Journal of Learning Disabilities*, **29**, 145–150.

Thomas, D. & Woods, H. (2003) *Working with People With Learning Disabilities: Theory and Practice*. Jessica Kingsley Publishers, London.

Turner, S. & Moss, S. (1996) The health needs of adults with learning disabilities and the health of the nation strategy. *Journal of Intellectual Disability Research*, **40**, 438–450.

Valuing People Support Team (2005) *Valuing People: The Story So Far*. Valuing People Support Team, London.

Walker, T., Stead, J. & Read, S.G. (2003) Caseload management in community learning disability teams; influences on decision-making. *Journal of Learning Disabilities*, **7**, 297–321.

Welsh Office (2001) *Fulfilling the Promises*. Welsh Assembly, Cardiff.

Chapter 15 Advanced Nursing Practice in the Community

Katrina Maclaine

Introduction

Over the past decade, the National Health Service (NHS) has experienced an unprecedented pace of change, providing both challenges and opportunities for nurses. Policy imperatives (Department of Health [DH] 2008a,b; NHS London 2007; Wanless 2007) and future plans for the NHS following its sixtieth year review, mean this trend is likely to continue apace. One key aspect that has enabled nurses to remain at the forefront of developments within the community, is the establishment of advanced nursing roles such as the nurse practitioner (NP), community matron and nurse consultant. However, despite proliferation in numbers, there remains significant debate regarding the nature of advanced practice in nursing, the meaning of the titles that are used and the underpinning education and assessment of competence that is needed to ensure that safe and effective advanced nursing practice is delivered in all of the settings that are embraced within community health care.

This chapter will therefore consider these issues, and with the aid of examples, provide key information that will enable the reader to appreciate the opportunities that are available to advance their practice within the community. Professional issues arising from advanced nursing practice will be highlighted and within this, the proposals for future regulation by the Nursing and Midwifery Council (NMC) reviewed.

Why advanced nursing practice?

There has always been an expectation that the nature and scope of community nurses' practice should evolve to meet the multiple demands that exist within primary care. With this context in mind, it is important to consider the key part that advanced nurses will play in the provision of community-based health care in the future, in addition to their value to the nursing profession as a whole.

When the United Kingdom Central Council (UKCC 1992) published the *Scope of Professional Practice*, the opportunity arose for nurses to extend and expand their practice. No longer were certificates needed to sanction every new activity or task. What mattered was the benefit to patients that could be offered by nurses providing a wider remit of care, as long as the nurse considered themselves to be competent to do so. This precipitated many of the new ways of working that we see in nursing today and was the real catalyst for many nurses to think outside the box regarding what was possible. Subsequently, frameworks to shape nursing careers in the future, such as *Modernising Nursing Careers* (DH 2006a), have identified advanced nursing roles as providing a much needed opportunity for nurses to continue their clinical career, rather than being limited to a choice of management, research or academic roles. The possibilities for new recruits into nursing have expanded to allow opportunities for practice that were unheard of a relatively short time ago, such as partnerships in general practice, truly nurse-led organisations such as walk-in centres (DH 1999a) and Personal Medical Services (PMS) (DH 1997) and nurse consultant positions (DH 1999b). The 'Maxi Nurse' report, produced by the Royal College of Nursing (RCN) and Department of Health (2007) captured the satisfaction that nurses working in advanced roles expressed with their ability to deliver more 'complete packages of care' for their patients as a result of the advancement of their clinical practice.

The trend to capitalise on the knowledge and skills of advanced nurses is also evident internationally. Although not necessarily labelled 'advanced nurses', countries such as Korea, Fiji, Jamaica and Botswana have long-demonstrated the significant roles played by nurses in providing care in areas where there is limited or no medical provision (Schober & Affara 2006). However, probably the main catalyst for global development was the success of advanced nursing roles in the USA. This originated with the development of clinical nurse specialists, nurse midwives and nurse anaesthetists in the 1950s, but it was the emergence of NPs in the mid-1960s that is cited as a key driver in much of the literature on advanced nursing.

The International Council of Nurses (ICN) recognised the global recognition afforded to the advanced practitioner (AP) role and established the International Nurse Practitioner/Advanced Practice Nurse Network (INP/APNN) in 2000 to provide a forum for sharing good practice, research, education and regulatory developments. This is testament to the global advancement of nursing, although it is notable that the nature of advanced nursing roles within individual countries is influenced by their nursing identity and values, the nature of their health care and socio-political context and current priorities. Nevertheless, a review of international developments by Schober & Affara (2006) demonstrated that it is possible to identify drivers that are common across the countries:

- The need to improve access to health care
- Shortage of doctors, particularly in inner city, rural areas and areas of deprivation
- Rising costs of health care
- Greater focus on prevention and community-based care
- Population trends such as an increasingly ageing population
- Epidemiological trends such as the escalating prevalence of long-term conditions such as heart disease and diabetes and the rising incidence of infectious diseases such as tuberculosis and human immunodeficiency virus (HIV)/acquired immune deficiency syndrome (AIDS).

- Inequalities in health and life expectancy
- Rising public expectations for health care
- Recognition of the limitations of applying a traditional 'medical model' to primary care
- Moves to achieve a collaborative patient-centred team approach to care
- The desire for professional advancement of nursing
- Emerging evidence, such as that produced by the World Health Organization (WHO 2002), that optimising the nursing contribution to health care through expanding their role is an effective strategy for improving health care services

These drivers can be applied equally to the UK. After 60 years of provision, the review of the NHS in 2008 (DH 2008a,b) has highlighted that access and availability of health and social care remain one of the main challenges as the complexity of patients needs grows. For example, people are increasingly living with multiple long-term conditions to an older age, meaning that assessment of any new problem cannot take place in isolation, but needs to incorporate consideration of their co-existing physical and psychological health issues, prescribed and over-the-counter medication, and the impact of their home environment, social circumstances and lifestyle. Patients and carers are also generally in a position to be better informed and able to access a variety of resources than ever before. This context demands that some nurses have and, will need increasingly to, develop a sophisticated ability to critically appraise and synthesise a range of information when providing patient care. This raises the important dilemma of what constitutes advanced nursing practice.

What is advanced nursing practice?

Advanced nursing has been discussed within literature and nursing policy since the origins of nursing; as nursing has evolved, so have perceptions of what constitutes advanced practice. It could be argued that in complex and dynamic health care systems, flexibility of approach is key, with variability in interpretation of 'advanced nursing' to be expected. However the

ICN has argued that definitions are fundamental to identifying and placing a profession and the boundaries of their practice within the health care system (Styles & Affara 1997). In acknowledgement of this, the ICN INP/APNN has therefore worked to achieve a consensus international definition for advanced nursing (to embrace NPs and other advanced nursing practice roles) that would foster common international understanding, support countries in the early stages of role development and foster unity around the emerging role. The ICN definition states that the NP/advanced practice nurse is:

'a registered nurse who has acquired the expert knowledge base, complex decision-making skills and clinical competencies for expanded practice, the characteristics of which are shaped by the context and/or country in which s/he is credentialed to practice. A master's degree is recommended for entry level.'

(ICN 2002)

The ICN has subsequently produced guidance – *The Scope of Practice, Standards and Competencies of the Advanced Practice Nurse* (ICN 2008) to support and inform international developments, in recognition of advanced nursing as a global phenomenon. However, this ICN work has not been formally adopted within the UK and a national consensus on advanced nursing practice remains elusive. Analysis of the literature and professional discourse suggests that there appear to be four strands of discussion within the on-going debate; the quest to establish the features of advanced nursing that differentiate it from first level nursing and the place of autonomous practice within this, the relationship between advanced and specialist practice, which nursing roles would be considered to fall under the advanced nursing umbrella and significantly, whether advanced nursing is in any way different from advanced practice exhibited by other health care professions.

Advanced nursing versus nursing

A review of the literature (such as Bryant-Lukosius *et al.* 2004; Daly & Carnell 2003; Distler 2006; Gardner *et al.* 2004; Hamric 2005; Maclaine

et al. Embracing nurse practitioners within the post-registration regulatory framework, 2004 [unpublished work]; Mantzoukas & Watkinson 2007; McGee & Castledine 2003; Ministry of Health New Zealand 2002; Roberts-Davis & Read 2001; Schober 2004) and some of the various models that have been proposed over the past couple of decades to conceptualise advanced nursing (for example Brown 1998; Hamric 2005; ICN 2008; Scottish CNO Directorate 2008) suggests that the following characteristics are key to advanced nursing practice:

- Depth and breadth of knowledge and experience
- Expertise in case management
- The extent and depth of assessment
- Critical thinking, appraisal and synthesis of information
- Application of clinical judgement
- Use of reflection and reflexivity to inform action
- Application and adaptation of advanced clinical and professional skills in complex and/or unstable situations
- Increased level of responsibility in decision-making
- Autonomous practice
- Referral to and acceptance of referrals from others
- Researcher role
- Evaluation of care delivered by self and others
- Acts in a consultancy capacity
- Educator role
- Provides leadership
- Acts as a role model
- Engages in professional and strategic health care activities
- Acts as a creative change agent and innovator
- And demonstration of an expanded range of competencies to reflect all of the above

Many of these authors describe the use of advanced comprehensive clinical assessment (incorporating history taking and physical examination), diagnostic, treatment planning, implementation (including making prescribing decisions) and evaluation skills, as fundamental to advanced nursing practice. Conway (1996) has previously described this perspective as the medical model approach to advanced nursing practice, which sees the adoption of traditionally medical knowledge and skills as being an indication of the advancement of nursing.

However, critics would suggest that this perpetuates the tradition of medicine handing down tasks to nurses under the guise of advancing nursing (Farmer 1995; MacAlister & Chiam 1995; Manley 1996). Indeed, Roberts (1983) would suggest that this is actually an indication of the continuation of the historical oppression of nursing by medicine, where medical knowledge is viewed as being more important that the more qualitative aspects of nursing knowledge. This stance is reinforced when one considers that many 'advanced nursing' roles have arisen out of a shortage of doctors and restrictions on junior doctors' hours. A common solution in response to the reduced availability of doctors hours has been delegation of 'medical' tasks to nurses, such as clerking in patients, administering intravenous therapy or providing night on-call cover. In this way nurses roles have been 'extended' in that the nurse remains dependent on the medical profession for sanctioning the delegation (Callaghan 2006; Davis 1992). Such nurses could be classed as 'doctor substitutes' or 'mini-doctors' rather than advanced nurses.

A contrasting perspective is held by nursing leaders such as Manley (1997), who have argued that advanced nursing is rooted in a reflective paradigm where the value of the nursing approach, the nature of the nurse–patient relationship, therapeutic use of self, use of advocacy, etc. are key. This has been described as 'expanded' practice in that such nurses would provide a higher level of practice that is routed in nursing (Davis 1992), but this change has occurred independent of and not for the benefit of another profession (Mitchinson 1996). This humanistic perspective of advanced nursing practice is captured within research to identify what is meant by nursing expertise. For example, Jasper (1994) and Conway (1996) have built on Benner's (1984) narrative explanations to suggest that nursing expertise is exemplified by possession of a specialised body of knowledge

or skill, extensive experience in the field of practice, highly developed levels of pattern recognition by synthesising theoretical and experiential knowledge in-action and recognition by others. However, Conway (1996) does usefully highlight that nursing expertise is not a definitive concept and does not exclude the use of technological knowledge such as that needed to form diagnosis, anticipate and monitor the trajectory of a patient's illness and recognise significant signs and symptoms both overtly and intuitively.

Adoption of both approaches has been described as producing a 'maxi-nurse' who is bilingual in both medicine and nursing (Walsh 2006). Research has indicated that this is entirely possible and enables advanced nurses to be more responsive to patients' problems (Barratt 2005; Seale *et al.* 2006). For example, in practice this means being able to fully assess a patient rather than passing them onto a medical colleague only for the patient to have to repeat their story over again. It also means that the advanced nurse can be a more effective educator as they can utilise their greater understanding of disease processes and treatment options to provide a explanations to the patient. It could be argued that this enables a truly holistic approach, and indeed Bates (1990) has highlighted the benefits to the therapeutic relationship that can be afforded by the conduction of a physical examination. Hamric (2000) has gone further to suggest that the incorporation of all the aspects of advanced nursing practice synergistically 'produces a whole that is greater than the sum of its parts' (p. 58), supporting the assertion by authors such as Bryant-Lukosius *et al.* (2004) and Walsh (2006), that purely clinical roles that extend beyond traditional boundaries of nursing practice cannot be categorised as advanced nursing.

Autonomous practice

One key distinguishing feature of advanced nursing practice that is common to all definitions of advanced nursing is that it involves highly autonomous practice. Various definitions of autonomy exist ranging from the 'right to self-govern, personal freedom and freedom of will' (Chiarella 2006) to 'professional practice which is defined, negotiated and developed by individual practitioners who are solely responsible and accountable to the patient and their professional body for their actions and omissions' (Mitchinson 1996). However, Callaghan (2006) has cautioned that autonomy is really a relative term because as Vaughan (1989) has suggested, 'there is a fine line between the freedom to practise autonomously and total freedom of action, which could degenerate into anarchy if we are not careful' (p. 54). Vaughan therefore defines autonomy as 'the freedom to act within the boundaries of competence, which in turn are confined by the boundaries of knowledge' (p. 54), a view that has been subsequently endorsed by writers such as Boyden & Edwards (2007).

One could also say that collaborative decision-making is now the goal involving the health care team and the patient, rather than any one individual independently determining what should or should not be done. However, autonomous practice is not just about what an advanced nurse does, but also their state of mind. Vaughan (1989) has described this as 'attitudinal autonomy' in that the advanced nurse needs to believe themselves to be free to exercise judgement in decision-making and be prepared personally to accept responsibility. This is strengthened by appropriate underpinning knowledge, competence and experience, and is also about self-perception and confidence (Chiarella 2006). Nurses have not traditionally been trained or socialised to manage the uncertainty that comes with operating at a higher level of clinical practice, nor to live with the risk of truly accepting the consequences for their actions (Dimond 2005). Thus nurses themselves may have been unconsciously perpetuating their own inhibitions (Cullen 2000). However, where advanced nurses have taken the risk to display attitudinal autonomy by trusting their judgement, they have felt empowered and motivated by the experience, and levels of job satisfaction have been higher (Cullen 2000; Mauksch 1991).

It is also worth highlighting another aspect of autonomy, namely 'structural autonomy' (Vaughan 1989). In today's reality all health professionals, even doctors, have boundaries to their practice determined by the professional regulation, legal requirements, employment arrangements, evidence-based guidelines, quality assurance processes and financial constraints. The views of the other team members and organisational hierarchy in relation to the health professional and what they should and should not be allowed to do can also be added to this list. Vaughan (1989) has described how a nurse would therefore need to use their judgement within the context in which they work, to be as autonomous as possible. Walsh (2006) illustrates this point with the significant barrier that lack of prescriptive authority placed on nurse's autonomy and therefore their ability to provide complete episodes of care 'independent' from the need for sanctioning of prescribing decisions by medical colleagues. Experienced advanced nurses, who have subsequently gained prescribing rights, have described the added dimension and job satisfaction that this now provides to their patient care. In this example, greater autonomy arose out of hard fought for legislative changes (DH 2004a ; Department of Health and Social Security [DHSS] 1986; Jones & Gough 1997).

Practice-based commissioning also provides opportunities for autonomous practice (DH 2007a). Overall the onus is also on advanced nurses to strive to negotiate to ensure that their employment and collaborative arrangements enable them to be as autonomous as is possible, and similarly to maximise the understanding of their role at all levels within their health care organisation and with all key external stakeholders.

Advanced versus specialist

Another dimension of the debate into advanced nursing practice is how advanced practice and specialist practice relate to each other. At first glance, it might seem relatively easy to differentiate what is meant by the term 'specialist'. As a survey by McGee & Castledine (1999) identified, the term specialist was most commonly used in the 1990s to indicate that the nurse was expected to perform care within a specific sphere, whereas the term advanced seemed to have broader connotations and be applied to new nursing roles where new ideas were being pioneered. Thus terms such as diabetic specialist and asthma specialist are used commonly within community nursing. However, the publication of the UKCC's definition of specialist practice in 1994 precipitated much of the subsequent confusion; it stipulated that this was exemplified by the ability to:

'exercise higher levels of judgement and discretion in clinical care … demonstrate higher levels of clinical decision-making and … be able to monitor and improve standards of care through supervision of practice, clinical nursing audit, developing and leading practice, contributing to research, teaching and supporting professional colleagues.'

(UKCC 1994)

Comparison of this content, with that proposed to denote advanced practice listed earlier, clearly demonstrates that fact that this definition confused a 'level' of practice with the 'specialty' in which care was provided. Many specialist practitioner programmes were subsequently developed on the basis of the UKCC definition. The UKCC at the time, tried to different advanced practice as:

'Advanced practice is concerned with adjusting the boundaries for the development of future practice, pioneering and developing new roles responsive to changing needs and with advancing clinical practice, research and education to enrich professional practice as a whole.'

(UKCC 1994)

However the differentiation between the two is very tenuous. They would appear to suggest that it would be possible to be a specialist and an advanced practitioner at the same time which raises the question; when we talk about advanced nurses are we meaning an advanced nurse who has advanced their practice within one specialty or a nurse who has a broader remit beyond one specialty, who in fact could be described as an advanced generalist, or could it encompass both?

The term 'advanced generalist' has been used to describe nursing roles where the practitioner is required to hold a high level of knowledge and expertise in relation to every system of the body, a very broad range of both acute and long-term problems that can impact on both mental and physical health, and of pharmacological and non-pharmacological interventions to manage a wide variety of conditions. For example, an advanced nurse working within emergency/urgent care, a walk-in centre or general practice could be said to fit this description because they do not focus on one specific disease or client group. In terms of advanced practice for specialist nurses, three different broad categories can be identified:

(1) Existing specialist nurses who wish to develop their practice to an advanced level within their specialism, e.g. asthma/chronic obstructive pulmonary disease (COPD) nurses who develop their knowledge and competence to an advanced level to be able to assess any patient presenting with a respiratory symptom in primary care, and to lead and provide complete packages of care for the majority of the patients with long-term respiratory conditions. Here, their existing expertise within the specialist area is developed further to a higher level to encompass all respiratory problems.

(2) Existing specialist nurses who also wish to develop their practice to an advanced level within their specialism, but in contrast to (1), this is to achieve a high level of expertise within a more specific area, e.g. a rheumatology nurse developing his or her practice to focus on assessment and management of joint pain or an older person's nurse choosing to specialise further to focus on assessing and managing patients with dementia and leading services to improve the care provided for this specific group.

(3) Existing specialist nurses who wish to develop their practice to an advanced level but instead of remaining within one specialist area, choosing to undertake competence-based education that will broaden their focus to develop their ability to function as an advanced generalist as outlined above.

What would be key here to saying that all three are functioning an advanced level, would that they are able to demonstrate the characteristics of advanced practice, listed earlier, within their practice, even though the area of application of these knowledge and skills would vary according to their focus. This illustrates that a core of advanced practice activities can be identified, by which to categorise existing and new nursing roles.

Which roles would come under the umbrella of advanced nursing?

Hamric (1996) has been a key advocate for the concept of a core of competencies that must be demonstrated by any nurse wishing to practise at an advanced level. This was the approach that was taken by the UKCC in its 'Higher Level of Practice' (HLP) project (UKCC 1999) in an attempt to establish a regulatory level beyond initial nursing registration. The competences and assessment criteria, identified by the HLP Steering Group, were tested with almost 700 nurses, midwives and health visitors who volunteered to produce the required portfolio, have their practice reviewed during workplace visits and participated in an interview by a panel of experts. The conclusions identified that a generic standard could be used to identify nurses and midwives working at a higher level of practice, however, questions were raised whether the focus of the standard was sufficiently clinical to serve as a threshold for ensuring safe clinical practice at a higher level (UKCC 2002).

The majority of subsequent discussion and proposed definitions for advanced nursing practice has centred upon the clinical aspects and competence required for that level of practice. This is not surprising, considering the potentially higher risk associated with the wider scope of practice. However, work such as that being conducted in Scotland, as part of the *Modernising Nursing Careers* activities, has highlighted that nurses who do not provide hands-on advanced clinical care as the main remit their role, such as nursing sisters/charge nurses, nursing researches, academics and managers, also demonstrate advanced nursing practice

(NHS Education for Scotland [NES] 2007). The 'Scottish Advanced Practice Toolkit' (Scottish CNO Directorate 2008) has articulated underlying principles to identify advanced practice in non-clinical roles include autonomous practice, critical thinking, high levels of decision-making and problem-solving, values-based care and improving practice. The directorate acknowledges that while it is only the clinical component that may require regulation, the other aspects of the role should also be recognised and valued.

Advanced nursing versus other advanced health care professionals

In reality, nurses are not the only professional that have or will expand their practice and contribute to the development and enhancement of patient care in ways that transcend traditional professional boundaries. Skills for Health (2005) has acknowledged this is its 'Careers Framework for Health', which has been designed to provide guidance for NHS and partner organisations on how roles can be categorised at different levels according to the skills and competences of the individual to thereby provide national consistency with maximum flexibility for local health organisations. The aim will be to demonstrate flexibility of career design and the ability of individual members of staff to progress in a direction that meets workforce, service and individual needs on a 'skills escalator'. Skills for Health (2005) defines an 'Advanced Practitioner' (Level 7) as:

> 'Experienced clinical professionals who have developed their skills and theoretical knowledge to a very high standard. They are empowered to make high-level clinical decisions and will often have their own caseload.'

The key here, as with all of Skills for Health work, is the skills associated with each level are not profession specific, but could apply to any clinically focused health professional, such as a radiographer, physiotherapist, health scientist or a pharmacist, or indeed any allied health professional and not just nurses. It is also worth noting that new roles such as the physician's assistant (DH 2006b) and the emergency care practitioner

(Skills for Health 2006) (as discussed in Chapter 20) have extended this debate in relation to whether their level of their practice should be regarded as advanced.

In acknowledgement of these wider developments, many universities now provide clinically focused advanced practice programmes that are multi-professional to enable health care practitioners to learn together and from each other (Association of Advanced Nursing Practice Educators [AANPE] 2007). This is consistent with the trend for increased opportunities for inter-professional learning (Quality Assurance Agency [QAA] 2000), with the intention that this will enable different professionals to understand each other better, counter existing reductionism and fragmentation of practice and facilitate the valuing of what each brings to collaborative practice, while overcoming negative stereotypes, and thereby ultimately improve practice and patient care (Barr 2002; Schober & McKay 2004; Sullivan 1998).

Do titles matter?

While the debate regarding advanced practice continues, the number of titles used within nursing in the UK continues to escalate, such as 'nurse practitioner', 'advanced nurse practitioner', 'specialist nurse', 'nurse clinician'. What's more, while many policy-makers have criticised nursing for this, they have then created their own titles such as 'modern matron', 'community matron', 'consultant nurse', 'first contact practitioner', 'physician's assistant' and 'primary care assistant practitioner'. The proliferation of titles has resulted in confusion not only for patients and carers, but also for the health professions themselves; precious time that could be spent on patient care and innovation can be lost explaining what the title means and justifying the scope of practice associated with it. However, the answer is not to do away with titles. They do convey meaning to patients and colleagues when used consistently and coherently to mean a specific set of competencies at a designated level of practice, as illustrated by three key advanced nursing roles: the NP, community matron and nurse consultant.

Nurse practitioners – history and development

It is widely recognised that the original pioneers of the NP role in the UK were Barbara Stilwell, who worked in two general practices in Birmingham in the mid-1980s (Stilwell *et al.* 1988), and Barbara Burke-Masters (1986), who worked with homeless men in East London. Both had been encouraged by the successful implementation of the NP role within the USA in the 1960s and the positive impact that this role had had on both patient services and perceptions of the scope of nursing practice. These factors were recognised within the Cumberlege Report (DHSS 1986) which recommended the introduction of NPs to neighbourhood teams of community nurses. The report suggested that NPs, who were appropriately qualified, would be able to receive and deal with direct referrals from the public and address the variety of physical, psychological and social needs experienced by patients presenting within primary care.

In a survey of NPs (Ball 2006) commissioned by the RCN NP association in 2006, results indicated that the majority of NPs who responded worked in general practice, however, NPs are now evident within PMS projects, walk-in centres, urgent care facilities, out-of-hours services, projects to address the needs of marginalised groups such as refugees and asylum seeks, and elderly care facilities, such as nursing homes. Some NPs have become Practitioners with a Special Interest (DH 2006c) in areas such as dermatology and heart failure, whereas others have combined their clinical work with an educational role as lecturer-practitioners. Similarly, nurse partnerships in general practice and new initiatives, such as social enterprise, appear to have provided further opportunities for NPs (Ball 2006). Many GPs have recognised the immense contribution that NPs can make within the community, indeed the British Medical Association (BMA 2002) recommended that NPs be the first point of contact for patients, and some have even advocated for a change in the traditional skill mix to accommodate more NPs within general practice (Bostock 2008). Proposals to extend general practice opening hours have provided a further catalyst for this new thinking.

By way of context, it is worth also noting that the NP survey provided evidence that the need to reduce doctors' working hours and improve continuity within the patient pathway (DH 2004b) has resulted in NP development within secondary and tertiary care settings. To illustrate, NP posts have now been established in emergency departments, minor injury units, medical assessment units, night services and within specialities such as paediatrics, neonates, cancer care, ophthalmology and orthopaedics (Ball 2006).

One of the drivers for on-going development of NPs within the UK has been overwhelmingly positive evidence generated by research. For example, a rigorous multi-site randomised controlled trial comparing NPs with GP provision by Venning *et al.* (2000) and two subsequent systematic reviews (Horrocks *et al.* 2002; Laurant *et al.* 2005) have evaluated the safety and effectiveness of NPs when delivering first contact services. The studies to date have concluded that NPs provide care that is of an equivalent standard to GPs and in some aspects better.

Defining the term nurse practitioner/ advanced nurse practitioner

Despite a growing body of research and proliferation in numbers of NPs within the UK non consensus on a definition has emerged, with extensive debate on-going (NMC 2005a, 2006, 2007; RCN, 2008; Walsh 2006; Willis & Maclaine 2004). The RCN has provided leadership in relation to NPs, with the setting up of the first NP programme in the UK in 1990, provision of a definition in 1996 (RCN 1996), followed by guidance on the standard of practice that should be expected of an NP and standards for accreditation of NP preparation programmes (RCN 2002).

Despite this activity many nurses use the title 'NP' without making any change in their existing role or having undertaken any additional education to enable them to practise safely at an advanced level. This is because the title 'NP' is not formally protected, resulting in widespread misuse by nurses and employers. Patients are not therefore guaranteed any minimum standards of care from a NP, and may in fact be cared for by a NP who is 'unconsciously incompetent' and not 'fit for practice'.

In 2005 the NMC Council concluded from an extensive consultation into the issues of post-registration nursing, that there was a case for establishing a sub-part of the nursing register for nurses who could demonstrate that their practice was of a specific standard, with the title 'advanced nurse practitioner' (ANP) to be adopted for nurses who successfully did so. The intention was not to imply that there should be two levels of NP practice, but rather was to denote specifically within the title, the advanced level at which a NP was expected to work (NMC 2005a). The NMC required approval from the Privy Council before these proposals could go ahead and at the time of writing, it is still waiting for a response. One reason for the apparent delay has been the subsequent review of medical and non-medical regulation following the actions of Shipman, leading to the publication of the White Paper *Trust, Assurance and Safety – the Regulation of Health Professionals* (DH 2007b). Through this, the discussion of regulation at an advanced level has widened to other health professionals.

In the absence of the implementation of a new regulatory framework the RCN (2008) has revised its guidance to make explicit links to NMC activities, such as moving to use of the title 'ANP'. They have defined an ANP, as outlined in Box 15.1, which compares favourably with early NMC work to formulate a 'patient-friendly' definition for an ANP for regulatory purposes. The content within this definition is expanded within the domains and competencies for ANPs (see Box 15.2), which provides a generic standard as the recommended minimum threshold for ANP's working in any health care setting and within all specialities within the UK, mapped against the Knowledge and Skills Framework (KSF) (DH 2004c). These domains and competencies arose from work published by the National Organisation of NP Faculties (NONPF) in the USA (NONPF 2001), which has a long history and extensive experience in formulation of NP competencies, development of standards for NP education and application of these within national frameworks (NONPF 2006a). The NMC, in turn, has utilised these competencies as the basis for its proposed standard for ANP regulation (NMC 2005b).

The competency standard described above have been used by many UK universities as the basis for determining the curricula required to develop ANP's to ensure that this threshold for delivery of safe and effective practice at an advanced level has been achieved and demonstrated by all programme graduates. This standard has also increasingly been used by nurses, other health professionals, employers and workforce planners as a standard that clearly articulates expectations in relation to clinical and professional practice at an advanced level. In this way, the standard has proved to be 'fit for purpose'.

Educational preparation

Early pioneers of the NP role relied on experiential learning to underpin their practice. However, Stilwell recognised the importance of establishing the first NP education programme in the UK, and successfully lobbied the RCN Institute to develop such a curriculum informed by the conclusions from her research into the benefits of the NP role (Stilwell *et al.* 1988). The first intake commenced in 1990, and such was the success of this programme that other universities followed suit by utilising a franchise model to produce graduates with the RCN Nurse Practitioner Diploma. Subsequently all of these NP programme providers went on to revalidate their programmes at BSc level to better reflect the nature of educational input and clinical skills development required commensurate with the RCN definition of an NP at that time (RCN 1996). This was later replaced by an accreditation model with the establishment of the RCN Accreditation Unit (RCN AU).

Accreditation of NP programme

Accreditation can be defined as 'a process of review and approval by which an institution, programme or specific service is granted a time-limited recognition of having met certain established standards beyond those are minimally acceptable' (ICN 1997, p. 41). With the development of the RCN AU in 2002, this model was implemented to make a statement about the quality of the educational preparation of NP graduates to patients, nurses, other health professionals and employers, when compared with 'NPs' who might have only completed a short course or brief in-house training. An international review by Schober & Affara (2006) has supported this approach as being the most commonly used mechanism for external quality assurance of NP education.

Initial RCN AU standards for NP programme accreditation (RCN 2002) were critically appraised (Maclaine, Critical appraisal and revision of the RCN accreditation unit standards for approval of programmes of preparation for nurse practitioners, 2006 [unpublished]) and further developed in 2008 in the light of increased use of distance and blended learning (QAA 2004), publication of NMC specialist community public health standards (NMC 2004), draft proposals for revised curriculum guidelines and programme standards for NP education (NONPF 2006a) and the NMC proposals for future regulation of ANPs (NMC 2005a,b, 2006, 2007). The resultant 15 standards and associated criteria (see Box 15.3) take a multi-faceted

---

> **Box 15.3   List of revised standards for RCN accreditation of ANP educational programmes (RCN 2008)**
>
> (1)   The higher education institution
> (2)   Research and development
> (3)   Meeting workforce requirements
> (4)   Curriculum
> (5)   Physical and learning resources
> (6)   Recruitment and admission
> (7)   Programme management
> (8)   Leadership of the ANP programme
> (9)   Staff resources
> (10) Staff development
> (11) Student support
> (12) Practice experience
> (13) Assessment
> (14) External examiners
> (15) Fitness for award

---

approach, in recognition that programmes have to meet not only academic standards but also professional and clinical requirements, to produce an ANP graduate who is able to demonstrate all of the competencies for practice (Castledine 2003; RCN 2008).

A key determinant of the 'fitness for purpose' of the programme and arguably the most important, given the autonomous approach to patient care, is whether graduates are 'fit for practice' and therefore able to deliver safe, effective patient care. The RCN AU standards try to ensure this by requiring application of both a performance outcome model and the traditional education competence model to the curriculum (Mitchell 2000), made explicit via mapping of the ANP competencies against course learning outcomes. This approach has been validated in a review of the effectiveness of strategies used in different countries where ANP roles and commensurate education have emerged (Schober & Affara 2006). It also endorses Masterson & Mitchell's (2003) recommendation that a combined approach ensures the focus is on what the students need to achieve in their clinical work, while also valuing traditional learning and bridging the oft-perceived gap between education and practice.

The literature emphasises that the process of development of competence for ANPs is also key. For example, Crumbie (2001) and Castledine (2003) have advocated the need for ANP education to develop not only the clinical elements of students' practice, such as history-taking and physical examination skills, but also higher-level reasoning skills and depth of reflective analysis. This might be achieved by using a case study of a presenting patient on which to frame student's learning activity (Neary 2000; Read & Roberts-Davis 2000; Ward & Willis 2007). Similarly, the importance of the clinical environment in which the students knowledge and skills are developed and utilised has been emphasised by the NMC (2004), the QAA (2001) and NONPF (2006a). These aspects highlight the importance of requiring that specific arrangements are utilised with an ANP programme to maximise the impact of practice based activities

(Inman 2003; Maclaine, Critical appraisal and revision of the RCN accreditation unit standards for approval of programmes of preparation for nurse practitioners, 2006 [unpublished]).

The NONPF (2006b) has more recently placed far greater emphasis on assuring competence through application of a range of assessment methods, with the rationale that public protection is paramount. ANPs in the UK have a duty to provide care for their patients that is of the equivalent standard to the professional who would normally provide that care, traditionally a doctor (Dimond 2005). The Bolam Test applies here (*Bolam* v. *Friern Hospital Management Committee* (1957) 2 All ER 118), namely 'the standard of the ordinary skilled man exercising and professing to have that special skill'. Thus the aspect of care provided by the ANP, e.g. patient presenting with a high fever and rash, would be compared with the standard provided by other advanced nurses given the same presentation and similarly with the clinician who would originally have performed the activity, i.e. a doctor (Dimond 2003). Similarly, no allowance is made in law for a lower level of practice just because the health care provider is a nurse (Callaghan 2006), inexperienced in the role (*Wilsher* v. *Essex Area Health Authority*, 1987), or still undergoing education to become an ANP (*Nettleship* v. *Weston*, 1971). This reinforces the fact that not only is it a professional requirement that an advanced nurse seeks the advice and help of someone more experienced when he or she judges that they are not competent to safely act to the appropriate standard (NMC 2008) but also that it is imperative that ANP educational standards ensure that the preparation and assessment of competence results in a graduate ANP who is competent to this standard (Walsh 2000).

Rigorous assessment of competence and safe practice is therefore required through demonstration of a matrix approach to the overall summative assessment strategy, that includes each of the following at appropriate stages of the programme; portfolio, minimum of one timed exam, written case study, OSCE (or equivalent), clinical facilitator feedback and patient feedback (RCN 2008). This requirement is underpinned by the recognition that use of more than one method to assess competency provides triangulation which adds rigour to the overall conclusion (Hand 2006; Stuart 2003).

Use of multiple methods is consistent with the approach taken at London South Bank University (RCN 2008). Students also undertake a health needs assessment, from which they develop a service proposal and explore a clinical dilemma in depth, using empirical research, ethical principles and personal reflection. These have immediate relevance to practice and ensure that the patients, organisation and service benefit from the student's development throughout the programme and not solely on their qualification.

First degree or master's level education

An additional key debate that is relevant to ANP education is the level of academic preparation for an ANP. The RCN (2008) stipulates a minimum of Honours degree preparation, however with the introduction of a graduate nursing workforce in Scotland, Wales and Northern Ireland, and its future introduction in England as part of *Modernising Nursing Careers* (DH 2006a), and stipulations within the banding criteria for *Agenda for Change* (DH 2004d), the association of advanced nursing practice with a master's level qualification has been reinforced. This is consistent with the international approach such as that taken in the USA (Towers 2005), Canada (Canadian Nurses Association 2002) and New Zealand (Nursing Council of New Zealand 2002). Similarly, in the NMC ANP regulation proposals (NMC 2005a), the requirement for nurses to demonstrate 'master's-level thinking' is stipulated and made manifest within the ANP competencies (NMC 2005b) by the incorporation of master's level descriptors (QAA 2001). However, a census by the Association of Advanced Nursing Practice Educators (AANPE) highlighted that a mixed picture of BSc and MSc provision exists (AANPE 2007), which may be reflective of the on-going debate regarding the association between master's awards and advanced nursing.

The community matron – history and development

A key challenge for the government was highlighted in April 2006 with the announcement of a new role, the 'community matron' (DH 2005). With estimates of 15 million people in England living with a long-term condition, such as diabetes, coronary heart disease, asthma, COPD, and their rising prevalence, the need for a coordinated personalised approach for vulnerable people at most risk was proposed. Community matrons would lead this by providing joined-up proactive case management which utilises a holistic approach to the commonly complex needs of these service users. A Public Service Agreement (PSA) target of reducing emergency bed days by 5% by 2008 was set, in an attempt to contain the significant NHS expenditure that results from 'reactive' care of this population.

These proposals arose from recognition of the significant impact that a 'proactive' approaches, such as the EverCare model and use of the Kaiser Pyramid, had made on the care of targeted patients within the USA and pilots within the UK (DH 2005; Toofany 2008). The UK model for the community matron, however, intended that these nurses would have advanced level nursing skills, articulated as a set of case management competences (NHS Modernisation Agency/Skills for Health 2005), subsequently supported by guidance on an education framework that was recommended for developing the competences (DH 2006c). Educational strategies used to develop practitioners for this new role have included individualised training needs analysis, personal development plans, portfolio development and action-learning groups (Board 2007; Lyndon 2006).

Original proposals relating to the role expectation for community matrons included an explicit focus on people identified as very high intensity users (over the age of 65), invariably with multi-pathology and complex health and social care needs. An expectation was also articulated that community matrons 'will have an expert knowledge base of physical, psychosocial, clinical and pharmacology and will provide a holistic generalist overview and care co-ordination for patients with multiple long term conditions. They will be making complex clinical decisions using expert clinical judgement' (DH 2005). Some NP graduates have gone on to assume 'community matron' roles and have anecdotally reported the benefits that their NP education brings to fulfilling the potential of this role.

Nurse consultant – history and development

The title 'consultant nurse' was announced by Prime Minister Tony Blair in 1998, largely in response to criticism that the invisibility of nursing leadership at higher levels accounted for the some of the perceived decline in the standards of care with the NHS at that time. The proposal seemed to be a original idea, however the concept of consultant nurses was debated in the 1970s (Ashworth 1975) and researched in the early 1990s (Manley 1997). The DH (England; 1999b) subsequently identified that the function of these posts would be:

- An expert practice function
- A professional leadership and consultancy function
- An education, training and development function
- A practice and service development research and evaluation function.

Recommendations indicated that these posts should all be firmly based in practice with at least half the working week spent in direct contact with patients, alongside opportunities for linkage with local universities to establish the academic and research side of the role (DH 1999b). NHS organisations were required to submit proposals for the new posts, with specific evidence to demonstrate that appointments were being based on recognised needs and to fulfil policy imperatives, parameters of the role had been identified and risks and accountability issues had been considered, and the post would be invested with professional and organisational autonomy and authority commensurate with its intended purpose.

Although use of the title was not regulated, the regional offices of the DH supervised the process of appointment, with some existing specialist nurses, in areas such as diabetes and respiratory care, being 'upgraded' and some brand new roles being established, such as those in primary and emergency care. This process prevented the adoption of the title 'consultant nurse' by any nurse or employer from the start and this has continued to be the case since approval was devolved to Strategic Health Authority level (Chief Nursing Officer 2003).

Early evaluation identified barriers that hampered the implementation of nurse consultant posts, such as the negative impact of insufficient administrative support and dedicated office space on performance (Guest *et al.* 2001). Questions as to the feasibility of fulfilling all of the aspects of the role have also been borne out (Guest *et al.* 2001; Read *et al.* 2001), echoing previous conclusions from evaluation of advanced practice nursing roles in the USA (Woods 2000) where Woods urged that the temptation to prepare an 'all-singing, all-dancing super nurse' should be resisted and tempered by the reality of clinical practice. Bryant-Lukosius *et al.* (2004) highlight such experiences are not unique to nurse consultants in the UK. They suggest that it is not that the multi-dimensional nature of advanced nursing is too broad, but rather that insufficient attention is often paid to defining and communicating role priorities and determining achievable goals for how components of the role will meet patient and health systems needs. It is worth noting that the research element has proved to be the most underutilised aspect of the role. This may be indicative of a lack of administrative and practical support to effectively conduct research, and it also highlights the deficits in many nurses knowledge, skills and experience to participate in research activities and even to evaluate the impact of their role (Guest *et al.* 2001; Read *et al.* 2001).

Despite these challenges, the nurse consultant is now widely recognised as the pinnacle of the clinical career pathway for nurses (Manley 2001). Many nurses have recognised that the creation of this role has provided a career opportunity that could never have been thought of in the past, and in many instances extended the higher pay scales for clinical nurses considerably. The majority of nurse consultants are required to posses a postgraduate level qualification at master's level.

Authors such as Manley (2001) have provided an underpinning rationale for the differentiation of a hierarchy between the nurse consultant and the level of practice expected of an ANP, community matron or a clinical nurse specialist. The functions of a nurse consultant encompass all of the facets of advanced nursing discussed earlier. However, Manley illustrates distinctions such as the level of operation; the primary purpose of the nurse consultant role is not about providing nurse-led services as a single agent, but about developing the quality of services strategically across interfaces so that person-centred, evidence-based and effective care can be provided by all in the service. Similarly the focus of nurse consultant activities is a cultural change through transformational leadership, facilitation, and consultancy to foster and nurture change and innovation, and the learning and effectiveness of themselves and others (Manley 2004). Here, consultancy crosses traditional professional boundaries and applies not just to matters arising from clinical practice, but also to research, education and practice development and would be described as the highest level, consultee-centred consultancy, in Caplan's (1970) hierarchy.

Conclusion

Advanced practice is now a feature of the nursing continuum within the UK and internationally that is here to stay. A host of opportunities are available for nurses who want to work in new and innovative ways, as core frontline providers of high quality, cost-effective health care. Unfortunately the benefits of advanced nursing practice are sometimes too readily overlooked in favour of a 'new' approach by policy and decision-makers and workforce planners. In the meantime, advanced nurses continue to expend considerable effort negotiating full implementation of their roles, overcoming resistance from many quarters and defending their worth. Time which could otherwise be focused on improving patient care. Establishing a critical mass of nurses working at an advanced level, with a clear identity and capacity to demonstrate positive impact, is now a priority and will only be achieved with sustained widespread investment in appropriate competence-based education and assessment, and equitable financial remuneration that values the clinical responsibility incumbent at this level of practice.

The discussion within this chapter has highlighted the lack of clarity and complexity surrounding advanced nursing practice. The nursing profession and the advanced nursing practice community must provide strong leadership by establishing consensus to communicate clearer messages about the scope and potential of advanced nurses and make their role in successful implementation of health policy and improved patient care explicit.

What is apparent is that advanced nurses within the community on an individual and local basis are making their mark. Whatever the will at a strategic level, it is probably true to say that the real on-going driver for advanced nursing practice in the community will continue to be the mutual benefit that is gained by being able to better meet the needs of patients and their families on a daily basis.

References

Association of Advanced Nursing Practice Educators (2007) *Membership Census Autumn 2007: Advanced Nursing Practice Courses Results.* Available at: www.aanpe.org/AANPEHome/tabid/448/Default.aspx (accessed 10 January 2008).

Ashworth, P. (1975) The clinical nurse consultant. *Nursing Times,* **71**, 574–577.

Ball, J. (2006) Nurse Practitioner Survey 2006. RCN Nurse Practitioner Association. Available at: www.rcn.org.uk/__data/assets/pdf_file/0005/78764/003183.pdf (accessed 2 February 2008).

Barr, H. (2002) *Interprofessional Education Today, Yesterday and Tomorrow: A Review, Occasional Paper No 1, Learning and Teaching Support Network (LTSN).* Centre for Health Sciences and Practice, Westminster University.

Barratt, J. (2005) A case study of styles of patient self-presentation in the nurse practitioner primary health care consultation. *Primary Health Care Research and Development,* **6**, 329–340.

Bates, B. (1990) Twelve paradoxes: a message for nurse practitioners. *Journal of the American Academy of Nurse Practitioners,* **22**, 136–139.

Benner, P. (1984) *From Novice to Expert: Excellence and Power in Clinical Nursing Practice.* Addison-Welsey, Menlo Park, CA.

Board, M. (2007) Education and support needs for the community matron role. *Primary Health Care,* **17**, 22–24.

Bostock, N. (2008) GPs to make nurse-led care a reality. *Independent Nurse,* **15**, 223–234.

Boyden, J. & Edwards, B. (2007) The advanced practitioner role in a community twilight service. *Journal of Community Nursing,* **21**, 10–12.

British Medical Association (BMA) (2002) *The Future Healthcare Workforce.* HPERU Discussion Paper 9. British Medical Association, London.

Brown, S. (1998) A framework for advanced practice nursing. *Journal of Professional Nursing,* **14**, 157–164.

Bryant-Lukosius, D. DiCenso, A., Browne, G. & Pinelli, J. (2004) Advanced practice nursing roles: development, implementation and evaluation. *Journal of Advanced Nursing,* **48**, 519–529.

Burke-Masters, B. (1986) The autonomous nurse practitioner: an answer to a chronic problem of primary care. *Lancet,* **i**, 1266.

Callaghan, C. (2006) The professional and legal framework for the nurse practitioner. In: *Nurse Practitioners. Clinical Skills and Professional Issues* (ed. M. Walsh) (2006). Butterworth Heinemann Elsevier.

Canadian Nurses Association (2002) *Advanced Nursing Practice: A National Framework, Revised.* Canadian Nurses Association, Ottawa.

Caplan, G. (1970) *The Theory and Practice of Mental Health Consultation.* Tavistock Publications, London.

Castledine, G. (2003) The development of advanced nursing practice in the UK. In: *Advanced Nursing Practice,* 2nd edition (eds P. McGee & G. Castledine) (2003). Blackwell Publishing, Oxford.

Chiarella, M. (2006) Advanced nursing practice. *Journal of Advanced Nursing,* **55**, 276–277.

Chief Nursing Officer (2003) *Approval of Nurse, Midwife and Health Visitor Consultant Posts.* Letter dated 22 May to all Lead Nurses, Strategic Health Authorities, PL CNO (2003)5. Department of Health, London.

Conway, J. (1996) *Nursing Expertise and Advanced Practice.* Mark Allen, Wilts.

Crumbie, A. (2001) Educating the nurse practitioner. In: *Nurse Practitioners: Developing the Role in Hospital Settings* (eds S. Reveley, M. Walsh, A. Crumbie) (2001). Butterworth Heinemann, Oxford.

Cullen, C. (2000) Autonomy and the nurse practitioner. *Journal of the RCN Nurse Practitioner Association, Nursing Standard*, **14**, 53–56.

Daly, W & Carnell, R. (2003) Nursing roles and levels of practice: a framework for differentiating between elementary, specialist and advancing nursing practice. *Journal of Clinical Nursing*, **12**, 158–167.

Davis, J. (1992) Expanding Horizons. *Nursing Times*, **88**, 37–39.

Department of Health (1997) *A Guide To Personal Medical Services Pilots Under the NHS (Primary Care) Act 1997.* Crown Copyright, London.

Department of Health (1999a) *NHS Primary Care Walk-in Centres.* HSC 1999/116. Department of Health, London.

Department of Health (1999b) *Making a Difference – Strengthening the Nursing, Midwifery and Health Visiting Contribution to Health and Healthcare.* Crown Copyright, London.

Department of Health (2004a) *Nurses' Prescribing Powers to be Expanded Even Further.* The Stationery Office, London.

Department of Health (2004b) *The NHS Improvement Plan.* The Stationery Office, London.

Department of Health (2004c) *The NHS Knowledge and Skills Framework and the Development Review Process.* Crown Copyright, London.

Department of Health (2004d) *Agenda for Change – Final Agreement, (December 2004).* Department of Health. Available at: www.dh.gov.uk/en/Publications andstatistics/Publications/PublicationsPolicyAnd Guidance/DH_4095943 (accessed 2 March 2008).

Department of Health (2005) *Supporting People with Long Term Conditions: Liberating the Talents of Nurses who Care for People with Long Term Conditions.* Department of Health, London. Available at: www.dh.gov.uk/en/Publicationsandstatistics/ Publications/PublicationsPolicyAndGuidance/ DH_4102469 (accessed 10 April 2008).

Department of Health (2006a) *Modernising Nursing Careers – Setting the Direction.* Chief Nursing Officer's Directorate, The Stationery Office, London.

Department of Health (2006b) *The Competence and Curriculum Framework for the Physician Assistant.* Department of Health, London.

Department of Health (2006c) *New Guidance– Implementing Care Closer to Home: Convenient Quality Care for Patients.* Department of Health, London. Available at: www.dh.gov.uk/en/Healthcare/ Primarycare/Practitionerswithspecialinterests/ DH_074419 (accessed 10 November 2007).

Department of Health (2007a) *Practice Based Commissioning: Guidance.* Department of Health, London. Available at: www.dh.gov.uk/en/Manag ingyourorganisation/Commissioning/Practice-basedcommissioning/DH_4127126 (accessed 10 November 2007).

Department of Health (2007b) *Trust, Assurance and Safety – the Regulation of Health Professionals. Department of Health, London.* Available at: www.dh.gov.uk/en/Publicationsandstatistics/ Publications/PublicationsPolicyAndGuidance/ DH_065946 (accessed 27 March 2007).

Department of Health (2008a) *High Quality Care For All: NHS Next Stage Review (Final Report – Lord Ara Darzi)*, July. Cm7432. London.

Department of Health (2008b) *Our NHS Our Future: NHS Next Stage Review – Leading Local Change. Department of Health, London.* Available at: www.dh.gov.uk/en/Publicationsandstatistics/ Publications/PublicationsPolicyAndGuidance/ DH_084644 (accessed 9 June 2008).

Department of Health and Social Security (DHSS) (1986) *Neighbourhood Nursing – A Focus for Care: Report of the Community Nursing Review Team (Cumberlege Report).* HMSO, London.

Dimond, B. (2003) Legal and ethical issues in advanced practice. In: *Advanced Nursing Practice* (eds P. McGee & G. Castledine) Blackwell Publishing.

Dimond, B. (2005) *Legal Aspects of Nursing*, 4th edition. Pearson Longman, London.

Distler, J.W. (2006) Critical thinking and clinical competence: results of the implementation of student-centred teaching strategies in an advanced practice nurse curriculum. *Nurse Education in Practice*, **7**, 53–59.

Farmer, E. (1995) Medicine and nursing: a marriage for the 21st century? *British Journal of Nursing*, **4**, 793–794.

Gardner, G., Gardner, A. & Proctor, M. (2004) Nurse Practitioner education: a research-based curriculum structure. *Journal of Advanced Nursing*, **47**, 143–152.

Guest, D., Peccei, R., Rosenthal, P., Montgomery, J. & Redfern, S. (2001) *Preliminary Evaluation of the Establishment of Nurse, Midwife and Health Visitor Consultants.* Report to the Department of Health, University of London, King's College, London.

Hamric, A.B. (1996) A definition of advanced practice nursing. In: *Advanced Nursing Practice: An Integrative Approach* (eds A.B. Hamric, J.A. Spross & C.M. Hanson). W.B. Saunders, Philadelphia.

Hamric, A. (2000) A definition of advanced nursing practice. In: *Advanced Nursing Practice: An Integrative Approach* (eds A. Hamric, J. Spross & C. Hanson). W.B. Saunders, Philadelphia.

Hamric, A.B. (2005) A definition of advanced practice nursing. In: *Advanced Nursing Practice: An Integrative Approach* (eds A. Hamric, J. Spross & C. Hanson). Elsevier Saunders, St. Louis.

Hand, H. (2006) Assessment of learning in clinical practice. *Nursing Standard*, **21**, 48–56.

Horrocks, S., Anderson, E. & Salisbury, C. (2002) Systematic review of whether nurse practitioners working in primary care can provide equivalent care to doctors. *British Medical Journal*, **324**, 819.

Inman, C. (2003) Providing a culture of learning for advanced practice students undertaking a master's degree. In: *Advanced Nursing Practice*, 2nd edition (eds P. McGee & G. Castledine) (2003). Blackwell Publishing, Oxford.

International Council of Nurses (1997) *An Approval System for Schools of Nursing. Guidelines.* International Council of Nurses, Geneva.

International Council of Nurses (2002) *Definition and Characteristics of Nurse Practitioners/Advanced Practice Nurses.* International Council of Nurses, Geneva.

International Council of Nurses (2008) *The Scope of Practice, Standards and Competencies for the Advanced Practice Nurse.* ICN Regulation Series. International Council of Nurses, Geneva.

Jasper, M.A. (1994) Expert: a discussion of the implications of the concept as used in nursing. *Journal of Advanced Nursing*, **20**, 769–776.

Jones, M. & Gough, P. (1997) Nurse prescribing – why has it taken so long? *Nursing Standard*, **11**, 39–42.

Laurant, M., Reeves, D., Hermens, R., Braspenning, J., Grol, R. & Sibbald, B. (2005) Substitution of doctors by nurses in primary care. *The Cochrane Library* (Issue 2). John Wiley and Sons, Chichester.

Lyndon, H. (2006) Developing the role of the community matron. The Cornwall experience. *Primary Health Care*, **16**, 14–17.

MacAlister, L. & Chiam, M. (1995) Why do nurses agree to take on doctors' roles? *British Journal of Nursing*, **4**, 1238–1239.

Manley, K. (1996) Advanced practice is not about medicalising nursing roles. *Nursing in Critical Care*, **1**, 3–4.

Manley, K. (1997) A conceptual framework for advanced practice: an action research project operationalizing and advanced practitioner/consultant nurse role. *Journal Clinical Nursing*, **6**, 179–190.

Manley, K. (2001) Consultant nurse: concept, processes, outcomes. Unpublished PhD Thesis, University of Manchester/RCN Institute London.

Manley, K. (2004) Transformational culture: a culture of effectiveness. In: *Practice Development in Nursing* (eds B. McCormack, K. Manley & R. Garbett). Blackwell Publishing, Oxford.

Mantzoukas, S. & Watkinson, S. (2007) Review of advanced practice: the international literature and developing generic features. *Journal of Clinical Nursing*, **16**, 28–37.

Masterson, A. & Mitchell, L. (2003) Developing Competences for Advanced Nursing Practice. In: *Advanced Nursing Practice*, 2nd edition (eds P. McGee & G. Castledine) (2003). Blackwell Publishing, Oxford.

Mauksch, I.G. (1991) Critical issues of the nurse practitioner movement. *Nurse Practitioner*, **3**, 35–36.

McGee, P. & Castledine, G. (1999) A survey of specialist and advanced nursing practice in the UK. *British Journal of Nursing*, **8**, 1074–1078.

McGee, P. & Castledine, G. (2003) Future directions in advanced nursing practice in the UK. In: *Advanced Nursing Practice*, 2nd edition (eds P. McGee & G. Castledine) (2003). Blackwell Publishing, Oxford.

Ministry of Health New Zealand (2002) *Nurse Practitioners in New Zealand.* Ministry of Health New Zealand, Wellington.

Mitchell, L. (2000) *Models of Competence.* Paper presented to the UKCC's Higher Level of Practice Steering Group, United Kingdom Central Council, London.

Mitchinson, S. (1996) Are nurses independent and autonomous practitioners? *Nursing Standard*, **10**, 34–38.

NHS London (2007) *Healthcare for London – A Framework for Action.* NHS, London.

NHS Modernisation Agency/Skills for Health (2005) *Case Management Competences Framework for the Care of Older People with Long Term Conditions. Department of Health, London.* Available at: www.dh.gov.uk/en/Publicationsandstatistics/Publications/PublicationsPolicyAndGuidance/DH_4118101 (accessed 10 April 2008).

NHS Education for Scotland (NES) (2007) *Pilot Succession Planning Development Pathway for Advanced Practice.* NHS Education for Scotland. Available at: www.nes.scot.nhs.uk/documents/publications/classa/131107Advanced_Practice_Succession_planning_draft_pathway.pdf (accessed 10 December 2007).

National Organisation of Nurse Practitioner Faculties (2001) *Draft One: Domains and Competencies of Nurse Practitioner Practice,* September. National Organisation of Nurse Practitioner Faculties, Washington.

National Organisation of Nurse Practitioner Faculties (2006a) *Draft Advanced Nursing Practice: Curriculum Guidelines and Program Standards for Nurse Practitioner Education.* National Organisation of Nurse Practitioner Faculties , Washington.

National Organisation of Nurse Practitioner Faculties (2006b) *Future Directions for the Educational Standards & Guidelines Committee. The Mentor* (The NONPF Newsletter), **17**, 5–6.

Neary, M. (2000) *Teaching, Assessing and Evaluation of Clinical Competence. A Practical Guide for Practitioners and Teachers.* Stanley Thornes, Cheltenham.

Nursing Council of New Zealand (2002) *The nurse practitioner: responding to the health needs in New Zealand.* Nursing Council of New Zealand, New Zealand.

Nursing and Midwifery Council (2004) *Standards of Proficiency for Specialist Community Public Health Nurses (Standards.04.04).* Nursing and Midwifery Council, London. Available at: www.nmc-uk.org/ aFrameDisplay.aspx?DocumentID=324 (accessed 14 July 2006).

Nursing and Midwifery Counci (2005a) *Implementation of a Framework for the Standard of Post Registration Nursing.* Agendum 27.1, December [Online]. Nursing and Midwifery Council, London. Available at: www. nmc-uk.org/aFrameDisplay.aspx?DocumentID=1669 (accessed 14 July 2006).

Nursing and Midwifery Council (NMC) (2005b) *Mapping of Competences to the Knowledge and Skills Framework.* Nursing and Midwifery Council, London. Available at: www.nmc-uk.org/ aArticle.aspx?ArticleID=2038 (accessed 14 July 2006).

Nursing and Midwifery Council (NMC) (2006) *Advanced Nursing Practice – update 4 July 2006.* Nursing and Midwifery Council, London. Available at: www.nmc-k.org/aArticle.aspx?ArticleID=2068 (accessed 23 September 2006).

Nursing & Midwifery Council (NMC) (2007) *Advanced Nursing Practice update –19 June 2007.* Nursing and Midwifery Council, London. Available at: www. nmc-uk.org/aArticle.aspx?ArticleID=2528 (accessed 10 March 2008).

Nursing and Midwifery Council (2008) *The Code: Standards of Conduct, Performance and Ethics for Nurses and Midwives.* Nursing and Midwifery Council, London.

Quality Assurance Agency(2000) *Code of Practice for the Assurance of Academic Quality and Standards in Higher Education, Section 7: Programme Approval, Monitoring and Review,* April. Quality Assurance Agency, Gloucester. Available at: www.qaa.ac.uk/ academicinfrastructure/codeOfPractice/section7/ default.asp (accessed 7 July 2006).

Quality Assurance Agency (2001) *The Framework for Higher Education Qualifications in England, Wales and Northern Ireland, January.* Quality Assurance Agency, Gloucester. Available at: www.qaa.ac.uk/ academicinfrastructure/FHEQ/EWNI/default.asp (accessed 7 July 2006).

Quality Assurance Agency (2004) *Code of Practice for the Assurance of Academic Quality and Standards in Higher Education, Section 2: Collaborative Provision and Flexible and Distributed Learning (including e-learning),* September. Quality Assurance Agency, Gloucester. Available at: www.qaa.ac.uk/academicinfrastructure/codeOfPractice/section2/default.asp (accessed 7 July 2007).

Read, S. & Roberts-Davis, M. (2000) *Preparing Nurse Practitioners for the 21st Century.* Executive Summary from the Report of the Project 'Realising Specialist and Advanced Nursing Practice: Establishing the Parameters of and Identifying the Competencies for "Nurse Practitioner" Roles and Evaluating Programmes of Preparation (RSANP)'. Sheffield University, Sheffield.

Read, S., Lloyd Jones, M. & Collins, K. (2001) *ENRiP: Exploring New Roles in Practice: Final Report.* King's Fund Development Programme, Bristol University.

Roberts, S.J. (1983) Oppressed group behaviour: implications for nursing. *Advances in Nursing Science,* **5**, 21–30.

Roberts-Davis, M. & Read, S. (2001) Clinical role clarification: using the Delphi method to establish similarities and differences between nurse practitioners and clinical nurse specialists. *Journal of Clinical Nursing,* **10**, 33–43.

Royal College of Nursing (1996) *Statement on the Role and Scope of Nurse Practitioner Practice.* Royal College of Nursing, London.

Royal College of Nursing (2002) *Nurse Practitioners – an RCN Guide to the Nurse Practitioner Role, Competencies and Programme Approval.* Royal College of Nursing, London.

Royal College of Nursing (2008) *Advanced Nurse Practitioners – An RCN Guide to the Advanced Nurse Practitioner, Role, Competencies and Programme Accreditation.* Royal College of Nursing, London.

Royal College of Nursing/Department of Health (2007) *Maxi Nurses: Nurses Working in Advanced and Extended Roles Promoting and Developing Patient-Centred Health Care*. Royal College of Nursing/Department of Health, London.

Schober, M. (2004) Global perspective on advanced practice. In: *Advanced Practice Nursing: Essentials for Role Development* (ed. L. Joel). F.A. Davis, Philadelphia.

Schober, M. & McKay, N. (2004) *Collaborative Practice in the 21st Century [Monograph]*. International Council of Nurses, Geneva.

Schober, M. & Affara, F. (2006) *Advanced Nursing Practice*. Blackwell Publishing, Oxford.

Scottish Chief Nursing Officer Directorate (2008) *Supporting the Development of Advanced Nursing Practice – A Toolkit approach*, June. Scottish Government.

Seale, C., Anderson, E. & Kinnersley, P. (2006) Treatment advice in primary care: a comparative study of nurse practitioners and general practitioners. *Journal of Advanced Nursing*, **54**, 534–541.

Skills for Health (2005) *What is the new Career Framework for Health?*. Skills for Health. Available at: www.skillsforhealth.org.uk/uploads/page/93/uploadablefile.pdf (accessed 9 June 2008).

Skills for Health (2006) *The Competence and Curriculum Framework for the Emergency Care Practitioner*. Department of Health, London. Available at: www.dh.gov.uk/en/Consultations/Responsestoconsultations/DH_078174 (accessed 10 April 2008).

Stilwell, B., Restall, D. & Burke-Masters, B. (1988) Nurse practitioners in British general practice. In: *The Nurse in Family Practice – Practice Nurses & Nurse Practitioners in Primary Healthcare* (eds A. Bowling & B. Stilwell) (1988). Scutari Press, London.

Stuart, C.C. (2003) *Assessment, Supervision and Support in Clinical Practice: A Guide for Nurses, Midwives and Other Health Professionals*. Churchill Livingstone, Edinburgh.

Styles, M.M. & Affara, F.A (1997) *ICN on Regulation: Towards a 21st Century Model*. International Council of Nurses, Geneva.

Sullivan, T.J. (1998) *Collaboration: Health Care Imperative*. McGraw-Hill, New York.

Toofany, S. (2008) Where are the cases? *Primary Health Care*, **18**, 36–39.

Towers, J. (2005) After forty years. *Journal of the American Academy of Nurse Practitioners*, **17**, 9–13.

United Kingdom Central Council for Nursing, Midwifery and Health Visiting (1992) *Scope of Professional Practice*. United Kingdom Central Council for United Kingdom Central Council for Nursing, Midwifery and Health Visiting, London.

United Kingdom Central Council for Nursing, Midwifery and Health Visiting (1994) *The Future of Professional Practice – The Council's Standards for Education and Practice Following Registration*. United Kingdom Central Council for Nursing, Midwifery and Health Visiting, London.

United Kingdom Central Council for Nursing, Midwifery and Health Visiting (1999) *A Higher Level of Practice. Report of the Consultation on the UKCC's Proposals for a Revised Regulatory Framework for Post-registration Clinical Practice*. United Kingdom Central Council for Nursing, Midwifery and Health Visiting, London.

United Kingdom Central Council for Nursing, Midwifery and Health Visiting (2002) *Report of the Higher Level of Practice Pilot and Project*. United Kingdom Central Council for Nursing, Midwifery and Health Visiting, London.

Vaughan, B. (1989) Autonomy and Accountability, *Nursing Times*, **85**, 54–55.

Venning, P., Durie, A., Roland, M., Roberts, C. & Leese, B. (2000) Randomised controlled trial comparing cost effectiveness of general practitioners and nurse practitioners in primary care. *British Medical Journal*, **320**, 1048–1053.

Walsh, M. (2000) *Nursing Frontiers: Accountability and the Boundaries of Care*. Butterworth-Heinemann.

Walsh, M. (2006) Development of the nurse practitioner role. In: *Nurse Practitioners, Clinical Skills and Professional Issues* (ed. M. Walsh) (2006). Butterworth Heinemann, Elsevier, Edinburgh.

Wanless, D. (2007) *The Wanless Report: Securing Good Health for the Whole Population*. HM Treasury, London.

Ward, H. & Willis, A. (2007) Student-centred teaching for educating nurse practitioners. *Nursing Times*, **103**, 30–31.

Willis, A. & Maclaine, K. (2004) Just what is a nurse practitioner? *The New Generalist*, **2**, 62–63.

World Health Organization (WHO) (2002) *Nursing and Midwifery Services: Strategic Direction 2002–2008*. WHO, Geneva.

Chapter 16 **Teamwork in Community Nursing**

Owen Barr

Introduction

The very nature of community-based health services requires nurses to work collaboratively with a range of other professional groups in order to effectively meet the needs of clients, patients and their families. This chapter provides an overview of the range of professionals who work in community health services and considers the developments in service provision that have highlighted the need for increasing the effectiveness of teamwork between a wider range of professionals who provide community-based health and social care services. The nature of teams is also explored to clarify the characteristics of effective teams and teamworking. Consideration is also given to the factors that potentially reduce the outcomes of teamwork and steps that might be taken to facilitate effective teamworking.

Potential team members in community services

The majority of people who use health services receive support from community-based services. There are a range of community nurses within the current configuration of services, including: district nurses, community nurses in learning disability, community nurses in mental health, community children's nurses and general practice nurses, as well as those community and public health nurses (public health/health visiting, occupational health and school nursing) now with Part Three of the Nursing and Midwifery Council (NMC) Register. Some other community nursing services have traditionally focused their work within specific settings such as schools or places of work, while yet other services have sought to meet the needs of people within their home and alternative community settings.

The services provided by staff within community health care nursing services include public health focused work with groups from local communities, including the provision of health advice aimed at maintaining the health of individuals, groups and communities. Community nurses are also involved in active health surveillance with members of the community ranging from young children (Gannon-Leary *et al.* 2006) to older people. Health surveillance is at the cornerstone of community practice and may be the point at which health needs are noted and further nursing responses identified to meet these needs. Community nurses are often involved in supporting people prior to their contact with acute hospitals services and they will usually be involved in providing ongoing support as part of a discharge plan for people with more complex health care needs. For other people, their contact with community health care nursing services may only commence following the conclusion of treatment in an acute or mental health hospital. However, it is important to note that the previous delineation between hospital and community services which viewed hospital care as acute- and community-based care as meeting continuing care needs is increasing becoming less distinct. Many people are now supported by community nurses across a range of services including children with complex health needs, people with acute exacerbations of chronic conditions, people with learning disabilities and people with mental health problems may received 'acute clinical care', for example, intravenous therapy, ventilator support, behavioural intervention or suicide risk assessment while in the community (Department of Health [DH] 2004c, 2005). These changes are reflected in the development of services which include community in-reach teams, intermediate care teams and crisis response teams.

Community health care nurses are one of a number of professional groups who are employed within statutory services to provide support for people with a range of health needs outwith hospital. Other professionals include nurses in specific posts, such as diabetes nurses and stoma care nurses or those who may have a role that straddles both hospital and community services as well as nurses who provide palliative care services and general practice nurses. In providing services to clients and their families community nurses work together with general practitioners, pharmacists, midwives, members of the allied health professions (including physiotherapists, speech and language therapists, occupational therapists). In addition, the services provided by social service departments, such as social work, domiciliary care, day services and residential care, may play a considerable role in supporting some people with complex needs in the community. Community health care nurses may also work across wider inter-agency networks involving education, housing, and independent sector providers.

Family carers usually provide the largest amount of support to relatives, and members of the community health care team have a key role to play in providing effective support to family members. Family members and other carers need to be included within inter-disciplinary networks at both an individual patient and carers organisational level in the process of organisation and delivery of care and support, however, this is still reported as problematic in several areas within the UK (Roulstone & Hudson 2007). Family members may also access support from independent sector services, comprising those provided by private and not-for-profit organisations. For some people these services could include the provision of nursing care at home or residential and nursing home provision, on an ongoing or respite care basis. The independent sector also has an important advocacy role in providing information to family carers and clients about health conditions and the availability

of services and their entitlements to services. Clients and family members may contact independent services directly, or such a service may be contracted by statutory service providers, for instance, as part of a case management package.

The need for effective collaboration between individual professionals and the services they are part of has long been advocated as the most effective way to deliver community-based services (DH 1989; Department of Health and Social Security [DHSS] 1991). More recently several developments in the role expansion of nurses and other in community service personnel, as well as the reorganisation of services, has further emphasised the need for the provision of effective teamwork (Glasby & Lester 2004).

The continuing need for effective teamwork

The view that the development of effective teamwork is the only framework for providing coordinated 'seamless services' is well established in health services within the UK (DH 1989; DHSS 1991; Hudson 1995; Towell & Beardshaw 1991). In addition to the health policy guidance on teamworking, the importance of working in collaboration with colleagues, clients and carers is stressed as a requirement for nurses, midwives and health visitors in guidance relating to their professional practice. The latest edition of the *Code of Professional Conduct* highlights the requirement of collaborating with those in your care, sharing information with colleagues (within the boundaries of confidentiality), working effectively as part of a team and delegating effectively (NMC 2008).

Teamworking has long been viewed as a strategy or conduit to coordinate the growing number of professionals who work within community services in order to encourage the delivery of more comprehensive services, bridge gaps in services and reduce duplication. The interest in teamwork within health and social care services had its origins in the health policy of the 1980s (DH 1989). Since that time, interest in providing effective team-based services has intensified as the pressure has increased to find ways in which health and social service staff can be encouraged to work more closely together than they did previously (Johnson *et al.* 2003).

The context in which health and social services operate is constantly changing as the expectations and needs of people using services and the structures within which services are provided alter (Glasby & Lester 2004). Five key changes in the context of community services have re-emphasised the need for effective teamwork within, and between, agencies. First, changes in service policy have emphasised the importance of people having the opportunity to live in their own home, complemented by the need to provide requisite support to clients and their families to facilitate this objective. The reconfiguration of hospital services that previously provided longer-term care for older people, people with learning disabilities, and people with mental health problems, has also emphasised the need for increased opportunities to live in community settings, such as supported living arrangements that provide as much flexibility and choice as possible (DH 2000a, 2001; Scottish Executive [SE] 2000). A move to providing support at home for people who are chronically ill or in need of palliative care has also been emphasised in the past few years (DH 2000b). In addition, revised policy in the form of the national service framework for children, often with complex health needs has highlighted the need to increase the support made available to children and their families in order to promote their inclusion (and protection) within society (DH 2004a).

Second, there is recognition of the increasing complexity of the needs of people who receive services in the community. People who may have previously been cared for in hospital settings are now being supported increasingly in their own home. This covers a wide range of people, from young children with complex health needs who live at home with the support of equipment such as intravenous therapies and ventilators only previously available in hospital settings (Lewis & Noyes 2007; Noyes 2007) to a growing number of older people, many of whom are healthy and yet need advice and support to remain so. There are also a growing number of people who present with complex health needs and require support from community services. Over the past few years there has been an increase in the number and range of services available for such people. Examples include the development of community children's nursing services and the provision of services that focus on people with specific health needs such as diabetes and epilepsy, and behaviour support services and support for people with dementia.

Third, there has been a change in emphasis in the domains of practice for community nurses. The future focus of community nurses in primary care services has been identified as centring on three key functions, namely:

- First contact/single case assessment, diagnosis, care, treatment and referral
- The provision of continuing care, rehabilitation, the management of longer-term conditions
- Public health/health protection and promotion programmes that improve health outcome and reduce inequalities

(DH 2002)

Alongside this, there have been developments in the role of nurses working in community settings, such as non-medical (nurse) prescribing. There has also been a growing emphasis on the need to bridge the perceived gap between community-based services and those provided within secondary, acute services. Developments in community-based services, for example, the evolving role of nurse practitioners, has seen community-based nurses involved in closer involvement with the referral of people to hospital services (Price & Williams 2003). Such developments have altered the equilibrium that existed previously between nurses and other professionals working within community teams.

Fourth, the focus of many teamwork developments has been on the actions that might be taken to increase the extent that teamwork occurs between individual practitioners. However, there is now a clear recognition of the need to develop more effective inter-agency working practices and emphasis has been given to the need to review how agencies work effectively together. This is particularly important given the development of PCTs and their associated counterparts in Scotland, Wales and Northern Ireland, requiring the need to formalise structures in which health and social services can be effectively coordinated (DH 2000a).

Finally, a series of national/judicial inquires into 'gross failures' to support some of the most vulnerable people in society have highlighted that at times fatal consequences may arise as the consequence of ineffective teamwork. Difficult lessons have to be learnt quickly from the frequent failures highlighted in such reports regarding the need for individuals and agencies to communicate openly if effective inter-agency teamwork is to develop. Unfortunately, a consistent finding across a number of these reports is a breakdown in communication between professionals within and across different teams, often complicated by a professional's narrow view of the remit of their role and lack of appreciation of the role of colleagues, for example in relation to child protection (DH 2003, 2004b; Eastern Health and Social Service Board/Western Health and Social Service Board [EHSSB/WHSSB] 2008; Mencap 2007).

Given the complexity of the needs among people who require support from community-based heath and social services, it is clear that no single professional group alone can provide comprehensive services to all people. Teamwork will therefore be an imperative that requires the coordination of complex community health and social service inputs. There continues to be an underlying assumption that teamwork is the most effective way to achieve this objective, and it has been argued that teamwork is essential between (and within) health and social services, if they are to remain intact and not become divisive, fragmented and profit-led (Leathard 1994). Such views have contributed to the current situation, which present inter-disciplinary teamwork as the most effective approach to provide maximum benefit to clients and team members (Glasby & Lester 2004; McLaughlin 2004).

However, despite the apparently clear rationale for developing teamwork in community

health and social services, there is much less clarity about what constitutes a team and the form it should take. Malin *et al.* (1999) capture this in their observation that 'it seems easier to agree that teams are a "good" thing' rather than to agree about what they are (p. 189).

The nature of teams

The word 'team' is widely used in everyday language and it appears that there is a common understanding of the term. However, when exploring the nature of teams it becomes clear that term may have a number of different meanings depending on the context in which the word is used. The meaning of the word may be clear when referring to one's favourite sports team, but when used within the context of health and social care the term is not so easily defined, nor its members listed. Indeed, it has been asserted that vagueness about exactly what constitutes a team within health and social care appears to have resulted in almost all forms of communication between colleagues and other professionals being described as multi-disciplinary teamwork (Ovretviet 1986).

The variation in the structure of 'teams' within local community services may also have contributed to the lack of clarity as to what constitutes a team. It is recognised that the number and professional backgrounds of the people who comprise the membership of health and social care teams will differ depending on several factors, including, the clients the team is seeking to support, the level of skills required of team members, the professionals available within that locality, and the other services available to the clients in that geographical area. The structure of teams working in community health and social services can include those developed to deliver individualised care packages to individual clients, such as those developed in case management. Equally so, more formal inter-disciplinary teams may provide services to a number of people with a diverse range of health needs across a specific geographical area (Ovretveit 1993). There is no 'right' team structures as the organisation of a team will vary depending on the service the team is required to provide. Each team structure has advantages and disadvantages; therefore it is important that decisions about team membership, processes and structures are made carefully. The team structure should be selected to meet identified client needs, both individually and across the locality the team serves. It can be a fundamental error to set up a team first, perhaps because funding has become available or for appearance purposes and then decide on its remit.

Indeed, in acknowledging the vagueness around the word 'team', it has even been suggested that the term should be dropped and replaced with the term 'integrated care', in order to focus on the needs of clients, rather than the members of a team (National Health Service [NHS] Executive 2000). Although, a range of definitions for teams can be found to exist in the health and social care literature, there is some degree of consistency about the characteristics that are present among team members and the structures in which they work. West (2004), for example states that in practice, teams have shared objectives among the team members in relation to their work and usually can be identified to belong to a 'team' by other members of their organisation. He also views teams as having a degree of autonomy and control to make decisions in order to achieve their corporate objectives and having responsibility and accountability for their work.

An important distinction has been made between 'teams' and what Hayes (1997) has referred to as a 'pseudo-team'. The former possesses the characteristics of teams as identified by West (2004). In contrast, some professionals or their managers may consider themselves, or a number of staff within their organisation to be a team. These people may well work in the same offices and be identified as a team within the local health and social care structures, but still lack the key characteristics of a team as identified by West. Although this collection of people may have the potential to become an effective team, if all they have in common is a location or collective name, then they do not possess the characteristics of a team. Hayes (1997) has referred to such groups as a 'pseudo team', which she defines as 'a group of people who are called, or

who call themselves, a team... but don't actually try to co-ordinate what they are doing or establish collective responsibility... in reality they act on a purely individual level and are concerned only with their own departments and responsibilities' (p. 129). In essence, such arrangements may have the structural attributes of a team, however, in practice they lack the level of functional integration and inter-dependence required to work effectively (Johnson *et al.* 2003).

The distinction between teams and pseudo teams is an important one, since the provision of effective support to clients is dependent upon the provision a 'functioning' team. Conversely, it is important to identify and either facilitate enhanced teamwork or disband those groups of people that function as teams 'in name only'. People who work in teams and those who manage services that are team based, need to remain alert to the emergence of factors that may limit the effectiveness of a team in order to ensure that these can be responded to promptly.

Teams do not work effectively when...

Teams may not always the most effective way of meeting the needs of people who use services or in achieving the objectives set by services providers. The perceived wisdom that bringing several professions involved in the provision of health and social care into an integrated team would increase the quality of services has not always been witnessed in practice. For example, people who use services and professionals who work in them continue to provide clear examples of how their experience with team members and teamworking did not result effective partnership and consequently in the delivery of better services (DH 2003; Malin *et al.* 1999; Roulstone & Hudson 2007). Unfortunately, and in part due to the unquestioning assumption that teamwork is effective, shortcomings in teamwork are not often openly discussed until failures have occurred on a major scale, resulting in an investigation into the working practices of the team and its members (DH 2003, 2004b; EHSSB/WHSSB 2008; Hudson 2002). Such problems highlight the need to provide closer attention to the indicators of ineffective teamwork and to take preventive action before difficulties arise. Three key issues frequently commented on in the literature are explored below.

Lack of investment in team development

In order to establish and maintain an effective level of functioning, teams require an investment of time. Managers of services seeking to develop teams need first to explore if a team is an appropriate way to achieve the identified objectives of care and then establish the nature of the team that may be required. Similarly care must be taken to guard against pressure that may be placed on services to develop complex team structures when more simple solutions would suffice (Hudson 2002).

In reality it is all too easy to bring a group of people together, set them a task to achieve and call them a team, creating the pretence that a team exists (McLaughlin 2004) This limited approach to team development often results in the presence of a group of people forming a team 'in name only' (a 'pseudo team'). Such teams fail to lead to the provision of effective teamwork since the focus has been placed on the structural integration of the team, without providing adequate attention to the development of strong inter-professional working (Johnson *et al.* 2003). This in turn can result in the absence of positive leadership for team members, which may increase their uncertainty over their own roles and the professional contribution that they bring to the work of the team (Bateman *et al.* 2003).

'Teams' set up in this way usually fail to achieve the objectives set for them (West 2004). However, all too often managers tend to focus attention on lack of teamwork by attributing failure to individual team members' reluctance to work together, rather than on the lack of investment of time and energy provided by them to establish an effective foundation from which the team might develop. While team members may have been provided with explicit objectives, the lack of discussion and opportunity to develop open communication between team members can result in people being reluctant to alter their previous ways of working and may strengthen their commitment to following their previous roles (Sheehan *et al.* 2007). This may be further complicated in larger teams by the emergence of contested leadership, when several leaders arise and groupings of team members around these people emerge within the team. Groupings may be formed on the basis of previous professional backgrounds; new allegiances may also develop as people seek to maintain or seek a favourable position within a team.

Teamwork may also result in stress, tension and conflict for team members. This is particularly evident when members are asked to change their working arrangements/practices when they are largely unsupported. Such situations could result in team members experiencing mixed emotions of anxiety, confusion, frustration, anger, fear, excitement and anticipation. Some members may need support to realise that although their hierarchical position and power position has altered, they are still important and valued members of the team. On a more practical level the impact and frustration that may result from the need to relocate offices, travel further to work, or share offices with other professionals or people with whom they may have had limited contact for the first time, should not be underestimated.

This may be a particular challenge when people from diverse organisations (e.g. community nursing, primary care, social services, housing services, local industry, advocacy groups), who have limited actual experience of working with each other, are brought together. In order to engage in open communication, the people involved need time to build up a picture of the functions, ideologies and culture of the other agencies and how that agency views their role (Fickel *et al.* 2007; Johnson *et al.* 2003).

Failure to promote opportunities for flexibility and creativity in providing services

Linked to the lack of investment in team development is the lack of flexibility and creativity within teamworking. When team members do not have the opportunity to reflect on their own professional contribution to the work of the team, they may seek 'security' by insisting on the development of rigid and complex decision-making procedures, sometimes proffered in the name of effective teamwork. This situation can be further complicated when people outwith the team seek to influence the development of these procedures (Hudson 2002). Similar conflict can occur when managers outwith the team continue to exercise control over team members, which may result in affected team members feeling that they are unable to make autonomous decisions, leading to frustration and a reduced commitment to the team. In reality the development of rigid procedures often has more to do with a desire to maintain previous hierarchical structures. Hence, the intensity with which some professional groups defend their perceived territory should not be minimised (Beattie 1995; Robinson & Cottrell 2005). Within such rigid structures the manner in which work is allocated to team members may have limited transparency and be perceived as originating from the assignation of roles based on people's position in the hierarchical structure, their previous status or perceived favouritism.

Inevitably difficulties might arise when rigid procedures are imposed on team members, which can be further compounded by the adoption of an authoritarian approach to leadership within which obedience to authority is the rule and those who comply are favoured within the team. From this viewpoint, there is no acceptance that conflict is an integral part of teamwork and any indicators of conflict among members are ignored or suppressed. This situation has been referred to as 'groupthink' and has been widely recognised within other social groups and teams (Hayes 1997; Janis 1983; Moorhead *et al.* 1991) and continues to be highlighted as a potential problem within teams in health and social services (West 2004). This can result in team members considering few alternatives when making decisions, failure to re-examine alternatives in the light of new information, and the lack of attention to, or rejection of, available evidence. This can lead to a firm belief in the certainty of the decisions taken to the extent that no consideration is given to the development of alternative or contingency plans (Moorhead *et al.* 1991). With a team environment characterised by groupthink, individual team members become fearful of making autonomous decisions due to the perceived or actual lack of support from other team members.

Lack of monitoring of team progress

Even when time and energy has been invested in facilitating the development of a team, ongoing support is necessary in order for the team to remain effective. New teams often emerge from the previous need to respond to changes in the needs of people who use the services, changing priorities in policy or the altering structures within organisations. As these factors continually evolve, there is a need for teams to monitor their success in remaining relevant to the services in which they operate.

Particular attention needs to be given to the operational culture and 'practice wisdom' as these evolve within teams. Operational culture has been described as 'the patterns of relationships and sets of assumptions which team members hold about themselves and their colleagues... the routine and often unspoken ways that members define their roles and their professional relationships' (Brown 1992, pp. 372, 377). This comprises the tacit knowledge of how things are done in the team, the unwritten rules and procedures. The 'operational culture' of a team is as important to successful team functioning as appropriate team structures and agreed team operational policies. Practice wisdom is the product of informal rather than formal theory and seeks to address the everyday concerns and realities of practitioners work. However, this is also rarely recorded, and often not officially recognised, and is therefore less often scrutinised (Hudson 2002).

A recognition of the importance of team culture requires managers and team members to invest time in open discussion about their perceptions/stereotypes of their own role and the role of other team members. Such discussions will provide opportunities for team members to get to know their colleagues as fellow professionals. Not doing so may lead to the situation outlined by Hattersly (1995) in which the failure to effectively monitor the performance of teams can result in a situation were they 'evolve gradually, without explicit review, and the resulting "monsters" can often establish their own demands for collaboration which exist only because of unnecessary division and barriers which have developed' (p. 261).

It is recognised that a number of problems can arise that will seriously impact on the effectiveness of a team in functioning to its full potential. These are not reasons for not pursuing teamwork, rather they emphasis the need for service managers and team members to take active steps to facilitate effective teamwork.

Teams work well when…

Team development is facilitated

People do not always work effectively together, as evidenced in the continuing interest provided by government departments on how the enhance the effectiveness of teams to support people with increasingly complex needs and the poignant lessons that must be learnt from the consequences of failures in teamwork (DH 2003, 2004b). The best opportunity to achieve successful teamwork is to build in and facilitate the growth of those factors that have been identified as contributing to effective teamwork.

Perhaps first among these is the need for prospective team members and their managers to accept that effective teamworking takes time to evolve (Tuckman & Jensen 1977). It is recognised that the collection of people who form the basis of a team need to work through the process of getting to know each other (Forming) and agreeing initial core objectives and acknowledging the role of other team members (Norming). These first two steps often occur without major difficulties and are usually assisted by the enthusiasm of people to make any new team a success. This process is assisted if the rationale for the team is clear to all involved and people have had the opportunity to shape the objectives of the team, rather then these being imposed on prospective team members (NHS Executive

2000). However, this apparent initial harmony and agreement is often disrupted for a period of time as team members start to provide services and face the challenges in doing so. Conflict is a key feature of this transition process to becoming a functioning team (Price & Williams 2003). These personal challenges often result in attempts to revise team objectives and roles. The core objectives of the team, as well as the role and value of team members may be directly and at times be forcibly questioned among team members (Storming). If these periods of discussion, and on occasions open disagreement among team members are facilitated, it usually results in further consensus developing among team members and this sets the scene for the team to provide effective services to clients (Performing).

The formative stages of teamworking require the opportunity for staff to meet with other team members regularly. This has been reported as assisting in developing effective approaches to working together (Nancarrow 2004). It also provides opportunities to develop creative ways of thinking and make decisions according the situation in which they are working, but that are flexible enough to be amended as the situation changes (Molyneux 2001). Managers in services have an important role to play in creating the time and space for these initial stages of development to take place before team members are expected to manage large case/workloads (Ovretveit 1997).

People in the team want to be 'team members'

The personal qualities of team members also have a major influence on the rate at which teamworking develops, as well as the emergence of flexibility and creativity that influences how team members undertake their roles. In particular the confidence of team members in their own role and their ability to undertake it, is crucial to the willingness and ability of professionals to engage in open communication about their work with other professionals (Molyneux 2001). It is through this process of dialogue that a language that can be clearly understood among team members is established. The development of a common language code is an integral component of people successfully explaining their perceptions of their own role and understanding roles of other team members.

Effective inter-disciplinary teamwork has been reported as being characterised by the use of inclusive language that encourages participation and discussion and the continual sharing of information between team members (Sheehan *et al.* 2007). This process of communication and the opportunity to more clearly understand the role of individual team members and getting to know more about people as individuals is important for team members to develop accurate knowledge about each other and to overcome stereotypes they may hold (Nancarrow 2004). This in turn facilitates the development of mutual trust and respect among team members and acknowledges the right of team members to make decisions based on mutual respect and professional and personal values or knowledge (although not all team members may agree with the decision made).

Teamwork requires people to work collaboratively, moving in the same direction and working with each other in order to achieve the objectives set for individual clients they are supporting and those of the overall team. Several of the factors noted above combine to form an environment in which collaborative working is possible. Such an approach is characterised by the sharing of power based on knowledge and expertise instead of role or title, and the provision of clear procedures for managing conflict within the team. Interaction between team members involves regular open and honest communication between all members, shared planning and decision-making, and cooperative endeavour in which team members are inter-dependent on each other for the successful achievement of agreed goals (Hennemann *et al.* 1995).

The development of collaborative working develops and becomes consolidated over time as team members become less concerned about the specific boundaries of their previous roles and start to work more flexibly with other team members (Price & Williams 2003). However, for this process to commence and flourish a number of antecedents have been identified as necessary, namely: individual readiness of all (or at least the majority of) team members, understanding and acceptance of one's own role and expertise, confidence in one's own ability and recognition the boundaries of one's own discipline. Furthermore team members need to function within an environment that is appropriately managed to facilitate effective group dynamics (communication skills, respect and trust), a team orientation, organisational values of participation, inter-dependence and a leader supportive of autonomy (Hennemann *et al.* 1995).

The work of the team members is made positive and reinforcing

West (2004) outlined three key aspects that need to be addressed in order that the commitment of team members is maintained. First, he asserts that teams should have 'intrinsically interesting' tasks to perform and that individual team members should have 'intrinsically interesting' tasks to perform. Team members do not need to find every task they undertake to be of significant interest, however both at team and individual levels some aspects of their work should be of particular interest. The interest of team members in the success of the team can be enhanced by their active involvement in the development of team objectives and an understanding of where the team fits into and is valued by other components of the overall service (Nancarrow 2004).

In seeking to motivate individual team members and make their job intrinsically interesting, it is important to develop an understanding of what each team member may find interesting and perhaps has a particular ability for, or areas in which they wish to learn new skills. By doing so the team leader is in a better informed position to coordinate the use of members' knowledge and skills to meet client needs in a way that the team member will find motivating to them. It is important that the needs and interests of all team members, including the role of secretarial and other support staff are considered in this process.

Second, not only should team members find their job (or at least some aspects of it) interesting, they should also feel that their individual contribution is important to the overall success of the team in achieving the agreed objectives. While it is important that people know the role they play in achieving the overall success of the team and the inter-dependence on the contribution of individual team members, care needs to be taken to value equally the contribution of all team members. For this reason it is important to ensure that each team member has an aspect of their role which they feel is their particular contribution. Once the team member accepts the new role and is aware of the requirements of that role, they should be afforded a degree of autonomy in how they undertake these activities and receive encouragement to develop that area of their work.

Finally, feedback on progress towards agreed objectives should be provided to team members individually in relation to their role and to all members of the team in respect of team's success and areas that might be considered for further development. Team members should also be made aware of the standards that will be used to evaluate both their individual role and that of the team. The involvement of team members in the negotiation of the areas to be focused on can further reinforce their value as a team member and the importance of their contribution to the team.

The value of 'conflict' is acknowledged and appropriately channelled

An underlying premise of inter-disciplinary teamworking is that by bringing together a group of people with different knowledge, skills and perspectives more comprehensive solutions may emerge to meeting the needs of people who are supported by that service. It is through the process of sharing information and ideas that increased flexibility and creativity emerges in comparison to what the thoughts of an individual or a team of people from one professional background may have produced.

Inherent in this process is the need for some degree of discussion and at times the emergence and sharing of disagreements. This is

to be encouraged and the creative energy that results should be channelled into the development of effective ways of working as a team. Disagreement is not a failing; indeed it is one of the few certainties the team will encounter as it evolves. Conversely, the absence of some level of disagreement from time to time may well reflect an unwillingness of team members to engage fully in the process of discussion and indicate the presence of some level of 'groupthink'. However, it is important that team members are aware of the limits of an acceptable disagreement and that clear procedures exist for dealing with differences between team members that cannot be resolved by discussion within the team. The presence of ground rules can enhance the development of trust and mutual respect among team members by providing a degree of certainty, predictability and fairness about how issues within the team are addressed. Such procedures need to acknowledge the need for discussion among team members and may vary between teams. However, procedures should be in place and agreed with team members shortly after the team is established, as it is likely to be more difficult to give adequate time and thought to develop the necessary procedures when a disagreement between team members has escalated at a later stage. As it is not possible to anticipate all eventualities, it is important that any strategies or procedures for dealing with conflict within the team are revised within regularly.

Conclusion

The pressure to find more effective ways of coordinating health, social services and other agencies is set to continue. In recognition of the multitude of factors that can impact on the health of people and communities, community health care nurses will find themselves needing to collaborate effectively with people from a wider range of agencies and services than they have traditionally worked with. More attention now needs to be given to the development of teamwork and collaborative working practices between individuals in order to balance the present focus on collaborative working at policy level. If these inter-agency policies are to materialise for people in their local communities, it is important that those people who will deliver services have the opportunity to develop the necessary knowledge, skills and competence to work together effectively. Individual community nurses also need to take steps through their continuing professional development to develop the necessary knowledge and skills to master the challenges required for effective inter-agency and inter-organisational teamworking.

As discussed in this chapter the process of ensuring successful collaboration is complex, and needs careful planning and ongoing attention from managers and team members. In addition to being aware of the factors that may facilitate effective teamwork, there is a need to remain vigilant and take action whenever dysfunctional team dynamics or practices are witnessed. Failure to address such issues at the very least may result in the insidious reduction of effective teamwork and an associated erosion of service quality to people who need the support of community nurses. However, it can have much more extreme consequences resulting in the catastrophic failures in services that result in fatal consequences for people who have depended on community services to meet their health care needs (DH 2003; EHSSB/WHSSB 2008).

References

Bateman, H., Bailey, P. & McLellan, H. (2003) of rocks and safe channels: learning to navigate as an interprofessional team. *Journal of Interprofessional Care*, **17**, 141–150.

Beattie, A. (1995) War and Peace among the health tribes. In: *Interprofessional Relations in Health Care* (eds K. Soothill, L. Mackay & C. Webb, pp. 11–30). Edward Arnold; London.

Brown, S. (1992) Profession in teams. In: *Standards and Mental Handicap, Keys to Competence* (1992) (eds T. Thompson & P. Mathais, pp. 371–385). Baillière Tindall, London.

Department of Health (1989) *Caring for People*. HMSO, London.

Department of Health (2000a) *The NHS Plan. The Government's response to the Royal Commission on Long Term Care*. CM 4818-II. HMSO, London.

Department of Health (2000b) *The NHS Cancer Plan. A Plan for Investment. A Plan for Reform*. HMSO, London.

Department of Health (2001) *Valuing People. A New Strategy for Learning Disability for the 21st century*. HMSO, London.

Department of Health (2002) *Liberating Talents – Helping Primary Care Trusts and Nurses to Deliver the NHS Plan*. HMSO, London.

Department of Health (2003) *The Victoria Climbié Inquiry*. HMSO, London.

Department of Health (2004a) *Disabled Child Standard, National Service Framework for Children, Young People and Maternity Services*. Department of Health, London.

Department of Health (2004b) *Harold Shipman's Clinical Practice 1974–1998: a Clinical Audit Commissioned by the Chief Medical Officer*. HMSO, London.

Department of Health (2004c) *National Service Framework for Children, Young People and Maternity Services*. HMSO, London.

Department of Health (2005) *National Service Framework for Long-term Conditions*. HMSO, London.

Department of Health and Social Services (1991) *People First*. DHSS, Belfast.

Eastern Health and Social Service Board/Western Health and Social Service Board (2008) *Report of the Independent Inquiry Panel to the Western and Eastern Health and Social Service Boards. Madeline and Lauren O Neill*. Eastern Health and Social Service Board, Belfast.

Fickel, J.J., Parker, L.E., Yano, E.M. & Kirchner, J.E. (2007) Primary care–mental health collaboration: An example of assessing usual practice and potential barriers. *Journal of Interprofessional Care*, **21**, 207–216.

Gannon-Leary, P., Baines, S. & Wilson, R. (2006) Collaboration and partnership: A review and reflections on a national project to join up local services in England. *Journal of Interprofessional Care*, **20**, 665–674.

Glasby, J. & Lester, H. (2004) Cases for change in mental health: partnership working in mental health services. *Journal of Interprofessional Care*, **18**, 7–16.

Hattersly, J. (1995) The survival of collaboration and co-operation. In: *Services for People with Learning Disabilities* (ed. N. Malin, pp. 260–273). Routledge, London.

Hayes, N. (1997) *Successful Team Management*. Thomson Business Press, London.

Hennemann, E.A., Lee, J.L. & Cohen, J.L. (1995) Collaboration: a concept analysis. *Journal of Advanced Nursing*, **21**, 103–109.

Hudson, B. (1995) A seamless service? Developing better relationships between the National Health Service and Social Services Departments. In: *Values and Visions. Changing ideas in services for people with learning difficulties* (eds T. Philpot & L. Ward, pp. 106–122). Butterworth Heinemann Oxford.

Hudson, B. (2002) Interprofessionality in health and social care: the Achilles' heel of partnership. *Journal of Interprofessional Care*, **16**, 8–17.

Janis, I.L. (1983) *Groupthink,* 2nd edition. Houghton Mifflin, Boston.

Johnson, P., Wistow, G., Schulz, R. & Hardy, B. (2003) Interagency and interprofessional collaboration in community care: the interdependence of structures and values. *Journal of Interprofessional Care*, **17**, 69–83.

Leathard, A. (1994) *Going Interprofessional. Working Together for Health and Welfare.* Routledge, London.

Lewis, M. & Noyes, J. (2007) Discharge management for children with complex needs. *Paediatric Nursing*, **19**, 26–30.

Malin, N., Manthorpe, J., Race, D. & Wilmot, S. (1999) *Community Care for Nurses and the Caring Professions.* Open University Press, Buckingham.

McLaughlin, H. (2004) Partnerships: panacea or pretence. *Journal of Interprofessional Care*, **18**, 103–113.

Mencap (2007) *Death by Indifference.* Mencap, London.

Molyneux, J. (2001) Interprofessional teamworking: what makes teams work well. *Journal of Interprofessional Care*, **15**, 29–35.

Moorhead, G., Ference, R. & Neck, C.P. (1991) Group decision fiascos continue. Space shuttle Challenger and a revised groupthink framework. *Human Relations*, **44**, 539–550.

Nancarrow, S. (2004) Dynamic role boundaries in intermediate care services. *Journal of Interprofessional Care*, **18**, 141–151.

NHS Executive (2000) *Making a Difference: Integrated Working in Primary Care.* Nursing, Quality and Consumers Directorate, NHS Executive, London.

Noyes, J. (2007) Comparison of ventilator-dependent child reports of health-related quality of life with parent reports and normative populations. *Journal of Advanced Nursing*, **58**, 1–10.

Nursing and Midwifery Council (2007) *Code of Professional Conduct,* 6th edition. Nursing and Midwifery Council, London.

Ovretviet, J. (1986) *Organisation of Multidisciplinary Community Teams,* London. The University of West London. A Health Services Centre Working Paper, Brunel.

Ovretveit, J. (1993) *Co-ordinating Community Care. Multidisciplinary Teams and Care Management.* Open University Press, Buckingham.

Ovretveit, J. (ed.) (1997) *Interprofessional Working for Health and Social Care.* Macmillan, London.

Price, A. & Williams, A. (2003) Primary care nurse practitioners and the interface with secondary care: A qualitative study of referral practice. *Journal of Interprofessional Care*, **17**, 239–250.

Robinson, M. & Cottrell, D. (2005) Health professionals in multi-disciplinary and multi-agency teams: Changing professional practice. *Journal of Interprofessional Care*, **19**, 547–560.

Roulstone, A. & Hudson, V. (2007) Carer participation in England, Wales and Northern Ireland: a challenge for interprofessional working. *Journal of Interprofessional Care*, **21**, 303–317.

Scottish Executive (2000) *The Same As You? A Review of the Services for People with Learning Disabilities.* Scottish Executive, Edinburgh.

Sheehan, D., Robertson, L. & Ormond, T. (2007) Comparison of language used and patterns of communication in interprofessional and multidisciplinary teams. *Journal of Interprofessional Care*, **21**, 17–30.

Towell, D. & Beardshaw, V. (1991) *Enabling Community Integration.* King's Fund College, London.

Tuckman, B. & Jensen, M. (1977) Stages of small group development revisited. *Group and Organisational Studies*, **2**, 419–427.

West, M. (2004) *Effective Teamwork: Practical Lessons from Organisational Research.* Blackwell Scientific Publications, London.

Chapter 17 Measuring Effectiveness in Community Health Care Nursing and Specialist Community Public Health Nursing

Elizabeth Porter

Introduction

The purpose of measuring effectiveness in the National Health Service (NHS) is to ensure that treatment, services and preventive care are of high quality and improve health outcomes for service users. This chapter will discuss the measurement of effectiveness, provide an overview and define and explore the term 'measurement of effectiveness in the NHS'. The aim is to demonstrate how clinical effectiveness links to a political imperative to drive up the quality of the service delivered by the NHS, reduce financial pressures, embrace new technologies and address increasing demands for more and better services where the emphasis is on improving both the cost-effectiveness and the quality of health services.

Approaches to the evaluation in health care will be discussed and NHS policy developments related to improving quality in the NHS. A sample of established evidence used to measure effectiveness in public health and primary care will be examined and the chapter will conclude with ongoing issues for the community health care nurse (CHCN) and specialist community public health nurse (SCPHN).

Throughout this chapter 'CHCN' refers to the district nurse, community mental health nurse, community learning disabilities nurse and general practice nurse. SCPHN refers to those in the role of health visitor school nurse and occupational health nurse (England and Wales),

occupational health nurse and family health nurse (Scotland).

The measurement of effectiveness in the NHS

The measurement of effectiveness in the NHS is the business of all workers in the NHS and is linked to the political agendas of government. For the past 25 years there has been a growing concern among health professionals and the public about variations in clinical practice and the uptake of research evidence in health care. In addition, financial pressures within the NHS, the development of new health technologies, and increasing demands for more and better services, have led to an emphasis on improving both the cost-effectiveness and the quality of health services. In 1996, the NHS Executive suggested that clinical effectiveness should focus on the extent to which specific interventions can improve health and deliver the best outcome for service users from available resources. Upton & Upton (2005) state that this drive for quality, formally implemented following the introduction of clinical governance, encompasses the twinned concepts of clinical effectiveness and evidence-based practice. These concepts have become increasingly important for CHCNs and SCPHNs as over the past 15 years they have provided them with a framework for developing best practice. By adopting this approach to developing clinical effectiveness they have been enabled to make clinical decisions based on and informed by up-to-date, relevant and robust evidence, thus producing professional effectiveness and accountability in all aspects of their practice.

Lord Darzi, in his *Next Stage Review of the NHS* outlined proposals for the development of a new quality and outcomes framework for primary and community services (Department of Health [DH] 2008). The proposed framework will incorporate best practice from the National Centre for Health and Clinical Excellence (NICE) and measure clinical effectiveness and user satisfaction through the use of patient reported outcome measures (PROMs, p. 45). Comparative quality information will also be generated by primary care trusts (PCTs) to help primary care professionals to understand and compare different areas of performance and identify areas for improvement. This approach will encourage greater transparency and public accountability and assist users to make informed choices about the selection of services and providers. Lord Darzi has also noted his intention to promote the use of accreditation schemes to drive quality improvement. Work will be undertaken in partnership with the Royal Colleges to identify performance measures that will generate a new system of independent/objective audit of general practice performance (DH 2008, p. 46).

Definition of clinical effectiveness
Clinical effectiveness is about providing evidence of what works (DH 2000) and is for nurses about doing the right thing in the right way and at the right time for the right patient with the right knowledge and skills (Royal College of nursing [RCN]1996).

Definition of evidence-based practice
Evidence-based practice is about using the best evidence in making decisions about the patient, based on skills which allow the nurse to find 'and critically appraise, analyse and interpret existing evidence in order to make decisions about best practice for groups of people or populations' (Reading [2008] cited in Coles & Porter [2008], p. 170).

As early as 1988, the NHS reforms following the White Paper *Working for Patients* (DH 1989) aimed to control costs and improve quality through a number of initiatives including the introduction of the internal market and managed competition, medical audit and the Patient's Charter (Paton 1996). The emphasis on measuring effectiveness and outcomes in the NHS continued throughout the 1990s (NHS Executive [NHSE] 1996, 1998). Subsequent policies of the decade (DH 1992, 1996) emphasised the need for specific, measurable health outcomes. Such outcomes were intended to enable the health service and the public to know whether health care interventions actually maintain and improve health, and whether they do so with the best use of resources.

Clinical governance
The introduction of clinical governance (DH 1998) provided a new framework at the time, through which NHS organisations became accountable for continuously improving the quality of their services and this has been the driving force for the first decade of the twenty-first century, where there is now an obligation to examine the effectiveness and quality of services throughout the NHS, including primary and community care provision.

Definition of clinical governance
Clinical governance can be defined as 'a system through which NHS organisations are accountable for continuously improving the quality of their services and safeguarding high standards of care, by creating an environment in which clinical excellence will flourish' (DH 1998, p. 17).

Measuring health gain
Section 45 of the Health and Social Care (Community Health and Standards) Act 2003 (Secretary of State 2003), sets out the legislative basis for the health care standards. *National Standards, Local Action* (DH 2004c) announces a new performance framework for the NHS and social care. The system is mainly driven by targets and measured by star ratings. In 2004, *Standards*

for Better Health (DH 2004a) introduced a series of key standards for the quality of care across the NHS. The aim was to set a common foundation for delivery of high-quality health care throughout England and to clarify what the NHS can and should be reaching for in its ambitions for the service user and health professionals. The standards fulfilled a responsibility placed on the Secretary of State for Health under the Health and Social Care Community Health and Standards Act 2003. Taking a user friendly approach (written for the user), the standards were developed within two categories, core standards, dealing with quality of care which can be expected by all users of the health service, and developmental standards to enable the quality of health care to improve as additional resources invested in the NHS took effect. These core and developmental standards covered the entire spectrum of health work from measures to improve health through to primary care services and specialist care. The purpose was to address real issues and the standards are capable of assessment through criteria set by the Commission for Health Care Audit and Inspection (CHAI). The standards built onto previous work in setting the framework for decentralising the management of the health service in order to shift the balance of power from central government to the NHS (DH 2001). From 2004, the adopted framework has considered the quality of health care and provides a measurement of performance. Assessment criteria have been developed for measuring how the standards should fit with performance ratings and how these assessment of performance ratings can best draw on the standards set and link into existing performance measures in the ratings system (DH 2004b). In 2006, these standards were revisited and *Standards for Better Health* (DH 2006e) set out new core and developmental standards to replace the previous star ratings and move away from a system that was mainly driven by national targets to one in which 'standards are the main driver for continuous improvements in quality… and all organisations locally play their part in service modernisation' (DH 2006e, p. 2). *Standards for Better Health* (DH 2006e) forms a key part of the performance assessment

by the Healthcare Commission of all health care organisations. Sale (2005) suggests the government implemented this revised quality assurance framework to consolidate the quality agenda within health care organisations to deliver safe, cost-effective care.

Within PCTs, governance leads set the agenda to implement national quality initiatives and local strategies to monitor and improve quality. The standards provide a common set of requirements applying across all health care organisations to ensure that health services provided are safe and of an acceptable quality. They also aim to provide a framework for continuous improvement in the overall quality of care people receive. The core standards (see Table 17.1) describe a level of service that is acceptable but the expectation is that the focus of the performance assessment by the Healthcare Commission will be on progress measured against the developmental standards. These standards reflect the direction set by the *NHS Improvement Plan* (DH 2004b) and stress the importance of organisations working together to provide a whole systems approach to delivering care that is tailor made to the individual patient. Measuring the effectiveness of this approach is discussed later in the chapter.

Development of research governance

Over the past 20 years, a number of instances of research misconduct and identified failures to improve the quality of health care led to lack of confidence in the NHS and spiralling costs of health care litigation claims. Childs (2008), cited in Coles & Porter (2008), reminds us that these failures included the trials of nurse Beverley Allittt (DH 1994), the Bristol Royal Infirmary Inquiry (2001) into the deaths of 23 children following cardiac surgery and the Harold Shipman inquiry (Smith 2004). The growing recognition that research activity needs to be supported and monitored in order to maintain public trust and participation in clinical research has led to the introduction of a framework for the governance of research undertaken in health and social

Table 17.1 The core standards set out by the government in 2006. Adapted from *Core Standards: Standards for Better Health* (DH 2006).

Seven domains	Domain outcome
Safety	Patient safety is enhanced by the use of health care processes, working practices and systemic activities that prevent or reduce the risk of harm to patients
Clinical and cost effective	Patients achieve health care benefits that meet their individual needs through health care decisions and services based on what assessed research evidence has shown provides effective clinical outcomes
Governance	Managerial and clinical leadership and accountability, as well as the organisation's culture, systems and working practices ensure that probity, quality assurance, quality improvement and patient safety are central components of all the activities of the health care organisation
Patient focus	Health care is provided in partnership with patients, their carers and relatives respecting their diverse needs, preferences and choices and in partnership with other organisations whose services impact on patient well-being
Accessible and responsive care	Patients receive services as promptly as possible, have choice in access to services and treatments and do not experience unnecessary delay at any stage of service delivery or of the care pathway
Care environment and amenities	Care is provided in environments that promote patient and staff well being and respect for patients' needs and preferences in that they are designed for the effective and safe delivery of treatment, care or specific function, provide as much privacy as possible, are well maintained and are cleaned to optimise health outcomes for patients
Public health	Programmes and services are designed and delivered in collaboration with all relevant organisations and communities to promote, protect and improve the health of the population served and reduce health inequalities between different population groups and areas

care settings (DH 2001). Table 17.1 identifies the accepted importance of this as research governance is one of the core standards for health care set out in *Standards for Better Health* (DH 2006e). The framework for the governance of research (DH 2001) sets out a model which was revised in 2005 (DH 2005b) with the aim of bringing together general principles of good practice 'to forestall poor performance, adverse incidents, research misconduct and fraud and to ensure that lessons are learned and shared when poor practice is identified' (DH 2005b, p. 3). Howarth *et al.* (2007) describe the main aim of the framework as one to enable organisations to develop a research culture through which 'robust and

scientifically rigorous research could be best supported' (p. 363). As with clinical governance, research governance involves bringing general performance up to that of those at the leading edge and can be defined as 'the attempt to derive, generalisable new knowledge by addressing clearly defined questions with systematic rigorous methods' (DH 2001, p. 4).

Clinical governance in primary care

The Royal College of General Practitioners (RCGP 1999) suggests that clinical governance in primary care is about developing people, teams and systems within primary care while protecting patients. Current developments in the NHS concerning quality and performance indicate that this is the case and the trend is set to continue (DH 2004a,b, 2006a; Hillier *et al.* 2007; NICE) 2008).

These developments build upon existing activity such as modification and implementation of professional regulation (Nursing and Midwifery Council [NMC] 2003, 2004, 2008) and continuing professional development (DH 2005a, 2007e); the development and implementation of guidelines and protocols (DH 2002, 2006b; NICE 2008); clinical audit (Healthcare Commission 2004, 2007a,b; HDA 2005); and evidence-based practice (DH 2003b; Heslehurst *et al.* 2007; Olds 2006). Nurses working in primary care trusts are already familiar with some or all of these activities. For example, clinical audit is often used by CHCNs and SCPHNs to examine their practice against agreed explicit standards and outcomes, and to modify practice where necessary (Pritchard & De Verteuil 2007).

Governance arrangements bring together all developments relating to clinical effectiveness and quality, with an emphasis on working interprofessionally with other practitioners and clinicians, and in partnership with users of the NHS (DH 2004b; Donaldson 2001). Therefore, in the context of these developments, CHCNs and SCPHNs must ensure that their practice is based on the best available evidence. In order to achieve this objective, they must be able to measure the effectiveness of their interventions in conjunction with other members of the primary health care team, public health team, patients, carers and all service users. This involves various activities (see Box 17.1) identified as stages in the 'clinical effectiveness process'. The CHCN and SCPHN therefore need to utilise critical thinking skills such as literature searching, critical appraisal, audit and research (Jones-Devitt 2007).

The arrangements for setting clear national quality standards through national service frameworks (DH 2002) and the NICE guidance (NICE 2005, 2008) are integral to a standards-based system and are key in supporting local improvements in service quality. They make this

---

Box 17.1 Stages in the clinical effectiveness process

(1) Identify the practice issue, question current practice and ask what evidence there is to support it
(2) Find the evidence through searching the literature, seeking expert opinion and using professional resources and networks
(3) Appraise, synthesise and interpret the evidence using critical appraisal skills
(4) Put the evidence into practice and implement changes where necessary
(5) Monitor and evaluate clinical change, for example through using audit
(6) Disseminate and share good practice

---

achievable by providing robust evidence and national guidelines upon which practice can be based at a local level. The NHS Library for Health (www.library.nhs.uk) provides a powerful medium for capturing and disseminating such evidence together with examples of good practice and methods of audit and evaluation.

The clinical effectiveness process, as described above, provides a systematic framework through which CHCNs and SCPHNs can evaluate their contribution to health and health care. It provides an opportunity for them to demonstrate the value of their contribution to the health of the population by revealing the evidence base for practice and clearly identifying health outcomes. Problems are sometimes witnessed with this approach, however, when applying it to practice. In some areas there is robust research evidence to support specific interventions, and guidelines for practice are clear, for example in pre-school surveillance services offered by health visitors to identify children with special needs in Sheffield (Foo & Chaplais 2008) and for the development of a community matron role in the management of long-term conditions in Leeds (Bee & Clegg 2006). However, sometimes the evidence to support practice is not available or does not provide clear guidance, such as with health screening programmes for older people (Illife & Drennan 2000). Additionally, health outcomes for CHCN and SCPHN interventions are not always easily identifiable or measurable, therefore using audit to measure effectiveness can be difficult (Barribell & Mackenzie 1993). These problems are not unique to community nursing and can be explained by examining approaches to clinical effectiveness and outcome measurement of health care.

Approaches to clinical effectiveness and outcome measurement of health care

There are concerns about the use of industrial management models in measuring outcomes of health care within the NHS. Campbell *et al.* (1995) suggest that an approach to clinical effectiveness and outcome measurement in the NHS, drawn from an industrial management model, offers a more predictable and objective context in industrial management than in health care. It may be possible to accurately measure inputs, outputs and end results in industry, but it is much more difficult in health care where the situation is complex, there are multiple influences on outcome and end results can be intangible. Over the past 20 years, there has therefore been a tendency to overemphasise outcomes in the assessment of the quality of health care (Martin & Henderson 2001). Campbell *et al.* (1995) stress the importance of outcome measurement but only as offering one part of an assessment of the quality of care. Seedhouse (2004) argues that the concentration on outcomes or end results means that much of the process (the complex activities and interactions involved in health care) is ignored. In fact, Donabedian's framework for the assessment of quality of health care, from which the concept of outcome measurement in health care is derived, does include measures of structure and process as well as outcome (Donabedian 1980). Donabedian proposes that a comprehensive evaluation of health care should include assessment of the environment and resources, and assessment of the intervention itself (what care is given and how), as well as the outcome.

Furthermore, some aspects and outcomes of health care are more easily quantifiable (such as survival rates or symptom relief) whereas others are more difficult to define and measure (such as raised self-esteem or quality of life). Seedhouse (2004), when looking at effectiveness in health care, concludes that there is a tendency to concentrate on the more easily measurable outcomes, which leaves the effects of many aspects of health care hidden and untested. He also points out that there are often different ways of assessing even the most apparently simple quantifiable aspects of a service. He argues that the methods chosen to assess the effectiveness of an intervention tend to favour outcomes that can be 'objectively witnessed' (for example, numbers of children immunised) rather than those which are more subjective or descriptive (such as parental levels of knowledge and understanding about side effects, or alleviation of anxiety). However, unintended and unexpected consequences of health care interventions can be as valid and worthwhile as outcomes that are predetermined. For example, a nurse treating a diabetic patient at home may be able to improve the quality of life of the patient as well as treating the physical condition, through identifying social isolation and organising opportunities to meet other people (Holmes & Griffiths 2002).

This simplification of information regarding effectiveness in health care has resulted in a tendency to focus on outcomes which can be objectively defined and measured, such as death and illness rates. However, the use of mortality and morbidity data as health outcomes presents further problems, as this suggests a narrow view of health as a purely biological function, with illness resulting as a consequence of pathological abnormality. This reflects a biomedical model, where health is defined as the absence of disease. Bowling (1991) advises that outcomes should be measured more comprehensively using a broad concept of 'positive health' which takes factors other than disease and disability into account, such as the ability to cope with stress; social support; morale; life satisfaction; and psychological well-being. Bowling reviews a number of 'quality of life' measurement scales which attempt to do this. Many of these methods involve the participation of patients or users of services in the assessment of health outcomes, yet the adoption of a biomedical model of outcome measurement militates against the involvement of service users in the evaluation of health care. User views do not fit neatly with the supposedly objective measurement of medical outcomes. This reflects a view of professionals as 'experts' who hold the power to make health care decisions on behalf of patients and lay people. However, the increase in public demand for information about health and health care, suggests a widespread belief that people should make their own, informed decisions about their health (DH 2007a). There is an increasing interest in and commitment to user involvement in quality and evaluation in health care and evidence that users of care are contributing measurable outcomes of care they themselves see as relevant (Tee [2008], cited in Coles & Porter 2008).

The domination of clinical effectiveness and outcome evaluation by a biomedical model is further strengthened by the continual drive for evidence based practice, whereby individual expertise is integrated with the best available evidence from systematic research (Sackett *et al.* 1996). This may be accounted for by the fact that this approach began with evidence-based medicine, which is based upon a scientific, experimental model of research with a hierarchy of evidence which favours quantitative rather than qualitative methods of data collection. For example, randomised controlled trials (RCTs) are seen as 'gold standard' evidence, followed by other robust experimental or observational studies (Greenhalgh 2006). Qualitative, descriptive studies may therefore be seen as less valuable or valid when considering the effectiveness of interventions. This poses problems, particularly for CHCNs and SCPHNs, who often use qualitative methods of evaluation. For example, it is argued that the SCPHN is not best served by using such quantitative research methods as RCTs, due to the ethical and practical difficulties of randomising people to experimental or control groups (Reading [2008], cited in Coles & Porter 2008). Kemm (2006) supports this view and argues that RCTs do not address the nature of public health interventions as the SCPHN is concerned with interventions for communities that exist in specific social contexts for

which there are unlikely to be matching controls. For the CHCN, quantitative methods of data collection go against the individualised nature of the therapeutic relationship between the CHCN and the patient, and do not account for the complexity of nursing interventions and the social and health care context in which they take place (Rolfe 1998; Schutz 1994; Shih 1998). Although many research and evaluation studies in the UK have been undertaken looking at the effectiveness and outcomes of nursing interventions (recent ones include Byles *et al.* 2002; Freeman & Peck 2006; Martin *et al.* 2007; Perry *et al.* 2008), Cullum (1997) states there are relatively few RCTs specific to nursing. The majority of those available appear to have been undertaken outside Europe (examples are Koehn & Lehman 2008; Lemstra *et al.* 2002; Marchionni & Ritchie 2008).

If the scientific, biomedical approach is to be viewed as a dominant one for evaluation in the NHS, the nursing profession will remain exposed to criticism for lack of objective evidence of effectiveness and outcomes. Fortunately for nursing, alternative approaches of evaluation are more prominent in the NHS today where a variety of qualitative and quantitative methods are accepted as appropriate. Such methodologies involve analysis of the process and quality of care delivery in addition to the measurement of health outcomes (Horta *et al.* 2007; Social Exclusion Task Force 2007). These approaches are reliant on the provision of service user feedback and place all service users at the centre of the evaluation process.

The nursing literature demonstrates how the application of outcome measurement based on the scientific method can be inappropriate and unsuccessful in describing and explaining the effectiveness of nursing interventions (Griffiths 1995). Evidence suggests that outcome measurement should include an analysis of the process of care and should use qualitative as well as quantitative methods of evaluation. Shih (1998) recommends the use of the qualitative approach in nursing research, but acknowledges that many authors are recognising the benefits of a combined qualitative and quantitative approach. The use of combined methods enables the nurse researcher to describe and conceptualise the 'multifaceted complexity of the human response to illness and various health care situations' (Shih 1998, p. 632).

Whilst Kemm (2006) identifies the unsuitability of RCTs for public health work, Macdonald *et al.* (1996) point to the unsuitability of quantitative methods to evaluate health promotion activities. They suggest that traditional epidemiological indicators of health and behavioural outcomes are often inappropriate when appraising the effectiveness of health promotion. The authors criticise the use of the experimental research design and believe it is rarely possible or desirable to use such a design in the evaluation of health promotion. The rationale for this relates to the acknowledgement of the practical problems that exist when applying an experimental design in a complex, naturalistic setting and with multifaceted programmes (such as experienced in community and primary care). They also point to the need for 'illumination' to gain insight into the processes involved in the implementation of health promotion programmes and the social and environmental context in which they take place. This involves a description in great detail of what occurs in the delivery of health promotion programmes, which enables reasoned judgements to be made about which particular features have been effective. Qualitative techniques are therefore needed to provide this 'thick, rich description' (Macdonald *et al.* 1996). There is evidence to show that the use of qualitative methods and the concentration on process as well as outcome evaluation is recommended and used in the field of health promotion (Bolam *et al.* 2006; Farquhar *et al.* 2006; Lomas & Mcluskey 2005).

Macdonald *et al.* (1996) advocate that approaches are needed which study programme development and process, including qualitative research, formative evaluation and naturalistic observation. Although such qualitative methods can be challenged as less robust by advocates of the experimental research design, there is evidence to suggest that the use of a number of different research methods and the combination and comparison of data from different sources,

or 'triangulation', can provide robust checks on the validity of conclusions drawn about effectiveness. In agreeing with this view, Naidoo & Wills (2004) advocate process or illuminative evaluation, which employs a wide range of qualitative methods and takes into account different stakeholders' views. They consider the use of these methods to overcome the problem of attribution with health promotion activities, thus validating that the results are due to the health promotion input, rather than to other variables. In particular they point to the strength of the case study (where a health promotion programme is intensively studied using a variety of methods) for demonstrating that identified effects reliably result from a programme.

The problems associated with the use of biomedical health outcomes as indicators of success are also identified in the field of health promotion. The use of 'indirect' and 'intermediate' indicators, such as the successful acquisition of teaching skills by health promotion workers (an indirect indicator) or changes in lifestyle (an intermediate indicator) is therefore recommended. Tones & Tilford (2001) describe outcome indicators, which can be used when measuring the effectiveness of health promotion programmes and suggest that the task of selecting indicators of effectiveness and efficiency is facilitated by the use of theories which not only suggest the appropriate strategies and methods to use in designing and running health promotion programmes but may also be employed to specify requirements for successful health promotion interventions.

Literature from the fields of nursing and health promotion combine to support the use of qualitative methods and the application of process indicators and intermediate outcomes in the evaluation of health care. Such an approach to evaluation takes account of social and environmental influences on health and may be more suitable for studies aiming to investigate the effectiveness of long-term interventions and interventions that are based on partnership with service users and have a community or public health focus. This approach can therefore be seen to be more appropriate for CHCNs and SCPHNs than the scientific approach previously described in this chapter. Concerns remain regarding the reliability and validity of such qualitative evaluation methods and outcome measures, particularly, if they are judged according to the 'rules' of the traditional scientific approach. However, the use of varied, rigorous methods in the development and measurement of outcome measures, the involvement of clients in the evaluation process, and the use of evidence to support the link between process, intermediate and final outcomes, can help to establish trustworthiness and rigor. The current policy context in the NHS appears to support this approach to evaluation, as evidenced by the emphasis placed on the involvement of service users and the examination of 'quality' issues, which include the effective delivery of, and fair access to, appropriate health care (DH 2007a).

NHS policy development and clinical effectiveness

Recent developments in government policy go some way towards changing the NHS's reliance on the use of quantifiable indicators of illness and disease and encouraging and validating qualitative approaches. Evidence of this is seen in current policy focus which provides opportunities to establish a means of evaluating health care that is based on a broader, social model of health, and which involve users as well as health professionals in the process (Wanless 2004). Policies relating to quality and performance in the 'new NHS' (DH 2006) propose a move away from 'counting numbers and measuring activity' and suggest an evaluation process which is based on a broader theory of health. As discussed earlier in the chapter, this performance framework considers access to services; effective delivery of appropriate health care; and patient/carer experience, as well as efficiency and health outcomes. Health improvement is seen as reflecting social and environmental factors and individual behaviour as well as health and social care services (DH 2006c). However, Wanless et al. (2007) suggest that it is hard to provide a full account of improvements in clinical care and

process since 2002 and thus harder to demonstrate links between the policies and their results. Nevertheless two conclusions can be reached. First, 'the government was right to introduce an explicit focus on quality of care, although that in itself does not guarantee that services will improve', and second, 'the evidence is not available to demonstrate how the various elements of clinical governance perform as a system and hence whether its design and implementation could be improved' (Wanless et al. 2007, p. 59).

The 1999 strategy for nursing (DH 1999b) identified the role for nurses, midwives and health visitors in contributing to, and leading the clinical governance/quality agenda, ensuring that it does not focus narrowly on medical interventions and outcomes. Furthermore, policies relating to public health and to services for communities, families and individuals demonstrate a change in underlying philosophy away from a biomedical approach, towards a public health approach, which considers public health as the 'science and art of preventing disease, prolonging life and promoting health through the organised efforts of society and informed choices of society, organisations, public and private communities and individuals' (Wanless 2004, p. 3). This public health definition acknowledges the importance of those social aspects of health problems which are caused by lifestyles. This was initially proposed in *Saving Lives: Our Healthier Nation* (DH 1999a), which recognised the influence of social and economic issues on health and proposed to improve the health of the population and reduce inequalities through promoting partnerships between government, local agencies, communities and individuals. This partnership theme is threaded through government policies designed to support families (DH 2003a; Department for Education and Skills [DfES] 2007). Many of the new initiatives build on programmes within which community health care nurses and specialist community public health nurses are regularly engaged. For example, *Supporting People with Long Term Conditions: Liberating the Talents of Nurses Who Care for People with Long Term Conditions* (DH 2005a) sees community matrons as key in delivering personalised, managed care to adults with complex long-term needs. *Choosing Health: Making Healthier Choices Easier* (DH 2004d) includes explicit recognition of the preventive work of health visitors 'with communities and families' (p. 48) in particular with reference to children's health, and other health improvement services.

There is continued recognition of the problems involved in the evaluation of public health interventions (HDA 2003). Furthermore, the need to widen the scope of research methods to establish the effectiveness of health programmes, thus reducing reliance on quantitative approaches to measuring health gain (HDA 2004; Heller 2005). Evaluation of health care cannot be solely based on biomedical health outcomes it has to encompass public health activity aimed at improving health gains. Such a focus provides opportunity for CHCNs and SCPHNs to demonstrate quality and effectiveness, through the development and use of more appropriate outcome measures based on a broad, holistic model of health and health care. Such measures relate, for example, to improving access to services, or to how they are delivered, and could be illustrated by the inclusion of subjective accounts of clients' experiences (Brooks & Barrett 2003; Dargie 2001; McHugh & Luker 2002).

Within specialist community public health nursing, there is also evidence to suggest that by taking on new and enhanced roles and responsibilities, health visitors and school nurses can be instrumental in delivering improvements in services to their client groups. Health visitors can play a vital part in reducing health inequalities through early childhood interventions (DH 2007b; Karoly *et al.* 2005), school nurses can make services more accessible to children and young people through the development of innovative service delivery (Ibarra *et al.* 2007; Sidebottam *et al.* 2008) and both can demonstrate improvement in the quality of care for clients (King 2006; Prothero *et al.* 2003; Wilson *et al.* 2008).

Although there is an increasing acceptance of different approaches and evaluative methodologies a tension between them is still evident in policy documents and indicative outcomes and targets continue to have a biomedical, quantitative focus. For example, hospital episode statistics for the NHS include information about patient treatment, death and surgery rates (DH 2007c) and targets based on reducing mortality rates (DH 2007d). It is therefore important that CHCNs and SCPHNs continue to develop outcome methods of evaluation which reflect both the public health activity and broader concepts of health and health care, and which focus on the experience of service users. If they fail to do this there is a danger that policy developments could be predominantly evaluated through the use of scientific, quantitative methods which have dominated health care evaluation in the past. The evidence to support this view is seen in the remit of the Audit Commission and in its review of PCTs in 2004 (Audit Commission 2004b).

As an independent watchdog the Audit Commission provides important information on the quality of public services. It is the driving force in the improvement of services and provides practical recommendations and spreads best practice. It is responsible for ensuring that public money is spent economically, efficiently and effectively, to achieve high quality local and national services for the public. The Audit Commission (2004a) review of PCTs' readiness to become proactive commissioners of primary care identifies the three key elements of the General Medical Services (GMS) contract (British Medical Association [BMA] & NHS Confederation 2003), supported by three funding streams:

- The global sum (funding for provision of essential primary medical services)
- The Quality and Outcomes Framework (a proportion of practice income is generated by the achievement of quality standards)
- Enhanced services (to enable the expansion of work carried out in primary care)

The relevance of this to measuring effectiveness within primary care is that it identifies that a substantial proportion of practice income will be generated by achievement of quality standards, achievement which will be assessed against 146 evidence-based standards that generate 1050 points if all are achieved (Audit Commission 2004a). The standards are drawn from the national service frameworks and from other evidence, establishing systems for quality assurance and an important role for PCTs in monitoring and supporting quality improvements. For the PCTs, there is a strategic risk that value for money may not be achieved through an increase in expenditure and an operational risk in ensuring systems are in place to report quality achievements. Findings from a study by the Audit Commission show how service redesign benefits patients (National Audit Office 2006), but in many PCTs it is still not a mainstream activity with sustainable outcomes.

Both service users and providers of services have a vested interest in the quality of primary care and service users expect their needs to be addressed. Since the 1980s their needs have been reviewed and analysed, and converted into functions met through the operation of the NHS (Martin & Henderson 2001). Today NHS providers offer choice in services and enter into a partnership with users of the service to design the service options (DH 2006b; DfES 2006). Users of the health service demand a quality service alongside one that is delivered at a lower cost, with greater accessibility, accountability, efficiency and effectiveness. They require access to information to enable them to make informed choices about their health, a right to know about the quality of the services, and assurance that the investment of resources is leading to demonstrable improvements in health care provision.

The work of the Commission for Health Care Audit and Inspection

The Commission for Health Care Audit and Inspection (CHAI) acts as an independent body and its involvement of service users in the audit and inspection of NHS services, signals a significant policy shift in prioritising the user experience as a central measure in the NHS assessment. CHAI provides a balanced and independent mechanism for championing clinical governance. The aim is to ensure that the user of the health services receives the highest quality of NHS care possible. In informing the systems and processes within the NHS, CHAI provides

a mechanism for monitoring and improving services so that they can deliver a user-centred approach that involves them in decisions about care and keeps them informed. It also has a commitment to quality, which ensures that health professionals are up to date in their practice and properly supervised where necessary and strive to promote continuous improvement to services and care within the NHS (National Audit Office 2006). It is proposed that CHAI will amalgamate with the Commission for Social Care Inspection (CSCI) and the Mental Health Act Commission (MHAC) to form a new unitary known as the Care Quality Commission in 2009 (DH 2006d).

Using benchmarks

'The essence of care patient-focused benchmarks for clinical governance' (DH 2003, 2006a, 2007) provides support to service improvement by offering patient-focused benchmarks for clinical governance and application guidance to practitioners. The patient-focused benchmarks aim to enable health care professionals to work with users of the NHS to identify best practice and to develop action plans to improve care. They adopt a qualitative approach, where patients, carers and the health professional work together to agree and describe good quality care and best practice. This is identified through areas of care relevant to all health and social care settings. Although patient experience is claimed to be the central tenet of the NHS, Ellis (2006) suggests that benchmarking activity appears to focus primarily on performance and process benchmarking with little mention of essence of care activity in Health Care Commission reviews. This demonstrates the tendency towards a 'continuing preoccupation in the health service with measurement that can support quantitative comparison and elements of competition' (Ellis 2006, p. 381).

Measuring health gain and outcomes in public health and primary care: established evidence

A selection of published examples of evaluation of practice reveal the application of a variety of qualitative and quantitative methods

---

Box 17.2   Published examples of evaluation in practice

- Audit Commission (1999): a review of district nursing services evaluated the effectiveness of community nursing interventions by examining some of the key processes that contribute to the quality of care, and outcomes in terms of users' experiences. Two specific conditions were selected to illustrate the process, leg ulcers and incontinence, because of their high prevalence and prominence in district nursing caseloads, the high cost to the NHS and the existence of evidence based clinical guidelines. As comprehensive, accurate assessment is acknowledged as a major determinant of patient outcomes in both these areas, assessment was taken as a key indicator of the quality of care.
- Baileff (2007): an audit of nurses' records pertaining to the administration or supply of medication using patient group directions. The assertion was that if record keeping was of a satisfactory standard, scrutiny of the records of patients who had received antibiotics would reveal to what extent the audit standards were achieved.
- Chamberlain et al. (1995): A multidisciplinary service evaluation project in the West Midlands used a range of outcome measures to evaluate the quality and cost effectiveness of community-based services for people with a learning disability across one health authority These included consumer outcome measures for Macmillan nurses, health visitors and learning difficulties nurses, such as the achievement of improved relaxation and personal control of terminal illness, the detection rate of mental health problems in children, and the percentage of the working day engaged in meaningful activities.
- Dennis et al. (2008): a qualitative investigation with parents and professionals using focus groups and semi-structured and narrative interviews to explore parents and professionals beliefs regarding the causes of attention deficit hyperactivity disorder and their perceptions of service provision.
- Health Development Agency (2002): School nurses have also used consumer outcome measures. *Coping with Our Kids* is a school-nurse-led research-based programme, designed to respond to an identified need to address the increasing numbers of children with behavioural problems, both at school and at home. It evolved in part as a result of a needs analysis and parental request and effectiveness is measured through the use of a pre- and post-course questionnaire given to parents.
- Potter (2005): a retrospective population-based survey of 273 women who initiated breastfeeding and whose babies were 6 months old. The survey measured the incidence of mastitis and the impact of the women's experience of managing mastitis on their reporting behaviour
- Sargent et al. (2007): a qualitative study to describe case management from the perspective of patients and carers in order to develop a clearer understanding of how the model is being delivered for patients with long term conditions. In-depth interviews were conducted with a purposive sample of patients and carers.
- Williams (2004): a non-randomised mini-review to establish if cleaning, dressing and removing crusts from external fixator or skeletal pin sites affected the risk of infection.
- Zabaleta & Forbes (2007): a criteria-based review of three controlled trials to determine the effectiveness of structured group-based diabetes education programmes in improving glycaemic control in adults with type 2 diabetes in primary care.

---

to measure a broad range of health gains and outcomes in public health and primary care (Box 17.2). Of particular relevance and in addition to the list of published examples in Box 17.2, is an earlier qualitative study undertaken by the Health Education Authority in 1997 (HEA 1997a). This study considered the use of process indicators for health promotion in community health

care nursing. The project aimed to develop a series of process indicators to use as quality measures of health promotion activities undertaken by nurses working in primary care. The quality indicators were developed as an exploratory exercise, which included observation, interviews and discussions with clients and with other stakeholders, including purchasers of primary health care nursing services, provider managers and primary health care nurses themselves. Six case studies were then used to refine and test these indicators in practice and to explore the relationship between quality indicators and health benefits or health gains for clients. Analysis of the case study data revealed many examples of primary health care nursing interventions that had made a difference to clients' lives, either in relation to short-term or intermediate improvements in health (health gain) or benefits which improved the way in which clients deal with health issues and problems (empowerment). This study has provided evidence of the tangible relationship between the quality of primary health care nursing interactions and subsequent health benefits for service users and their families. It has demonstrated how qualitative research methods can illuminate positive health outcomes through the examination of process and intermediate health indicators, and has emphasised the importance of involving the service user in the monitoring and measurement of quality and outcome. The authors concluded that gaining the service user's view is essential, in order to validate professional perceptions of whether health gain and quality care have actually been achieved. The indicators were operationalised into a 'guide to quality indicators for commissioners' (HEA 1997b) and included relevant research evidence to support the link between the indicators and outcomes.

New process and intermediate health outcome indicators are being developed all the time to measure the effectiveness of interventions by CHCNs and SCPHNs with service users. Increasingly studies are aggregating data about individual or family outcomes at a caseload, GP practice or community level, in order to examine the effectiveness of interventions which have a public health or population focus. For example, the effect of innovative Trailblazer Sure Start initiatives in tackling child poverty or in overcoming inequalities and social exclusion may only be visible when information is collected from a large population (Northrop *et al.* 2008). This was confirmed in an earlier study by Kelsey (2000), who regarded the aggregation of data as a solution to the problems associated

with outcome measurement in health visiting. She described two approaches to collecting and using aggregated data. The first refers to a population approach, based on the compilation of an accurate and detailed community profile that is maintained and regularly updated. CHCNs and SCPHNs are increasingly using such profiles to identify needs and to plan and evaluate services (Mischenco *et al.* 2004; Rowland & Buckingham 2002). The second approach involves the aggregation of outcomes that have been individually negotiated with clients, around issues such as nutrition, child behaviour, sleep, smoking, rest and recreation and family finances. In both cases, it is important that the information collected is accurate and comparable. For example when collecting information about breast-feeding rates, the definition of breast-feeding and the schedule for data collection must be clearly stated and adhered to if comparisons are to be made locally, regionally and nationally (Unicef 2003). However, as Kelsey points out, there is a danger that standardisation of data collection may reduce sensitivity to local issues therefore it is important to ensure that clients are actively engaged in the development and use of outcome measures. The HEA project (HEA 1997a) described earlier is an example where standardised indicators have been developed which can be adopted and applied to the local situation. Successful local adaptation is dependent on the provision of a qualitative approach that includes client participation and takes into account the complexity of practice in the community setting.

Ongoing issues for CHCNs and SCPHNs

An approach to clinical effectiveness and outcome measurement based on a scientific, biomedical model continues to present particular problems for CHCNs and SCPHNs. These problems are related to the context of practice as well as to the nature of nursing itself. For example, public health and health promotion activities are often long term and health gains may not be visible for many years. The social and environmental setting in the community is very complex, with numerous social, psychological and economic influences on health, and various different health and social care workers involved. This therefore creates difficulties in isolating the contribution of CHCNs and SCPHNs to health outcomes. Furthermore, the complexity of interventions creates problems with measuring outcomes. CHCNs and SCPHNs often address multiple health and social care needs at an individual, family and community level, and practice is often client-led and unpredictable.

These problems have been widely documented over the past 20 years, for example, Barribell & Mackenzie (1993), noted that the outcome of preventive work may be more difficult to measure than other inputs, as results are often long term and may also be influenced by social and environmental factors beyond the control of health professionals. They also identify the problem of isolating the contribution of nursing interventions to outcomes, as CHCNs and SCPHNs practise within a multi-disciplinary setting. Mckenna *et al.* (2004) identified barriers to evidence-based practice in primary care and Kelsay (1995) discussed the problems associated with the different definitions of health and the methods of measurement in relation to health visiting. The issue of health visitors, adopting a broad concept of health, which aims to maintain and improve health in the general population, means that changes in health status are more difficult to detect than, for example, health improvements for patients in hospital. Furthermore, tests are not always available to measure all the varied dimensions of health, and quantitative research methods may not be appropriate. Baseline measurements of health status are also difficult, as health visitors often first meet clients around the time of major life events (such as during the ante-natal period). Kelsay (1995) pointed to the risks of fragmenting practice and over-simplifying outcomes, as outcome measures do not always recognise the wide range of health visiting skills which may be needed to achieve a particular change in health status. Pressure to concentrate on simple, easily measurable outcomes could result in health visitors focusing on one aspect of health,

such as improving immunisation status, at the expense of trying to improve the overall health of their clients.

Almond's study (2001) of approaches in decision-making and child protection issues supported the view that the complexity of health visiting practice means that conventional measures of outcome could be and are often inappropriate. There is a dearth of literature on decision-making in health visiting and it is possible that the gap exists because psychosocial situations do not lend themselves readily to rational approaches. The suggestion is made that rational approaches are more suited to structured situations where there is often a right or wrong answer and a phenomenological and ethical approach are more suited to exploring the nature of decision-making in health visiting.

Methods of monitoring and evaluating community health care nursing and specialist community public health nursing performance therefore tend to concentrate on easily measurable outcomes and quantitative statistics such as activity numbers (number and 'type' of clients contacted). CHCNs and SCPHNs argue that the data produced is meaningless and fails to describe the quality or effectiveness of their interventions (Cowley 1994; Macdonald *et al.* 1996). Additionally, the review of district nursing services in England and Wales (Audit Commission 1999) found that services were generally commissioned using numbers of patient contacts or numbers of staff required by individual GP practices. Therefore in many cases, the award and design of contracts was not based on the needs of the local population or on the desired outcomes of care. The commission concluded that 'contact figures are inadequate for monitoring patient care… because they ignore the purpose, appropriateness and length of visit' (Audit Commission 1999, p. 16). This view is further supported by evidence produced by health visitors who noted that their service had come to focus almost entirely on a mechanistic monitoring of child health and target achievement (HEA 1997a). This example indicates that using inappropriate statistics to monitor performance in community nursing actually may be influencing and changing practice, as activities become restricted to areas which can easily be measured.

It could be argued that a tension therefore appears to exist between the practice of community health care nursing and specialist community public health nursing and the dominant approach to, and methods of measuring effectiveness in health care. The scientific method, which emphasises the objective analysis of predictable phenomena, is not always able to capture the complexity of practice. It emphasises quantitative outcomes and does not value qualitative information which captures the 'processes' of care and consumer perspectives. While CHCNs and SCPHNs are still required to collect information on biomedical health outcomes and are evaluated using quantitative statistics, only part of their role and perceived effectiveness is actually measured and recorded. However, policy developments and developments in research and practice reveal opportunities, ideas and strategies that can be adopted and applied more appropriately to measure the effectiveness of community health care nursing and specialist community public health nurses practice.

Conclusion

This chapter has focused on the particular issues that require consideration by CHCNs and SCPHNs when measuring the effectiveness of their practice. The emphasis on evidence-based practice and monitoring and improving the quality of health care through clinical governance provides opportunities for those working in primary care and public health within community settings to demonstrate their positive contribution to the health of individuals, families and communities. However, a dominant, scientific approach to measuring effectiveness in the NHS is inadequate and inappropriate for evaluating the complexity of CHCNs and SCPHNs interventions within the context of a dynamic social care environment. Nevertheless, alternative methods of evaluation do exist and are being used. These incorporate qualitative and quantitative techniques. Such combined approaches examine processes as well as outcomes of care and

involve service users and carers in the evaluation process. These evaluative methods complement and are supported by government policies and strategic developments. With appropriate education and support for the use of these approaches to evaluation, CHCNs and SCPHNs are able to measure effectiveness in a meaningful way, rather than relying exclusively on statistics and outcomes that measure only a small part of their work with clients, families and communities.

References

Almond, A. (2001) Approaches to decision-making and child protection issues. *Community Practitioner*, **74**, 97–100.

Audit Commission (1999) *First Assessment. A Review of District Nursing Services in England and Wales.* Audit Commission, London.

Audit Commission (2004a) *Quicker Treatment Closer to Home. Primary Care Trusts' Success in Redesigning Care Pathways.* Audit Commission, London.

Audit Commission (2004b) *Transforming Primary Care. The Role of Primary Care Trusts in Shaping and Supporting General Practice.* Audit Commission, London.

Baileff, A. (2007) Using patient group directions in walk-in-centres. *Primary Health Care*, **17**, 36–39.

Barribell, K.L. & Mackenzie, A. (1993) Measuring the impact of nursing interventions in the community: a selective review of the literature. *Journal of Advanced Nursing*, **18**, 401–407.

Bee, A. & Clegg, A. (2006) Community matrons implementation: meeting the challenge in Leeds. *British Journal of Community Nursing*, **11**, 64–67.

Bolam, B., McLean, C., Pennington, A. & Gillies, P. (2006) Using media to build social capital for health: a qualitative process evaluation study of participation in the CityNet Project. *Journal of Health Psychology*, **11**, 297–308.

Bowling, A. (1991) *Measuring Health. A Review of Quality of Life Measurement Scales.* Open University Press, Buckingham.

Bristol Royal Infirmary Inquiry (2001) *Learning from Bristol Royal Infirmary Inquiry. The Report into the Public Inquiry into Children's Heart Surgery at Bristol Royal Infirmary 1884–1995.* HM The Stationery Office, London.

British Medical Association & NHS Confederation (2003) *New GMS Contract: Investing in General Practice.* BMA & NHS Confederation, London.

Brooks, N. & Barrett, A. (2003) Identifying nurse and health visitor priorities in a PCT using a Delphi technique. *British Journal of Community Nursing*, **8**, 376–380.

Byles, J., Francis, L. & McKernon, M. (2002) The experience of non-medical health professionals undertaking community based assessments for people aged 75 years and over. *Health and Social Care in the Community*, **10**, 67–73.

Campbell, F., Cowley, S. & Buttigieg, M. (1995) *Weights and Measures. Outcomes and Evaluation in Health Visiting*. London Health Visitors Association (HVA).

Chamberlain, P., Hipwell, R., Samuel, R. & Stevenson, J. (1995) Measuring the quality of service in the community. *Nursing Times*, **91**, 36–37.

Coles, L. & Porter, E. (2008) (eds) *Public Health Skills: A Practical Guide for Nurses and Public Health Practitioners*. Blackwell, Oxford.

Cowley, S. (1994) Counting practice: the impact of information systems on community nursing, *Journal of Nursing Management*, **1**, 273–278.

Cullum, N. (1997) Identification and analysis of randomised controlled trials in nursing: a preliminary study. *Quality in Health Care*, **6**, 2–6.

Dargie, L. (2001) Primary care trusts: an agenda for change. *Primary Health Care*, **11**, 16–18.

Dennis, T., Davis, M., Johnson, U., Brooks, H. & Humbi, A. (2008) Attention deficit hyperactivity disorder: parents and professionals perceptions. *Community Practitioner*, **81**, 24–28.

Department for Education and Skills (DfES) (2006) *Every Child Matters: Change for Children, Making it Happen, Working Together for Children, Young People and Families*. DfES publications, Nottingham.

Department for Education and Skills (DfES) (2007) *Governance Guidance for sure Start Children's Centres and Extended Schools*. DfES publications, Nottingham.

Department of Health (1989) *Working for Patients*. HMSO, London.

Department of Health (1992) *The Health of the Nation: A Strategy for Health in England*. HMSO, London.

Department of Health (1994) *The Allitt Inquiry (Clothier, C, Chair)*. HM The Stationery Office, London.

Department of Health (1996) *The National Health Service: A Service With Ambitions*. Department of Health, London.

Department of Health (1998) *A First Class Service. Quality in the New NHS*. Department of Health, London.

Department of Health (1999a) *Saving Lives: Our Healthier Nation*. The Stationery Office, London.

Department of Health (1999b) *Making a Difference, Strengthening the Nursing Midwifery and Health Visiting Contribution to Health and Health Care*. The Stationery Office, London.

Department of Health (2000) *The NHS Plan*. The Stationery Office, London.

Department of Health (2001) *Research Governance Framework for Health and Social Care*. The Stationery Office, London.

Department of Health (2002) *National Service Frameworks: A Practical Aid to Implementation in Primary Care*. The Stationery Office, London.

Department of Health (2003a) *Tackling Health Inequalities: A Programme for Action*. Department of Health, London.

Department of Health (2003b) *Essence of Care: Patient-Focused Benchmarks for Clinical Governance*. Modernisation agency, Department of Health, London.

Department of Health (2004a) *Standards for Better Health: Health Care Standards for Services Under the NHS, A Consultation*. Available at www.dh.gov.uk/en/Consultations/Closedconsultations/DH_4082361 (accessed 2 December 2008).

Department of Health (2004b) *NHS Improvement Plan: Putting People at the Heart of Public Services*. HMSO, London.

Department of Health (2004c) *National Standards, Local Action, Health and Social Care Standards and Planning Framework, 2005/6–2007/8*. Department of Health, London.

Department of Health (2004d) *Choosing Health: Making Healthier Choices Easier*. HMSO, London.

Department of Health (2005a) *Supporting People with Long Term Conditions: Liberating the Talents of Nurses Who Care for People with Long Term Conditions*. The Stationery Office, London.

Department of Health (2005b) *Research Governance Framework for Health and Social Care*, 2nd edition. HMSO, London.

Department of Health (2006a) *Health Reform in England: Update and Commissioning Framework*. HMSO, London.

Department of Health (2006b) *Essence of Care Benchmark for Promoting Health*. Available at: www.dh.gov.uk/en/Publicationsandstatistics/Publications/PublicationsPolicyAndGuidance/DH_075613 (accessed 11 April 2008).

Department of Health (2006c) *Our Health, Our Care, Our Say: A New Direction for Community Services*. HMSO, London.

Department of Health (2006d) *The Future Regulation of Health and Adult Social Care in England*. The Stationary Office, London.

Department of Health (2006e) *Standards for Better Health*. HMSO, London.

Department of Health (2007a) *Our NHS, Our future: NHS Next Stage Review. Interim Report*. HMSO, London.

Department of Health (2007b) *Government's Response to Facing the Future: A Review of the Role of Health Visitors*. HMSO, London.

Department of Health (2007c) *Hospital Episode Statistics*. HMSO, London.

Department of Health (2007d) *Reducing MRSA and Other Healthcare Associated Infections in Renal Medicine*. HMSO, London.

Department of Health (2007e) *Essence of Care: Benchmarks for the Care Environment*. London.

Department of Health (2008) *NHS Next Stage Review: Our Vision for Primary and Community Care*. The Stationary Office, London.

Donabedian, A. (1980) *Explorations in Quality Assessment and Monitoring: The Definition of Quality and Approaches to its Assessment*. Health Administration Press, Ann Arbor, MI.

Donaldson, D. (2001) *The Report of the Chief Medical Officer's Project to Strengthen the Public Health Function*. The Stationery Office, London.

Ellis, J. (2006) All inclusive benchmarking. *Journal of Nursing Management*, **14**, 377–383.

Farquhar, S., Parker, E., Schulz, A. & Israel, B. (2006) Application of qualitative methods in program planning for health promotion interventions. *Health Promotion Practice*, **7**, 234–242.

Foo, A. & Chaplais, J. (2008) Efficacy of pre-school surveillance services in identifying children with special needs. *Community Practitioner*, **81**, 17–20.

Freeman, T. & Peck, E. (2006) Evaluating partnerships: a case study of integrated specialist mental health services. *Health and Social Care in the Community*, **14**, 408–417.

Greenhalgh, T. (2006) *How to Read a Paper: The Basis of Evidence Based Medicine*, 3rd edition. British Medical Journal Publishing, London.

Griffiths, P. (1995) Progress in measuring nursing outcomes. *Journal of Advanced Nursing*, **21**, 1092–1100.

Healthcare Commission (2004) *Acute Trust Performance Indicators*. London.

Healthcare Commission (2007a) *Investigations into the Service for People with Learning Disabilities Provided by Sutton and Merton PCT*. Commission for Health Care Audit, London.

Healthcare Commission (2007b) *A Life Like No Other. A National Audit of Specialist In-Patient Healthcare Services for People with Learning Difficulties in England*. Commission for Health Care Audit, London.

Health Development Agency (2002) *National Healthy School Standard. School Nursing*. Health Development Agency, London, pp. 33.

Health Development Agency (2003) *Public Health Intervention Research*. Health Development Agency, London.

Health Development Agency (2004) Nine steps to health development. *Community Practitioner*, **77**, 50.

Health Development Agency (2005) *Clarifying Approaches to Health Needs Assessment, Health Impact Assessment, Integrated Impact Assessment, Health Equity Audit and Race Equality Impact Assessment*. Health Development Agency, London.

Health Education Authority (1997a) *The Developing Quality Indicators Project. Phase 2, Final Report*. Health Education Authority, London.

Health Education Authority (1997b) *Promoting Health Through Primary Care Nursing. A Guide to Quality Indicators for Commissioners*. Health Education Authority, London.

Heller, R. (2005) *Evidence for Population Health*. Oxford University Press, Oxford.

Heslehurst, N., Ellis, L.J. & Simpson, H. (2007) Trends in maternal obesity incidence rate, demographic predictors and health inequalities in 36,821 women over a 15 year period. *British Journal of Obstetrics and Psychology*, **114**, 187–194.

Hillier, D., Caan, W. & McVicar, A. (2007) Research training and leadership for midwives and health visitors. *Community Practitioner*, **80**, 28–33.

Holmes, V. & Griffiths, P. (2002) Self monitoring of glucose levels for people with type 2 diabetes. *British Journal of Community Nursing*, **7**, 41–46.

Horta, B.L., Bahl, R. & Martino, J.C. (2007) *Evidence on the Long Term Effects of Breastfeeding: Systematic Reviews of Meta-Analysis*. World Health Organization (WHO), Geneva.

Howarth, M., Kneafsey, R. & Haig, C. (2007) Centralization and research governance: does it work. *Journal of Advanced Nursing*, **61**, 363–372.

Ibarra, J., Fry, F., Wickenden, C. & Olson, A. (2007) Overcoming health inequalities by using the bug busting 'whole school approach' to eradicate head lice. *Journal of Clinical Nursing*, **16**, 1955–1965.

Illife, S. & Drennan, V. (2000) Primary care for older people: learning the lessons of history. *Community Practitioner*, **73**, 602–604.

Jones-Devitt, S. (2007) *Critical Thinking in Health and Social Care*. Sage, Oxford.

Karoly, L.A., Kilburn, M.R. & Cannon, J.S. (2005) *Childhood Interventions. Proven Results, Future Programme*. Rand Corporation, Santa Monica, CA.

Kelsay, A. (1995) Outcome measures: problems and opportunities for public health nursing. *Journal of Nursing Management*, **3**, 183–187.

Kelsey, A. (2000) The challenge for research. In: *The Search for Health Needs* (eds J. Appleton & S. Cowley). Macmillan Press, London.

Kemm, J. (2006) The limitations of evidence based public health. *Journal of Evaluation of Clinical Practice*, **12**, 319–324.

King, A. (2006) Age-paced parenting newsletters: delivering healthy messages. *Community Practitioner*, **79**, 89–92.

Koehn, M. & Lehman, K. (2008) Nurses perceptions of evidence based nursing practice. *Journal of Advanced Nursing*, **62**, 209–215.

Lemstra, M., Stewart, B. & Olszynski, W. (2002) Effectiveness of multidisciplinary intervention in the treatment of migraine: a randomized clinical trial. *Headache*, **42**, 845–854.

Lomas, L. & McLuskey, J. (2005) Pumping up the pressure: a qualitative evaluation of a workplace health promotion initiative for male employees. *Health Education Journal*, **64**, 88–95.

Macdonald, G., Veen, C. & Tones, K. (1996) Evidence for success in health promotion: suggestions for improvement. *Health Education Research*, **11**, 367–376.

Marchionni, C. & Ritchie, J. (2008) Organizational factors that support the implementation of a nursing Best Practice Guideline. *Journal of Nursing Management*, **16**, 266–274.

Martin, G., Hewitt, G., Faulkner, T. & Parker, H. (2007) The organisation, form and function of intermediate care services and systems in England: results from a national survey. *Health and Social Care in the Community*, **15**, 146–154.

Martin, V. & Henderson, E. (2001) *Managing Health and Social Care*. Routledge, London.

McHugh, G. & Luker, K. (2002) User perspectives of the health visiting service. *Community Practitioner*, **75**, 57–61.

McKenna, H., Ashton, S. & Keeney, S. (2004) Barriers to evidence based practice in primary care. *Journal of Advanced Nursing*, **45**, 178–189.

Mischenco, J., Cheater, F. & Street, J. (2004) NCAST: tools to assess caregiver-child interaction.

Naidoo, J. & Wills, J. (2004) *Public Health and Health Promotion Developing practice*. Baillière Tindall, London.

National Audit Office (2006) *Driving Improvements in Out-of-Hours Care*. HMSO, London.

National Health Service Executive (1996) *Promoting Clinical Effectiveness: A Framework for Action in and Through the NHS*. NHS Executive, London.

National Health Service Executive (1998) *The New NHS, Modern and Dependable: A National Framework for Assessing Performance*. NHS Executive, London.

National Institute for Health and Clinical Excellence (2005) *Statins for the Prevention of Cardiovascular Events*. National Institute for Health and Clinical Excellence, London.

National Institute for Health and Clinical Excellence (2008) *Improving the Nutrition of Pregnant and Breastfeeding Mothers and Children in Low Income Households*. National Institute for Health and Clinical Excellence (NICE), London.

Northrop, M., Pittam, G. & Caan, W. (2008) The expectations of families and patterns of participation in a trailblazer Sure Start. *Community Practitioner*, **81**, 24–28.

Nursing and Midwifery Council (2003) Radical restructure: a new look register. *NMC News*, Autumn 2003 Number 3.

Nursing and Midwifery Council (2004) *Standards of Proficiency for Specialist Community Public Health Nursing*. Nursing and Midwifery Council, London.

Nursing and Midwifery Council (2008) *Guidelines on the Administration of Medicines*. Nursing and Midwifery Council, London.

Olds, D. (2006) The nurse family partnership: an evidence-based preventive intervention. *Infant Mental Health Journal*, **27**, 5–25.

Paton, C. (1996) *Health Policy and Management*. Chapman Hall, London.

Perry, L., Grange, A., Heyman, B. & Noble, P. (2008) Stakeholders perceptions of a research capacity development project for nurses, midwives and allied health professionals. *Journal of Nursing Management*, **16**, 315–326.

Potter, B. (2005) A multi-method approach to measuring mastitis incidence. *Community Practitioner*, **78**, 169–173.

Pritchard, C. & De Verteuil, B. (2007) Application of health equity audit to health visiting. *Community Practitioner*, **80**, 38–41.

Prothero, L., Dyson, L., Renfrew, M.J., Bull, J. & Mulvihill, C. (2003) *The Effectiveness of Public Health Interventions to Promote the Initiation of Breast Feeding*. Health Development Agency, London.

Rolfe, G. (1998) The theory practice gap in nursing: from research based practice to practitioner based research. *Journal of Advanced Nursing*, **28**, 672–679.

Rowland, L. & Buckingham, M. (2002) Developing an assessment device and service. *Community Practitioner*, **75**, 223–226.

Royal College of General Practitioners (1999) *Clinical Governance: Practical Advice for Primary Health Care in England and Wales*. Royal College of General Practitioners, London.

Royal College of Nursing (1996) *National Health Manifesto*. Royal College of Nursing, London.

Sackett, D.L., Rosenberg, W.M., Gray, J.A., Haynes, R.B. & Richardson, W.S. (1996) Evidence based medicine: what it is and what it isn't [editorial]. *British Medical Journal*, **312**, 71–72.

Sale, D. (2005) *Understanding Clinical Governance and Quality Assurance. Making it Happen*. Palgrave, London.

Sargent, P., Pickard, S., Sheaff, R. & Boaden, R. (2007) Patient and carer perceptions of care management for long-term conditions. *Health and Social Care in the Community*, **15**, 511–519.

Schutz, S.E. (1994) Exploring the benefits of a subjective approach in qualitative nursing research. *Journal of Advanced Nursing*, **20**, 412–417.

Secretary of State for Health (2003) *Community Health and Standards Act*. Department of Health, London.

Seedhouse, D. (2004) *Health Promotion; Philosophy, Prejudice and Practice, 2nd edition*. John Wiley, Sussex.

Shih, F. (1998) Triangulation in nursing research: issues of conceptual clarity and purpose. *Journal of Advanced Nursing*, **28**, 631–641.

Sidebottam, A., Harrison, P., Amidon, D. & Finnegan, K. (2008) The varied circumstances promoting requests for emergency contraception at school based clinics. *The Journal of School Health*, **78**, 258–263.

Smith, J. (2004) *The Shipman Inquiry 4th Report Regulations of Controlled Drugs*. HMSO, Norwich.

Social Exclusion Task Force (2007) *Reaching Out: Think Family. Analysis and Themes from the Families at Risk Review*. Cabinet Office, London.

Tones, K. & Tilford, S. (2001) *Health Promotion: Effectiveness, Efficiency and Equity, 3rd edition*. Nelson Thornes, Cheltenham England.

Unicef UK Baby Friendly Initiative (2003) *Public Health Strategies for Breast Feeding Initiatives*. Unicef Baby Friendly Initiative, Geneva.

Upton, D. & Upton, P. (2005) Knowledge and use of evidence based practice of GPs and hospital doctors. *Journal of Evaluation of Clinical Practice*, **12**, 376–384.

Wanless, D. (2004) *Securing Good Health for the Whole Population*. HMSO, London.

Wanless, D., Appleby, J., Harrison, J. & Patel, D. (2007) *Our Future Health Secured. A Review of NHS Funding and Performance*. King's Fund, London.

Williams, H. (2004) The effectiveness of pin site care for patients with external fixators. *British Journal of Community Nursing*, **9**, 206–210.

Wilson, P., Furnivall, J., Barbour, R. & Rosabre, S. (2008) The work of health visitors and school nurses with children with psychological and behavioural problems. *Journal of Advanced Nursing*, **61**, 445–455.

Zabaleta, A.M & Forbes, A. (2007) Structured group based evaluation for type 2 diabetes in Primary Care. *British Journal of Community Nursing*, **12**, 158–162.

Chapter 18 **Non-Medical Prescribing**

Helen Ward, Dr Jaya Ahuja, Amanda Tragen and Sandra Horner

Introduction

The Department of Health ([DH] 2003a,b, 2006) has provided the health service with various legislation specifying new types of prescribing for health care professionals other than doctors and dentists. Some nurses have had the authority to prescribe from a limited nurse prescribers' formulary since 1994. However, in recent years this has been extended to give independent prescribing rights to nurses and pharmacists and supplementary prescribing rights to nurses, pharmacists, physiotherapists, radiographers, optometrists and podiatrists. Hence the title of this chapter: Non-Medical Prescribing.

The road to prescriptive authority for nurses has been a long and complicated one. This chapter will focus on non-medical prescribing for nurses. The existing forms of prescribing, administration and supply of medicines will be discussed and the history of nurse prescribing within the framework of a modern national health service will be explored. The educational programmes available for role preparation as a nurse prescriber and the maintenance of this competence will be described in detail. The chapter will also examine the role of non-medical prescribing in the current context, while keeping in mind the accountability and legal issues relevant to non-medical prescribing.

Medicines management: prescription, supply and administration of medicines

Modern management of illnesses often involves drug treatments. Consequently, health care professionals, including community nurses, contribute to the process referred to as 'medicines management'. Medicines management can be understood as a broad concept that encompasses a comprehensive range of activities and procedures from the development of new drugs through the choice of medicines by a prescriber to the use of medicines by a patient. The NHS health care professionals are closely involved in those parts of the process referred to as prescribing, supply and administration of medicines.

The terms prescribing, supply and administration of medicines all relate to each other. However, they are not synonymous and the distinction should be clearly understood. When prescribing, the prescriber makes a choice of medication to be taken or used by the patient, based on the initial assessment of the patient, ideally in concordance with the patient, and in light of the best available current evidence. The prescriber then issues a prescription. A prescription is a legal order requesting supply of a medicine(s) and gives instructions on its administration (by a patient, carer or a health care professional). A health care professional involved in supply of medicines makes the prescribed medicine(s) available to a patient, carer or other health care professional so that the medicine(s) can be administered. Further distinction can be made between the supply and dispensing of medicines.

Dispensing not only includes supply but also encompasses other activities aimed at ensuring safe and effective use of medicines. Administration means giving a medicine as intended to a patient either into the body (for example tablets, injections) or on the body (external preparations). Medicines can be administered by a health care professional, carer or a patient (self-administration). A health care professional who supplies and/or administers medicine(s) has to do so as instructed by a prescriber, or as directed by a Patient Group Direction (PGD). PGDs have been defined as 'written instructions for the supply or administration of medicines to groups of patients who may not be individually identified before presentation for treatment' (DH 2000d). Therefore, supply and administration under PGDs is different from prescribing. The health care professional supplying or administering a medicine cannot change the drug, its formulation, dose or dose regimen; the medication has to be supplied or administered exactly as advised on the prescription, or as directed by a PGD.

Pharmacists have traditionally been involved in supply/dispensing of prescription-only medicines (POM). The role of a nurse would normally include administration of medicines (and supply in secondary care). However, since the late 1980s, these traditional health care professional roles in the UK have changed and nurses have been prescribing since the early 1990s, followed by other non-medical health care professionals in the early years of the twenty-first century. New terms such as 'independent' and 'supplementary prescribing' and 'prescribers' have been introduced to name and describe these new roles. Currently there are three non-medical prescribing options available to nurses:

- *Nurse Prescribers' Formulary* (NPF) for district nurses/health visitors (community practitioners)
- Nurse independent prescribing from all the drugs within the *British National Formulary* (BNF) within the scope of nurse's competence
- Nurse supplementary prescribing, where the nurse can prescribe any medicine (including controlled drugs and off-licence) within the patient-specific clinical management plan (CMP)

The DH defines *independent prescribing* as 'prescribing by a practitioner responsible and accountable for the assessment of patients with undiagnosed or diagnosed conditions and for decisions about the clinical management required, including prescribing', and *supplementary prescribing* as 'a voluntary prescribing partnership between an independent prescriber and a supplementary prescriber, to implement an agreed patient-specific clinical management plan with the patient's agreement'.

History and background of non-medical prescribing

Non-medical prescribing: the origins

The government's strategy document *The NHS Plan* (DH 2000a) integrated the main principles of the modernisation of the NHS, initiated in the late 1990s. The principal aim of the reform was to provide high-quality, accessible health care, designed and delivered around the needs of its users. An important part of the reform, and one of the tools designed to achieve its aims, was the goal to redesign the NHS workforce and to develop and better utilise skills and abilities of the NHS staff.

The Chief Nursing Officer defined ten key roles for the profession and these included prescribing (DH 2000a). Following *The NHS Plan*, the DH, in collaboration with professional bodies, detailed changes to the National Health Service (NHS) workforce in a range of specific documents (DH 2000b, 2001, 2002); nurses and other allied health professionals were encouraged to expand their clinical roles, particularly in chronic disease management, and were empowered to prescribe medicines (DH 2000c).

Towards independent prescribing

In developing the non-medical prescribing agenda, the government has built on the prescribing experience acquired by nurses who possessed the district nurse (DN) and health visitor (HV) qualifications. DNs and HVs have been prescribing since 1994, following eight years of political and profession negotiation. The Committee headed by Baroness Cumberlege in 1986 stated:

'The Department of Health and Social Security (DHSS) should agree a limited list of items and simple agents which may be prescribed by nurses as part of a nursing care programme, and issue guidelines to enable nurses to control drug dosage in well-defined circumstances.'

(DHSS 1986)

Specific recommendations to the government on prescribing by DNs and HVs were made by the Advisory Group on Nurse Prescribing in 1989 (Crown Report I; DH 1989). The necessary legislation enabling nurse prescribing was provided in the Medicinal Products: Prescribing by Nurses etc. Act passed in 1992 and implemented in 1994. DNs and HVs have since been able to prescribe a limited range of products approved by the DHSS/DH and listed in the BNF, the NPF and Part XViiB(i) of the Drug Tariff.

Educational preparation for non-medical prescribing is now integrated into university-based specialist practitioner programmes and is known as the V100 programme (DH 2004a). V100 is the code used to record the qualification with the Nursing and Midwifery Council following successful completion of the course. In late 2005, eligibility to undertake the V100 was extended to all registrants undertaking the Specialist Practice Qualification Award (community pathway) and the Specialist Community Public Health Nursing (SCPHN) Degree. For the first time school nurses, general practice nurses, community children's nurses and occupational health nurses could join this programme, which prepares the specialist practitioners to prescribe from the *Nurse Prescribers' Formulary for Community Practitioners* (NPF) only (NMC 2005). Following changes in relevant legislation, educational programmes for nurse prescribers were extended, although the V100 course remained as a programme to enable specialist practice community nurses to prescribe from the NPF. NMC circular 31/2007 is clear in directing that it is no longer mandatory for health visitors to take the V100 programme as previously undertaken. As with the other pathways in the SCPHN programme it became optional from the end of October 2007.

The NPF for DNs and HVs or 'limited' NPF was been criticised by nurse prescribers as well as doctors (Luker 1997), and these reactions led to the extension of prescribing rights. Following the second Crown Report (DH 1999), recommendations were made to extend nurse prescribing. After a lengthy consultation process, a formulary was drawn up from four areas of clinical practice: minor injury, minor ailments, health promotion and palliative care. Eighty medical conditions and 180 POMs were selected for nurses to prescribe

for from a nurse's formulary known as the *Nurse Prescribers Extended Formulary* (*NPEF*). This programme was known as the V200 and was offered as a stand-alone unit for nurses, midwives and health visitors selected by their employing organisation and who had a medical assessor who was willing to clinically support the nurse while undertaking the programme.

Nurse independent prescribing and supplementary prescribing
Following further public consultation a proposal was made to introduce supplementary prescribing for nurses and pharmacists. In 2003 alterations were made to the NHS regulations and the POMs order to allow implementation of supplementary prescribing via the establishment of CMPs (DH 2003a).

From 1 May 2006, the *NPEF* was discontinued and all independent nurse prescribers received prescriptive authority to prescribe any drug from the BNF (including some control drugs), providing it was within their scope of professional practice (DH 2006).

Currently, nurses and midwives who undertake the non-medical prescribing programmes successfully have a recordable qualification with the NMC as a nurse independent/supplementary prescriber; this programme is currently known and recorded as the V300 award. Changes have occurred in subsequent programme titles to reflect changes in the recordable qualifications (see Table 18.1 for the timeline relating to these changes for nurse prescribing).

Supplementary prescribing and clinical management plans
Supplementary prescribing is based on a voluntary agreement between a medical independent prescriber (doctor/dentist), the patient, and the supplementary prescriber (nurse) (DH 2003). This agreement is recorded as a CMP. The CMP is a legal document that has to be complied, agreed and signed by both the independent prescriber and the supplementary prescriber before supplementary prescribing can take place. Each patient for whom supplementary prescribing is to be used has to have their own CMP, although each CMP

Table 18.1 Timeline for nurse prescribing (NMC 2006)

1994 onwards	2002	2003	From May 2006
Nurse Prescribers' Formulary (NPF) for district nurse/health visitor			NPF for all specialist practice qualification community practitioner nurse prescribers
		Nurse Prescribers' Extended Formulary (NPEF)	*British National Formulary* for nurse independent prescribers and supplementary prescribing using CMPs
		Supplementary prescribing using clinical management plans (CMPs)	

can encompass a number of disease states. Several key factors have to be incorporated into the CMP to fulfil the legal requirements. These include clinical outcomes, name(s) of the medication(s), when the patient should be referred, review dates (at least annually by the independent prescriber), and plan for reporting adverse drug reactions. The ideal CMP should consider evidence-based prescribing, clinical governance and the supplementary prescribers level of competency. The CMP can be cancelled at any time, either by the health care team or by the patient.

It is important to recognise that the CMP differs from a PGD. PGDs are drawn up for groups of patients; these are usually patients with a common complaint (presenting with pain) or in a common clinical situation (presenting for vaccination, smoking cessation, emergency contraception, etc.). In this way PGDs deal with the situation, not the individual patient (DH 1999). In contrast, the CMP is specific to an individual patient, based on a full patient assessment undertaken by an independent prescriber.

Education and training

Nurses wishing to gain prescriptive authority as an independent/supplementary nurse prescriber or a community nurse prescriber are required by the NMC to undertake a specific programme of education and training. There are currently three separate programmes for nurse prescribers. The programme for independent/supplementary prescribing is known as the V300, the programme for specialist community practice nurses is known as the V100 and the programme for community nurses wishing to prescribe from

the *Nurse Prescribers' Formulary*, but who do not have a Specialist Practice Qualification, is known as the V150. The standards for all three of these programmes are set by the NMC and can be found in the *Standards of Proficiency for Nurse and Midwife Prescribers* (NMC 2006). The differences in the formulary from which nurses can prescribe reflect the different practice needs, although there are significant overlaps. Table 18.2 shows the salient features of each of these programmes.

V100

The first programme developed for the training of nurse prescribers was implemented in April 1993 as a short course that comprised 15 taught hours, an open learning pack and a final examination (English National Board 1992). This course was delivered by selected accredited higher education institutions (HEIs) and prepared nurse prescribers in eight limited NPF pilot sites. The programme content for this programme was stipulated by the United Kingdom Central Council for Nursing, Midwifery and Health Visiting in 1991.

Following the success of the pilot study, a programme was initially designed to prepare DNs and HVs to prescribe from a limited NPF and was delivered as a stand alone module. This programme was formally introduced in 1994 and then rolled out nationally. This is now available as V100.

V150

In December 2007, the NMC approved the standards of proficiency for nurse prescribers without a Specialist Practice Qualification to prescribe from the *Community Practitioner Formulary*. This programme is known as the

Table 18.2   Requirements for the prescribing programmes

Programme	Number of taught days	Hours in supervised practice	Course duration	Prescriptive authority
V100	5	Normally included in the practice supervision of the specialist qualification	1 year	From the *Nurse Prescribers' Formulary* (NPF) for community practitioners
V150	10	65	Usually 6 months	From NPF for community practitioners
V300	26	78	Usually 6 months	From the *British National Formulary* as nurse independent prescribing/ supplementary prescribing

V150. In order to undertake this programme nurses must have been practising as a registered nurse for a minimum of two years and identify an area of clinical need where prescribing from the NPF will improve patient care and service delivery. In addition, nurses must be able to study at a minimum of degree level and have employer support to undertake the programme.

Supervision in practice as part of education

Nurses undertaking this programme also need to identify a practising community practitioner nurse prescriber who will agree to provide clinical supervision for the duration of the programme. It is the responsibility of the sponsoring trust to ensure that the student has an identified nurse prescriber who has agreed to support the student and provide 65 hours of supervised training.

Progression from V150 to V300

Nurse prescribers who have previously studied the V150 programme and have the qualification recorded by the NMC, may accredit (Accreditation of Prior Experiential Learning [APEL]) their earlier learning against the V300 programme award standard.

V300 (education and training for nurse independent prescribers/nurse supplementary prescribers)

The NMC (2006) *Standards of Proficiency for Nurse and Midwife Prescribers* forms the structure of the non-medical prescribing programme. The programme of educational preparation for nurse and midwife prescribers is delivered by HEIs and is approved by the NMC to ensure educational quality assurance. Programmes can be offered at level H (undergraduate level) or level M (post graduate level) and are often delivered as integrated programmes with other non-medical prescribers such as pharmacists, physiotherapists, radiographers and podiatrists. The educational programme providers are required to meet with local key stakeholders to ensure that nurse prescribers are meeting with the health care needs of the local populations. The DH (2006) guidance requires nurse prescribers to:

- Study at least at level H (degree level)
- Have three years' post registration experience, with one year in the area in which they will be prescribing
- Be competent to undertake a history/clinical assessment/make a diagnosis
- Have a designated medical practitioner (DMP) willing to supervise the 12 days (78 hours) of learning in practice
- Have an identified 'need and opportunity' to act as a nurse prescriber
- Have access to a budget to meet the cost of prescriptions
- Have access to continuing professional development (CPD)
- Work within a robust clinical governance framework

The key principles that should be considered when selecting nurses to undertake the non-medical prescribing programme are: patient safety, benefit to patient in terms of quicker and more efficient access to medicines and a better use of a nurse's skills (DH 2004a). Examples of nurses undertaking the programme include: nurse-led services such as NHS walk-in centres, advanced nurse practitioners working within primary care services, nurse-led clinics within the hospital setting, family planning services, and nurses working with the homeless and palliative care nurses (DH 2008).

Educational programmes for non-medical prescribing can be delivered as either a face-to-face programme or as a distance learning programme. All nurses undertaking this programme must complete both the independent and supplementary components. The face-to-face programme consists of a minimum of 26 taught days with an additional 12 days (78 hours) of supervised learning in the clinical area. For distance-learning programmes, there must be a minimum of eight face-to-face taught days with an additional 12 days (78 hours) of supervised learning in clinical practice. The programme documentation must clearly demonstrate how the learning outcomes are to be met.

All educational preparation for prescribing programmes must be completed within one academic year and all nurses undertaking the programme must complete it within one year, unless there are exceptional circumstances and then it must be completed with two years. If a registrant does not successfully complete all the assessment components within this time frame, the whole programme, including the assessments must be undertaken again. Throughout the programme all students are required to apply the principles of prescribing to their practice and reflect on this through a learning log or portfolio. However, they may not prescribe until they have successfully completed the programme and the relevant qualification has been recorded with the NMC (NMC 2006).

Supervision in practice as part of education

Supervised clinical practice is a crucial element of the non-medical prescribing educational programme. Each student is required to identify a Designated Medical Practitioner (DMP), a doctor or a dentist, who will provide the student with supervision, support and the opportunities to develop the competencies required to become a safe, cost-effective and competent prescriber. At London South Bank University, the DMP must sign a written statement agreeing to take on the role of clinical mentor. They must be a medical practitioner who meets the government's criteria for fulfilment of this role. This includes at least three years spent in the relevant field of practice and some experience as a trainer/teacher in clinical practice (DH 2004b).

The time spent with the DMP and the range of activities undertaken within the 78 hours of supervised clinical practice will depend on the individual student and their relevant experience. However, as guidance, time should be spent observing consultations with patients, discussion of differential diagnoses, clinical reasoning in relation to the patient presentation and discussion and analysis of the patient management plan using a case study approach. Nurse prescribers who have achieved prescriptive authority as a result of successfully completing the nurse independent/supplementary programme must aim to maintain their standard of competence.

Prescribing for children

The NMC (2006) state that only nurses with the relevant knowledge, competence, skills and experience in nursing children should prescribe for children. This is important for primary care services such as out-of-hours provision, walk-in-centres and GP practices, as children are frequent attendees of these services. Anyone prescribing for children in these settings must be able to demonstrate competence to prescribe for children or refer to another prescriber (NMC 2006). In 2006, the NMC stipulated that all non-medical prescribing programmes must incorporate additional learning outcomes to ensure that all nurses undertaking the programme can take a history, undertake a clinical assessment and make an appropriate diagnosis or refer, having considered the legal, cognitive, emotional and physical differences between children and adults. Nurses planning to prescribe for children within these settings must ensure that they have adequate training in the assessment of children. If not, it is advised that they seek further training. In these settings the DMP is required to confirm demonstration of competence.

Maintaining competence in practice and CPD

Health care professionals have a duty of care and are responsible for the well-being of their patients. There are measures in place to support them to do this successfully, such as clinical governance frameworks (DH 1997). Clinical governance is a well-embedded tool which the government uses to achieve the aims of *The NHS Plan* (DH 2000c) to provide safe and effective, high-quality patient-centred care. The government defines clinical governance as a:

'system through which NHS organisations are accountable for continuously improving the quality of their services and safeguarding high standards of care, by creating an environment in which clinical excellence will flourish.'

(DH 2004d)

Organisations and their employees are responsible for ensuring that their work conforms to principles of clinical governance. Thus, this has clear implications for non-medical prescribing practice.

Clinical governance principles should be well-integrated into prescribing practice. This is achieved by the provision of high-quality education and training, followed by CPD. Non-medical prescribing practice should also be subjected to regular audits and evaluations and be part of risk assessment frameworks established by employer organisations (DH 2004a). The national Clinical Governance Support Team is available to help with aspects such as audit (NHS Clinical Governance Support Team 2007) and local resources in trusts should also be accessible and utilised by practitioners. High standards of clinical excellence can only be achieved by non-medical prescribers who are competent in their area of practice and who are able to achieve and maintain appropriate skills and knowledge, supported by their organisation.

Employing NHS organisations have a duty to support their staff in expanding and maintaining their competence. Clinical governance is what Halligan (2006, p. 7) calls the 'organisational conscience'. There should be a partnership between employer and employee striving to maintain professional competencies and improve care based on evidence-based practice. This is very important in prescribing practice with new evidence emerging constantly and the influence of cost becoming increasingly important.

It is also important that non-medical prescribers have the opportunity to reflect on their practice both as individuals and with their teams. One tool which they can use is structured reflection. Reflection facilitates an evaluation of one's own practice, identifies gaps in knowledge and areas for development. There are many models to choose from and practitioners need to select one which best meets their needs and personality (Burns & Bulman 2004; Johns 2004). Leading on from this is the need for regular clinical supervision; this is a support structure which has been in place for more than ten years. Clinical supervision helps practitioners to expand their knowledge base, become clinically more proficient, and gain confidence in their practice settings (Winstanley 2000). Research studies exploring nurse prescribers' practice experiences suggested that workplace peer support, mentoring and clinical supervision are important factors in maintaining nurses' prescribing competence in practice (Basford 2003; Humphries & Green 2000; Otway 2001).

In order to maintain competence and keep abreast of current research, practitioners should implement the skills acquired during their prescribing course. Critical appraisal skills are particularly useful in evaluating the validity and usefulness of newly published research before considering its implementation. It is important to join with other practitioners in prescribing forums, study groups and professional teams to assess evidence also. Developing critical appraisal skills comes with practice and peer support is also valuable. Sharing opinions and experience is invaluable.

A variety of evidence-based resources exist for prescribers to use, including a range of national service frameworks, which all support good practice in particular areas such as mental health or coronary heart disease. The National Institute for Health and Clinical Excellence (NICE) produces evidence-based guidelines for use by prescribers on a regular basis. On a more local level, health trusts produce formularies and clinical guidelines for practitioners to use. Once they become confident, non-medical prescribers can participate in the development of such tools as clinical guidelines (Chapman 2007). A pharmacy lead in a primary care or an acute trust can be very helpful in offering guidance on local prescribing issues, especially around local formulary usage. Financial data can be obtained in the form of PACT (prescribing analyses and cost) through the employing NHS organisation. This provides information about individual prescribing patterns, trends and costs. PACT is also available electronically from ePACT.net. This gives non-medical prescribers access to their prescribing patterns and the opportunity to use tools to analyse the data through their NHSnet accounts (Garrett 2008).

Finally the National Prescribing Centre (2001) also offers learning support to newly qualified practitioners. This is particularly important when practitioners are unable to gain peer or professional support easily.

Professional and legal accountability

The NMC (2008) states that accountability is the professionally recognised term for responsibility for doing something to someone. It means that practitioners must be able to give an account of their actions with rationale and reason. It also involves the obligations and liabilities that arise from within regulation. Since accountability is an integral part of professional practice, the nurse prescriber is accountable for: prescribing, recommendation of over-the-counter (OTC) products, assessment, decision-making and ensuring that the prescribed/recommended item is applied or administered correctly by either the patient or a carer to whom the task is delegated (Beckwith & Franklin 2007).

Professional accountability is defined by the *Code of Professional Conduct* (NMC 2008b). The code defines the criteria of appropriate nursing practice and serves as a bench mark against which allegations of misconduct in practice are considered. When considering allegations of drug errors, the NMC takes care to discriminate between cases where the error was the fault of reckless or incompetent practice and was concealed and those where the error was a result of serious pressure of work and where there was honest disclosure (NMC 2002). Professional accountability covers a range of issues, including, respect for the patient, informed consent, confidentiality, cooperation with other professionals, the maintenance of professional knowledge and competence, and the identification and minimising of risk to patients.

Legal accountability

There are several statutory documents that define the legal framework for non-medical prescribing. These have mostly been discussed earlier in this chapter. Significantly, the *Medicines and Human Use (Prescribing) (Miscellaneous Amendments) Order May 2006* enabled nurse independent prescribers to prescribe any licensed medicine from the BNF within their area of competence. Legally such practitioners must be first-level registered nurses/midwives whose name appears on the NMC register with an annotation saying that they have successfully completed the training (McHale & Tingle 2007).

Any form of breach of the enactments of the Medicines Act 1968 or other relevant legislation makes the prescriber liable to prosecution. When prescribing drugs, the nurse will be judged by the standard of the experienced nurse undertaking such a role. The nurse will also be held personally accountable in court, should harm result to a patient. The DH (2006, para 85) states that:

'Prescribers are accountable for all aspects of their prescribing decisions. They should therefore only prescribe those medicines they know are safe and effective for the patient and the condition being treated. They must be able to recognise and deal with pressures (e.g. from pharmaceutical industry, patients, colleagues) that might result in inappropriate prescribing.'

The Bolam test (1957) also applies:

'When you get a situation that involves the use of some special skill or competence, then the test as to whether there has been negligence or not is the standard of the ordinary skilled man exercising and professing to have that special skill.'

Thus the negligence standard for nursing practice is determined by the standard of the ordinary skilled nurse (Dimond 2005, p. 42). Nurses should only write a prescription for a patient for whom they have personal responsibility. In addition, they should only write a prescription on a prescription pad bearing their unique number (this includes private prescriptions).

Prescribing within the area of competence

All nurses are accountable to civil law with regard to the scope of their practice and must prescribe only in areas that they are deemed to be competent. In cases where a nurse may want to expand the scope of clinical practice by increasing their area of competence, it is important that this is done within the framework of clinical governance as explained earlier in this chapter.

Consent

Patient consent is a fundamental principle of health care law and is based on the legal and ethical principles that a patient has a right to decide what will happen to their body. Provision of information is core to the consent process and it is the nurse prescriber's responsibility to provide the patient with correct information regarding any treatment that is prescribed. Nurse prescribers should confirm that their patients know and understand what their treatment is for, how it works and any risks or possible adverse reactions. Patients should also be given advice as to what to do if they experience any adverse reactions.

Record keeping

Nurse prescribers are encouraged to adopt good record keeping practice and maintain records that are 'unambiguous and legible' (DH 2006). Records should contain details of the prescription as well as a documented record of the consultation. Ideally, any information given to the patient should be documented in the patients' notes. Neighbour (1987) described this as 'safety netting' and considers it to be an integral part of the consultation process. This should include advice given to patients about when and how to seek further medical attention if symptoms deteriorate. Records should be written immediately after the consultation or as soon as possible afterwards (NMC 2005).

Professional indemnity

Vicarious liability in health care means that health care professionals have legal exemption from liability for damages or claims made by patients and resulting from performing duties specified in their job description. However, despite this level of indemnity, nurses should ensure that they have personal professional indemnity insurance through professional organisations such as the Royal College of Nursing and ensure that their job description reflects any extended role, including prescribing.

Although indemnity protects the prescriber in case of patient legal claims, any claims would be reviewed with respect to contractual law. This demands that practitioners adhere to all policies and procedures laid down by their employer. Practitioners must then act within the context of these policies and within the parameters of their employment contract and job description. Expanded prescriptive authority is a good example of how advanced nursing is developing. However, through expansion of responsibility there is also the risk of the expansion of liability.

Current practices in nurse prescribing

While non-medical prescribers are set to make a significant contribution to the health care economy in the UK, there is variation in their practice and impact. For example, only 0.8% of the total prescriptions written in 2006 were from nurses or other non-medical prescribers (DH 2007). Clearly the number of prescriptions will rise as numbers of non-medical prescribers increase, but there is room for further development.

Future expansion of the number of non-medical prescribers will depend on the provision of responsive support and learning facilities for trainee practitioners Indeed the findings of an audit conducted in Staffordshire and Shropshire (Ring 2005) of the organisational structures required to support non-medical prescribing practice, noted health care organisations must be ready even before candidates are selected for training. In other words, support must be in place and non-medical prescribing must be integral to long-term planning and funding streams. Of equal importance are the benefits that can be realised following investment in the appointment of a proficient prescribing lead. Such leads can make a significant difference to the professional development and activity of these prescribers.

Those non-medical prescribers who have consolidated their practice and demonstrate that they are capable of integrating their role within mainstream practice, offer positive role models to others. A nurse consultant in dermatology, for example, is leading the way in Nottingham University Hospitals Trust by helping to deal with increased demand for services (DH 2008). Keele University has developed decision support systems that are particularly useful for nurses who prescribe, using evidence-based practice as part of their work with patients with long-term conditions, such as diabetes (Chapman 2008).

Role of supplementary prescribing for nurses in the current context

The process involved in designing, agreeing and implementing a CMP is complex and time consuming. A recent survey (Courtenay & Carey 2008) has confirmed that implementation of the CMP is the greatest barrier to supplementary prescribing and the NMC (2008a) has highlighted that with the new role of nurses as independent prescribers the need for supplementary prescribing may alter. Currently there is still a requirement for a CMP to be used when prescribing the majority of controlled drugs and all unlicensed medication, as these cannot be prescribed by a nurse independent prescriber. In addition, using a CMP would be of benefit for those newly qualified prescribers wishing to develop expertise and for teams of prescribers looking to create uniformity.

At present supplementary prescribing is being used successfully in a wide range of clinical areas, in particular those focusing on treating people with longer-term conditions, such as mental health. This area has all the characteristics (team approach, long-term care pathways and use of controlled drugs) that make it ideal for supplementary prescribing to be deployed, supported by experienced of mental health nurses and psychiatrists, with patients showing positive outcomes (Jones *et al.* 2007).

Conclusion

This chapter has explored the history, legislation, education and legal and professional issues that surround the complexity of nurse prescribing in the twenty-first century. The road to prescriptive authority for nurses has been a long and arduous one which is not yet complete. The future may see nurse prescribing as an integral component of pre-registration nursing and become the norm for every day nursing practice. However, before this can be achieved, the pioneers of nurse prescribing will need to have their prescribing habits evaluated and audited to ensure that nurse prescribing is improving the health outcomes and meeting the needs of the patients.

Nurses have been responsible for the administration of medicines as an important part of their nursing role since nursing began, but it is the new role of nurse prescribing that is challenging. The different programmes and formularies that encompass non-medical prescribing are complex and have the potential to be very confusing for the patient. The added accountability and responsibility that nurses have as prescribers can be daunting at first. However, with confidence develops competence and as the numbers of nurse prescribers increase attitudes towards nurse prescribing will become more positive.

Although nurse prescribing has evolved from a need for the provision of more efficient care in the community, it is also developing within the secondary care setting. Nurse-led clinics, for example, form a vital component of the health service provided for patient care. As prescriptive authority for nurses continues to be evaluated, the DH is also considering extending the prescribing rights of independent nurse prescribing to include more controlled drugs. This is an exciting time for nurses as they are beginning to develop new roles, focussing on prescribing. These roles have clearly benefited patients and contributed significantly to the expanded role of the nurse and promoted the image of nursing as a primary profession (DH 2008).

References

Basford, L. (2003) Maintaining nurse prescribing competence: experiences and challenges. *Nurse Prescribing*, **1**, 40–45.

Bolam v Friern Hospital Management Committee (1957 – 1 WLR. 583) – cited in Robertson, G.B. (1988); Whitehouse v Jordan: Medical Negligence Retried, 44, *Modern Law Review*, pp. 457–481.

Beckwith, S. & Franklin, P. (2007) *Oxford Handbook of Nurse Prescribing* Oxford University Press, Oxford.

Burns, S. & Bulman, C.H. (2004) *Reflective Practice in Nursing*. Blackwell Publishing, Oxford.

Chapman, S. (2007) Developing decision support systems for nurse prescribers. *Nurse Prescribing*, **5**, 251–255.

Chapman, S. (2008) Making decisions about prescribing in diabetes. *Practice Nursing*, **19**, 128–131.

Courtenay, M. & Carey, N. (2008) Nurse independent prescribing and nurse supplementary prescribing practice: national survey. *Journal of Advanced Nursing*, **61**, 291–299.

Department of Health (1989) *Report of the Advisory Group on Nurse Prescribing*. Department of Health, London.

Department of Health (1997) *The New NHS, Modern and Dependable*. The Stationery Office, London.

Department of Health (1999) *Review of Prescribing, Administration and Supply of Medicines. Final Report (Crown Report II)*. The Stationery Office, London.

Department of Health (2000a) *Health Service Circular 2000/026*. Department of Health, London.

Department of Health (2000b) *Pharmacy in the Future: Implementing the NHS Plan*. Department of Health, London.

Department of Health (2000c) *Lord Hunt Announces Proposals to Extend Prescribing Powers for Around 10 000 Nurses. Press release 2000/0611*. Media Centre, Department of Health, London.

Department of Health (2000d) *Health Service Circular 2000/026*. Department of Health, London.

Department of Health (2001) *The NHS Plan: An Action Guide for Nurses, Midwives and Health Visitors*. Department of Health, London.

Department of Health (2002) *Liberating the Talents Helping Primary Care Trusts and Nurses to Deliver The NHS Plan*. Department of Health, London.

Department of Health (2003a) *Supplementary Prescribing by Nurses and Pharmacists within the NHS in England. A Guide to Implementation*. Department of Health, London.

Department of Health (2003b) *A Vision for Pharmacy in the New NHS*. Department of Health, London

Department of Health (2004a) *Extending Independent Nurse Prescribing within the NHS in England. A guide for Implementation*, 2nd edition, Department of Health, London.

Department of Health (2004b) *Supervision in Practice for Nurse and Midwife Independent Prescribers and Nurse and Pharmacist Supplementary Prescribers*. Department of Health, London.

Department of Health (2006) *Improving Patients' Access to Medicines: A Guide to Implementing Nurse and Pharmacist Independent Prescribing within the NHS in England*. Department of Health, London.

Department of Health (2007) *Statistical Bulletin*. Department of Health, London.

Department of Health (2008) *Case Studies of Pharmacists and Nurse Independent Prescribers*. Department of Health, London.

Department of Health and Social Security (1986) *Neighbourhood Nursing: A Focus for Care (Cumberlege Report)*. HMSO, London.

Dimond, B. (2005) *Legal Aspects of Nursing*, 4th edition. Pearson Longman, Harlow, England.

English National Board for Nursing, Midwifery and Health Visiting (1992) *Open Learning Pack for Nurse Prescribers*. English National Board, London.

Garrett, D. (2008) Non-medical prescribers in primary care: practitioners or policemen? *Nurse Prescribing*, **6**, 106–109.

Halligan, A. (2006) Clinical governance: assuring the sacred duty of trust to patients. *Clinical Governance: An International Journal*, **11**, 5–7.

Humphries, J.L. & Green, E. (2000) Nurse prescribers: infrastructures required to support their role. *Nursing Standard*, **14**, 35–39.

Johns, C. (2004) *Becoming a reflective practitioner*, 2nd edition. Blackwell Publishing, Oxford.

Jones, M., Bennett, J. & Lucas, B. (2007) Mental health nurse supplementary prescribing: experiences of mental health nurses, psychiatrists and patients. *Journal of Advanced Nursing*, **59**, pp. 488–496.

Luker, K. (1997) Patients' views of nurse prescribing. *Nursing Times*, **93**, 51–54.

McHale, J. & Tingle, J. (2007) *Law and Nursing*, 3rd edition. Butterworth Heinemann, Edinburgh.

National Prescribing Centre (2001) *Maintaining Competence in Prescribing. An Outline Framework to Help Nurse Prescribers*, 1st edition. National Prescribing Centre, Liverpool.

Neighbour, R. (1987) *The Inner Consultation. How to Develop an Effective and Intuitive Consultation Style*. Libra Pharm Ltd. MTP Press, Lancaster.

Nursing Midwifery Council (2002) *Guidelines for the Administration of Medicines*. Nursing and Midwifery Council, London.

Nursing and Midwifery Council (2005) *Guidelines for Records and Record Keeping*. Nursing and Midwifery Council, London.

Nursing and Midwifery Council (2006) *Standards of Proficiency for Nurse and Midwife Prescribers*. Nursing and Midwifery Council, London.

Nursing and Midwifery Council (2008a) *Clinical Management Plans Advice Sheet*. NMC, London.

Nursing and Midwifery Council (2008b) *Code of Conduct*. Nursing and Midwifery Council, London.

Otway, C. (2001) Informal peer support: a key to success for nurse prescribers. *British Journal of Community Nursing*, **6**, 586–591.

Ring, M. (2005) *An Audit of the Organisational Structures and Systems in Place to Support Non Medical prescribing In Shropshire and Staffordshire*. Shropshire and Staffordshire Strategic Health Authority.

NHS Clinical Governance Support Team (2007) *What is Clinical Audit?* Available at: www.cgsupport.nhs.uk/downloads/What_Is_Clinical%20Audit_international.pdf (accessed 15 April 2008).

Winstanley, J. (2000) Manchester clinical supervision scale. *Nursing Standard*, **14**, 31–32.

Chapter 19 Public Health Nursing – Strategic Directions for Future Development

Liz Plastow

Introduction

This chapter identifies some of the challenges for the future and offers suggestions that reflect changes in government policy across the UK and the changing commissioning arrangements for children's services and primary care. It identifies the tensions that exist between individualised practice and population-based approaches to health needs assessment and prevention, the role of specialist services versus universal provision, and the dilemma of health promotion versus public health. The chapter also challenges the reader to define what is meant by health visiting and the challenges public health nursing faces in today's political climate, where function as opposed to title defines service provision.

Public health policy context

There are two main strategic drivers that underpin the current focus on public health interventions. First, the increase in health inequalities which has led to a greater focus of attention being given to the role of public health practice in reducing inequality, and, second, the need to consider the financial impact that changes in demography and technological advances in health care have made which has led to increased demand on scarce resource.

Over the past two decades, it would appear that continued investment in clinical care only brings diminishing returns, and this has led to a renewed interest in public health policy. Public health practice is multi-faceted, yet most definitions include within them, the contribution to the assessment of health and health needs, policy formulation and assurance of the

availability of services (Institute of Medicine 1988; Stoto *et al.* 1996), the latter being the most controversial, as current policy encourages outcome-focused service provision.

Acheson (1998) defined public health as the:

'science and art of preventing disease, prolonging life and promoting health through the organized efforts of society.'

This definition clearly embeds public health in the business of the wider community and inextricably links the well-being of individuals to societal influence. This argument is revisited in contemporary public health literature and strengthens the need for consideration of the individual within the context of the wider determinants of health and the impact of poverty and deprivation on health (Department of Health [DH] 1999a, 2002, 2007a; Ellefsen 2001). The paradox has been the difficulty in developing a common understanding of public health among political players and the population and contributes to the ongoing debate as to whether resources are targeted to an individual family focused service or whether public health nursing should be more broadly defined and targeted to tackling the wider determinants that impact on individual health.

In England the political context for the development of public health services within the National Health Service (NHS) was promoted by the DH White Papers *The New NHS: Modern, Dependable* (1997), *Making A Difference* (1999b), *The NHS Plan* (2000), *Choosing Health* (2005) and, more recently, *Our Health, Our Care, Our Say* (2006). These key government papers outlined the challenges for public health within

England and a commitment to target inequalities so that everyone would have the same life chances and the ability to make informed decisions about their own health. Similarly across the three devolved administrations, the Scottish Executive's Health Department (SEHD) White Paper *Partnership for Care* (2003), *Delivering for Health* (2005) and *Delivering Care, Enabling Health* (2006b), the Welsh Assembly Government (WAG) Paper *Designed for Life: Creating World Class Health and Social Care for Wales in the 21st Century* (2005); and the Department for Health, Social Services and Public Safety, Northern Ireland (DHSSPSNI) Paper *A Healthier Future: A Twenty Year Vision for Health and Well -being in Northern Ireland 2005–2025* (2005) and *The Review of the Public Health Function in Northern Ireland* (2004) have all set out their own political agendas and time frames for change with a major emphasis on strengthening public health practice.

Furthermore, the DH has demonstrated a commitment to funding public health through the recommendations of the Wanless Report (2004), which placed increasing emphasis on public health and the social and environmental aspects of ill-health. The report expressed concern at the deterioration in the quality of population lifestyles, particularly those of minority groups and the potential impact that this could have on health services in the future. Importantly, Wanless identified that the future of health services in England were unsustainable unless individuals took greater personal responsibility for their own health. This is described as the 'fully engaged' scenario and Hunter (2003) described this as having 'championed' the cause of public health.

Since the enactment of *The NHS Plan* (DH 2000), there has been a concerted effort in policy to encourage the individual to take increasing responsibility for their own health, and also to encourage providers of services to listen to the public in redesigning service provision. It could be argued that this is in response to technological developments, access to the internet, increasing public expectations and a greater voice to the consumer. A counter-argument could be that by encouraging the public to have a greater say, providing care closer to home and increasing

the plurality of providers merely takes the responsibility away from the state and places it onto the individual, while contestability ensures that cost is kept to a minimum with each provider undercutting its competitors. Whichever view is correct, the reality is that most of us would prefer to be nursed in familiar surroundings at home if we had choice and that we would prefer to choose from a number of providers than just one. The challenge here is the shift in provision from secondary to primary care.

UK-wide policy issues

Since devolution in 1999, the four governments of the UK have determined their own health policies on the basis of what is considered best to meet the needs of each country and fits with the political ideology of each country. However, they all struggle with the dilemma of increasing public expectation, demographic change, and increased life expectancy leading to large numbers of the population surviving longer with long-term conditions, and advancing technologies resulting in increased health care and treatment options and also with increasing delivery costs.

What is possible to see is that all four countries, in response to recommendations from the Wanless Report (2004), have opted to consider a model which puts prevention first, a health service as opposed to an ill-health service, characterised by a service whereby all health professionals are health-promoting practitioners, and individuals are encouraged to take responsibility for their own health. Each country is at a different point in the journey, with England having moved a considerable way along the journey of practice-based commissioning and the provider commissioner split.

In Scotland it has been recommended that the disciplines of district nursing, public health nursing (school nursing and health visiting) and family health nursing should be absorbed into a new single discipline of community health nursing. This is seen by some as further dismantling the traditional role of the health visitor and leading to fears that the public health elements of the role will be lost at the expense of acute nursing need (SEHD 2006a). The paper also advocates for the introduction of community nurse consultants, who would lead teams of workers in specialist areas of practice, including public health, working with the most challenging, complex families or leading the Child Health Promotion Programme. The role of the family nurse has been proposed in Wales, focusing on work with children of school age within the context of the family. The outcome of the ongoing review of public health nursing in Northern Ireland is expected in the summer of 2009.

Vision for health reform

Closer inspection of the strategic direction of policy across the UK indicates the following common key themes:

- More choice and voice
- Care closer to home
- Stronger commissioning – better services with better value for money
- Freedom for providers to innovate and improve services
- More opportunities for other sectors – voluntary, private and social enterprise
- Frontline staff driving forward change

The Darzi review in England (DH 2008) takes the Wanless 2004 agenda one step further in making recommendations 'for action to improve physical, mental and emotional health and well-being and to reduce health inequalities'. Thus, by developing a culture of prevention rather than one that prioritises the treatment of ill-health, it is anticipated this will contribute to long-term improvements in the population's health. This will depend on the creation of a more explicit and strengthened role for public health practice that focuses on the empowerment and enablement of individuals in taking responsibility for their own health, the role of health professionals being to assist people in making informed choices about their health and well-being, arguably a role that has always been a key function of public health nursing practice.

The development of public health nursing

Public health nursing has its origins in health visiting. The role emerged in response to societal

and political issues of the day including over-crowding, poverty and high infant mortality, issues that in relative terms remain a challenge for public health nurses today (DH/Department for Children, Schools and Families [DfCSF] 2007).

There is little doubt that during the first half of the twentieth century health visiting activity focused on maternal and child health from a more individualised perspective. By 1956 (Jameson Report), health visiting roles were extended to include mental health and the care of the older person, yet health visitors maintained responsibility for raising public awareness of health needs as well as influence health policy (Mason 1995). It is possible to see at this stage in the evolution of the profession that there was increasing tension between individualised- and population-based approaches to practice. In spite of the tensions, over the past ten years, the role of the health visitor has been identified as pivotal to achieving a number of policy initiatives (Acheson 1998; DH 1999a,b, 2001; Home Office 1998) and health visiting has been consistently encouraged to modernise to enable practice to further develop in response to policy directives.

Policy focus has since emphasised the need to reduce health inequalities and to target resources to those most in need. The Acheson Report (1998) for example specifically recommended that health visitors should further develop their role in providing social and emotional support for parents and their children in disadvantaged circumstances. The report identified the need to target the least well off in society in order to reduce health inequalities and, very importantly, considered that improving the health of women and children would have the most influential effect on the health of future generations.

Addressing health inequalities may be addressed by targeting hard-to-reach individuals, and also by addressing disadvantaged populations. This requires commissioners and our public health colleagues to adopt insight into the impact that both individual and aggregated population interventions might have on the reduction of health inequalities. *Saving Lives: Our Healthier Nation* (DH 1999a) further strengthened the role of health care to address health inequalities, and identified health visiting as being pivotal to the achievement of this strategy. Health visitors were encouraged to respond effectively to the government's agenda by developing 'a family-centred public health role, working with individuals, families and communities to improve health and tackle health inequality' (DH 1999a, p. 132). This in turn reflected a shift back to a population-focused service delivery.

In spite of the need to modernise health visiting, and introduce skill mix and delegation of duties, practice continued to focus on the tradition of an individual practitioner working with individuals, families and communities to offer health promotion and preventive health care to all age groups (DH 2001). The fact that practice was often at an individual level, but embedded within a population context was never clearly articulated by the profession or understood by the commissioners. Such misconceptions have led to the role being a target for rationalisation by cash-strapped health trusts. However, the public health role was gaining prominence and the profession rose to the challenge by publishing new standards for public health nursing practice.

In 2004, the Nursing and Midwifery Council (NMC) published its new *Standards of Proficiency for Specialist Community Public Health Nursing*, which incorporated the Faculty of Public Health competencies for public health practice and steered the profession to a much wider population-focused public health role. In 2007 the DH published its review of health visiting (DH 2007a), which recommended once more a role focused on the individual, working with families and addressing parenting issues, attachment and child development. The policy direction (DH 2007a) supported the value of home visiting and recommended that all families should benefit from receipt of a universal home visiting service.

Specialist community public health nursing

In 2002 the United Kingdom Central Council for Nursing (UKCC) was reformed to become the Nursing and Midwifery Council, mandated under the Nursing and Midwifery Order 2001. Under the (Transitional Provisions) Order of Council, 2004, a new nursing register was opened which came into force on 1 August 2004. The legislation allowed only for the provision of regulation for nurses and midwives as two separate professions. The order in effect removed the title health visitor. So while contemporary government policy appeared to further confirm endorsement of the unique and distinct nature of health visiting practice, the subsequent Nursing and Midwifery Order 2001 appeared to be at odds with this. Following lengthy consultation and significant effort by the health visitors on the council at the time a third part, the specialist community public health nursing part of the Register was opened in August 2004. All health visitors who were originally on Part 11 of the 'old UKCC register' were automatically migrated to this new part of the register and had their registration marked with the title health visitor. Under the rules it is only possible to be registered as a specialist community public health nurse if the registrant is already registered on either the nursing or midwifery parts of the register.

Since the opening of the register a number of other discrete groups, namely school nurses, occupational health nurses and sexual health nurses, who have been identified as working in specialist community public health nursing and having been seen to meet the competencies required to practise in this field, have also migrated to become registered on the new part of the register as specialist community public health nurses (SCPHN). The NMC (2004) defined specialist community public health nursing as:

'Specialist community public health nursing aims to reduce health inequalities by working with individuals, families and communities promoting health, preventing ill-health, and in the protection of health. The emphasis is on partnership working that cuts across disciplinary, professional and organisational boundaries that impact on organised social and political policy to influence the determinants of health and promote the health of whole populations.'

Hence the birth of the SCPHN, whose primary function is to:

'To safeguard the health and well-being of persons using or needing the services of registrants'.

(NMC 2002)

Registration on the SCPHN part of the Register has been undertaken as a staged approach, with increasing numbers of public health practitioners, who met all of the prescribed NMC, SCPHN standards, joining the register. This started initially with discrete groups, e.g. sexual health nurses, and proposals are that individual practitioners will follow. So, for example, a district nurse who works with the homeless and clearly meets all the competencies would also be eligible to register.

Modernising nursing careers

Recognised post-registration education for community practitioners in the UK is currently divided into two discrete groups:

- Specialist Practice Qualification (district nursing, community children's nursing, practice nursing, community mental health nursing, community learning disability)
- Specialist Community Public Health Nursing (health visiting, school nursing, occupational health nursing, health protection nursing, sexual health nursing)

Specialist Practice Qualifications were introduced in 1995 by the UKCC, followed by the NMC's implementation of the SCPHN qualification in 2004. Since that time much has changed in terms of the direction of policy, society, demography and technological advances, requiring the design of new contemporary courses and programmes to equip the current workforce to meet specific targets as defined by government policy. The four UK Chief Nursing Officers embarked on a major review of nursing careers in 2006 – *Modernising Nursing Careers* (DH, DHSSPSNI, SEHD, WAG 2006). The review sets out to define the principles to underpin a ten-year direction to prepare the future

nursing contribution to health care. It has four principles:

- Developing Career Pathways
- Improving image of nursing
- Flexible, competent workforce
- Nursing workforce that is 'Fit for the future'

Concurrently, the government's has reviewed its strategy for health, with its focus on health promotion, preventive care and reducing inequalities in health, placing public health and primary health care centre stage. Policy leaders have advised that they seek a confident and quality focused workforce that is more responsive, flexible and able to provide services that are closer to patients' homes. In order to respond to this agenda, it is essential that both SCPHNs and specialist practice community nurses (district nursing, community children's nursing, practice nursing, community mental health and community learning disability) work together to redefine their roles and contribution. Focus should be placed on addressing health inequalities, preventing ill-health and targeting those most in need. Practitioners will also be required to discharge increasingly complex care and support to acutely ill people back in the community. It is therefore timely that all groups of community nurses think strategically about how best to adapt and develop their skills, knowledge and competence to respond to new health reform requirements (Queen's Nursing Institute [QNI] 2006).

Early indicators suggest that future educational provision will be modularised, providing sequential development opportunities to enable practitioners to advanced practice standards. It is also anticipated that education will follow clinical pathways to support patients with acute care needs and longer-term conditions. As these care needs are prioritised there is a danger that public health will lose its prominent focus, as emphasis is placed on 'clinical' outcomes (concentrating advanced practice skill acquisition in areas, for example such as diagnosis and nurse independent prescribing). However, a nurse working in public health would be better equipped to function as advanced practitioner if she undertook further study in areas such as advanced epidemiology and strategic partnership working.

Current students of specialist practice and SCPHN programmes are entering an exciting period, characterised by new health care reforms and new patterns of educational provision. They are well placed to influence future educational design and provision, but they must be united in their vision and be prepared to lobby for the way forward.

Title versus function

There is little doubt that health visitors have made a significant contribution to enhancing the health of the nation, particularly through their role and function with children and public health, even if the 'title' is no longer recognised in the legislation of the Nursing and Midwifery Order 2001.

In 1977, the Council for the Education and Training of Health Visitors (CETHV 1977) formulated principles of professional practice based on a belief in the value of health which reflected the process of health visiting, These health visiting principles were revisited in 2006 (CPHVA 2006) and were seen to be as relevant today as they were when they were first written in 1977. The challenge for contemporary public health nursing, however, is to map these principles into modern policy requirements and at the same time reflect how the health visitor's role impacts on health outcomes for children and families. A further challenge will be to ensure that any future role mapping reflects the wider public health nursing role, including that of school nursing, health protection, occupational health nursing and sexual health nursing.

Despite political attempts to remove the title 'health visitor', the workforce now has more opportunities to be employed across a range of care groups, which require access to a range of public health nursing skills. However, it is also true to say that this has sometimes confused the specific role of the health visitor, resulting in concerns about the future direction of the 'health visiting' profession and its associated role and function.

Facing the future: a review of the role and function of health visiting

In spite of ongoing support for the heath visiting function by 2006, health visitors were calling to redefine their role in recognition of the need to respond more effectively to the government's emergent public health agenda. At the same time, the Secretary of State (England) in 2006, commissioned a review of the role of the health visitor (DH 2007a), its purpose being to 'sharpen, clarify and revitalise the health visitor's role' (Lowe, 2007). Although the review was undertaken in England, its recommendations have been considered by the other three devolved administrations to assist in the development of their own policies for the provision of early years children's preventative services. Following significant consultation, with frontline practitioners, managers, commissioners, parenting groups, users and professional bodies, a number of recommendations have been made that describe a renewed role for health visitors that (DH 2007a):

- Delivers measurable outcomes for individuals and communities and provides a rewarding and enjoyable job for nurses
- Has the support of families and communities
- Primary care trusts (PCTs) and practice-based commissioners will commission
- Delivers government policies for children and families, improving health and reducing inequalities and social exclusion
- Fits the new system of providing choice and contestability through new providers, that promotes self care, service integration, improved productivity and local decision-making
- Can adapt and respond to changing needs and aspirations
- Attracts a new generation to the profession

A number of other key messages arose from the review; the most controversial being that health visitors should only work with children and families, rather than to provide a 'cradle to the grave' service, underpinned by the rationale being that they could make the most impact on health outcomes at this stage of life. The review, however was not prescriptive and did not state that practitioners should not work with other age groups, but it was implicit in its recommendation that health visitors should target their interventions with the under-5s. Other recommendations included a proposal that existing health visiting services should be redesigned to form a fully integrated preventive service for children and families within a public health context. There was also a key statement to advise that to deliver future public health policy would require not simply the provision only health visitors doing the same work, but rather there should be well trained and competent teams led by a health visitor to ensure that a universal preventive service could be efficiently and effectively delivered to all families with young children. This builds explicitly on existing policy direction (DH 1999b) and on the skills outlined in the *Health Visitor Practice Development Resource Pack* (DH 2001).

The report recommended that the primary role of the health visitor should be either to lead and deliver the Child Health Promotion Programme using a family-focused public health approach, or to deliver intensive programmes for children originating from society's most complex and challenging families. The English government accepted the recommendations arising from this review and have since undertaken further work on updating Standards 1 and 2 of the *National Service Framework for Children, Young People and Maternity Services* (DH/DfES 2004). Twenty pilot sites have also been identified to 'test' a new model of intensive home visiting to families, known as the Family Nurse Partnership model, which originated in the USA (Olds 2006). This sets the direction of travel back from a wider public health focus one that concentrates on the individual child within a broader family context. The recommendations, while welcomed by many, marked a move away from the health visitor's broader public health practice role, in which they strove to address health inequalities. At the same time the NMC published new standards of proficiency for specialist

community public health nursing, which supported practice within a broader public health context as opposed to individual focused practice. Recommendations arising from a further review (DH 2007a) also strengthened the family-focused role of the practitioner within a public health context.

By delineating the two key roles, first, to lead local Child Health Promotion Programmes, and, second, to work with the most complex families, could lead potentially to the implementation of a two-tier service, with those working with the most complex families being seen as elite practitioners requiring additional skills, while those who work with services users in more deprived or unmet need areas being devalued for their contribution.

Taking the focus back to evidence-based parenting programmes and working with the most complex and challenging families is clearly following a much needed direction, but is one that also poses the risk of trying to stretch scarce resource even more thinly.

Workforce implications

The shifting policy agendas across the four devolved administrations of government have led to concerns for practitioners that their roles will no longer be transferable across the UK. However, closer scrutiny indicates that all four UK country policies are broadly similar, underpinned by a shift in emphasis from ill-health to preventive health care, increasing the voice of patients, promoting choice and accessibility and promoting closer working relationships with social care and education. Similarly all four countries have called for workforce change to support evolving integrated children's services. As such local PCTs have been invited to review the skills and competencies required to work with local children (Department for Education and Skills [DfES] 2005, 2006; Skills for Health and Public Health Resource Unit [SfH & PHRU] 2008) with the aim of strengthening integrated working practice across all services. Similarly, emphasis on promoting positive public requires the development of strategic level partnerships that collaborate to sustain service change.

This clearly has an impact on the knowledge and skills possessed by the present workforce, in addition to its shape, role and function.

In 1999, the DH (England) published a strategy for nursing, midwifery and health visiting to respond positively to the modernisation agenda (DH 1999b), which re-stated the workforce components required of health visitors. It also placed greater emphasis on the development of a leadership role for health visitors, recommending them to lead teams of nurses, nursery nurses and community workers in partnership with local communities and vulnerable groups to identify and tackle their own health needs. This has been further supported in the latest review of health visiting (DH 2007a).

It is evident from these recommendations that while an important component of the health visitor's role continues to be supporting families with young children, they are also expected to lead teams and to seek opportunities to work with other groups in the community. The publication of the *Health Visitor Practice Development Resource Pack* (DH 2001) and *Looking for a School Nurse?* (DfES/DH 2006) offered a framework and guidance for practitioners, their colleagues and managers to develop a 'reformed' way of working with families and communities, working together to accomplish common priorities, such as national service frameworks. Furthermore these tools have recognised that health visitors and school nurses are public health practitioners and have suggested that they need to refocus their professional practice from routine task orientated activities towards responding to those priorities that have been identified through community health needs assessment.

Leadership is a core function of specialist practice (UKCC 2001), yet for the majority of practitioners the ability to use and develop these skills is limited. A number of health visitors who work in children's centres or at a strategic level are able to further develop their leadership role. However, many work single handedly or within a team of health practitioners working at the same level and therefore have limited opportunity to develop their leadership skills.

However, skill mix in local health visiting teams has increased over the past ten years, which has resulted in an increasing need for leadership skills, delegation and risk assessment. However, some professionals remain reluctant to accept changes in practice and the impact that demographic change has on the health workforce, choosing to see skill mix purely as a cost cutting exercise (Keys 1997).

Other key leadership skills include, motivational interviewing, health needs assessment at an individual level as well as preparation for the coordination, management and delivery of parenting programmes and brief intervention therapies. These changes have significant implications for contemporary health visiting practice (as set out by the NMC 2004) and reflect both public health skills and competences required for child- and family-focused practice. The development of the Public Health Career Pathway (SfH & PHRU 2008) provides evidence of one attempt to map differing professional skills and competencies in public health practice with the aim of encouraging shared flexible career paths across the four countries of the UK.

Public health nurses or public health practitioners?

Public health nursing has been clearly delineated from the generic nursing profession but differences also remain between the role of the SCPHN and other public health practitioners. Apart from a few leaders in the field the majority of public health nurses are registered solely with the NMC, although there are a number of nurses who have completed competence-based portfolios of evidence to entitle them to register on the UK Voluntary Public Health register. Such recognition by the wider family of public health practice really promotes the role of SCPHNs within the wider family of public health practitioners.

Skills for Health, in conjunction with the Public Health Resource Unit, has developed a competency framework resulting in a career pathway for public health practice. This was published in 2008 and opens up opportunities for nurses and midwives to develop a career in public health (SfH & PHRU 2008). The United Kingdom Voluntary Public Health Nursing Register has also been afforded powers to register all public health practitioners and although in its infancy, it does give health visitors and other public health nurses the opportunity to consider an alternative career pathway and the chance to further their profession and to explore opportunities for registration as a public health practitioner.

Future development and challenges for practice

Opportunities exist for public health nurses to use their leadership skills differently and to influence local commissioning teams to ensure the provision of a universal early years preventive service is accessible in response to need as it arises. Such changes will require a shift in thinking by the current workforce if they are to create a service that is responsive to need, has the flexibility to continue to provide home visiting as well as providing a range of assessments and interventions in several other settings that are accessible to the local population.

In their capacity as team leaders the public health nursing workforce has a responsibility to apply evidence received from the analysis of the early years team workload to review work patterns, to prioritise interventions and to evaluate the effectiveness of their own practice. Information acquired from health needs assessments and public health databases should be critically analysed, acknowledging both their strengths and weakness, to support primary care trusts in the implementation of local public health action plans and to commission relevant services. As health care professionals skilled in community profiling and epidemiology, public health nurses should consider marketing this aspect of their role, and consider what routine elements of their role may be delegated to others to free their time to deliver on this key function.

Challenges exist if SPCHNs are to make a smooth transition from existing service provision to respond positively to future service demands. In England, the greatest challenge might be associated with the need to develop advanced competencies in commissioning. The government, in its document *World Class Commissioning* (DH 2007b) has identified that health service commissioners will be charged with responsibility to determine future systems of service provision. Furthermore, as service provision is increasingly commissioned to meet localised need, wide variances in the universal provision of public health nursing have been witnessed across the country. In addition, emphasis has been placed on the implementation of integrated working in England, requiring a strategic joint needs assessment between the health, local authority and education sectors to be undertaken (DH 2007b). Such collaborative working will provide many opportunities for SCPHNs to extend their skills and competencies. However, there is a larger pool of workers who could possibly carry out some of the functions of the health visitor's role, which adds to the need for the profession to define its contribution to the public health agenda and to articulate clearly what aspects of their role may only be undertaken by a public health nursing professional.

Public health priorities

Key public health priorities include: reducing the number of people who smoke, encouraging sensible alcohol consumption, reducing illegal drug taking and reducing teenage pregnancy rates. Health visitors strive to stimulate health needs awareness and to facilitate health enhancing activities amongst the local population, in particular with some of the most hard-to-reach families, and in so doing undertake a key function in the drive to reduce heath inequalities. More recently, advances in our understanding of early years interventions indicate that a number of public health priorities would be better tackled through early years intervention, which in turn will go some way to addressing generational cycles of deprivation.

Modern day concerns relate to the increasing range health inequalities encountered across the UK, characterised by regional variances that provide further evidence of the need to maintain prevention as a primary function of the health visitor's role and function. Although infant mortality in England and Wales has substantially decreased over the last quarter of the twentieth century, largely due to falling neonatal mortality (Maher & Mcfarlane 2004), it remains a government priority. This is evidenced by the government's focus on early start programmes such as those outlined in the publication *Starting with Children Under One Year*, which sets out plans to reduce the present gap in mortality between the 'routine and manual' groups and the population as a whole by at least 10 per cent by 2010 (HM Treasury 2007). Health visitors have a key role to plan with this agenda by engaging with children and families to identify a number of risk factors that impact on infant mortality, including smoking and poverty. They are also ideally placed to promote protective (and bonding) factors, such as breast-feeding and positive parenting regimens.

Childhood obesity presents another major challenge for practitioners (DfCSF/DH 2008). Although the rise in obesity is worldwide (Lobstein & Jackson 2007), the prevalence has more than doubled in the past 25 years in the UK. In England, nearly a quarter of adults and about 10% of children are now obese, with a further 20–25% of children overweight (Canoy & Buchan 2007). Foresight extrapolations suggest that we can anticipate some 40% of Britons being obese by 2025 (Government Office for Science 2007). The number of obese people is rising as a result of societal changes, with major changes in work patterns, transport, food production and food sales, exposing an underlying biological tendency, possessed by many people to both put on weight and retain it. If the ratio of total costs of overweight and obesity to health service costs remain similar to today, by 2050 the overall total cost to the NHS of overweight and obesity per annum will be in the region of £45.5 billion at today's prices (McPherson *et al.* 2007). Although there are significant gaps in the evidence base for effective interventions for obesity prevention, what is clear is that there are a number of critical opportunities for interventions to be provided during an individual's lifespan

including the impact of maternal nutrition on the fetus, increasing the number of women who breast feed, weaning advice, and encouraging physical activity in individuals and families as both individual and group activities.

Children's policy context

If the focus of health visiting and school nursing services for the future in England is to be on children within the context of family-focused intervention, it is important to consider some of the policy drivers that are currently influencing children's services. *The Children's Plan: Building Brighter Futures* (DfCSF 2007) was published in December 2007 and has an ambitious aim to make England the best place in the world for children and young people to grow up. It builds on the foundations set by *Every Child Matters* (2004) and is underpinned by five principles:

- The government should do more to back parents and families in their quest to promote better lifestyle opportunities for their children
- All children have the potential to succeed
- Children should enjoy their childhood and grow up prepared for adult life
- Services should be shaped and responsive to children and families and not designed around professional boundaries
- Acceptance of the fact that it is always better to prevent failure than to tackle a crisis later in life

Emphasis has also been placed on the involvement of fathers and in strengthening of the role of Sure Start children's centres to provide improved outreach services to families, including provision of more intensive support to the neediest families. The government has outlined six key objectives (DfCSF 2007), the first two of which relate to the potential future role that health visitors might play to better secure the health, safety and well-being of children. To this end the government published *Staying Safe: Action Plan* (DfCSF 2008), which was designed to respond to the specific needs of vulnerable children. A series of publications, *Aiming High for Children: Supporting Families* (DfES\HM Treasury 2007), further stress the need for collaborative working in improving health outcomes with a focus on parenting, responding intensively to those most in need and developing integrated services that are responsive to local need as identified by children and families.

Embracing the challenge of change

Health care policy has repeatedly reinforced the fact that all nurses have a role to undertake public health practice (DH 2006), which leads to questions as to the meaning of public health nursing. Health visiting has always struggled to define its role and as the health visitor's input is targeted to long-term outcomes, some have advised that the profession has been disadvantaged in not being able to demonstrate its true worth. However, in recent years health outcomes have been broken down into short-term measurable outcomes, which enable practitioners to measure the outcome of their interventions.

Arguably those working in preventive health care, namely health visitors and school nurses should feel most at ease with change for this has been the philosophy of their work since the profession was established back in the late 1800s. However, for many this has not been the case, with fears that there has been an erosion of their role as increasing numbers of health care workers take on components of their role (e.g. child health and early years workers etc). For example, the advent of Sure Start in England, with its principles broadly mirroring the role of health visiting services, has been welcomed by practitioners who have been able to utilise their health visiting skills to the full, but for others this has not been the case. The initial roll out of Sure Start children's centres in the most deprived areas of the country led to debates as to whether or not health inequalities were reduced or not. The expansion of services and the ongoing significant investment in children's centres have provided evidence to confirm that a well-resourced service that utilises health visiting skills does impact on reducing health inequalities and supporting children to meet their true potential (Barlow *et al.* 2007).

The modernised role for the health visiting function of the future will be to identify the high level skills that only a qualified health visitor can undertake, delegating other elements of the role to early years workers and leading early intervention and prevention teams. This represents a significant shift for many practitioners and though leadership has always been seen as a core function of the health visitors role, many have not had the opportunity to exercise such skills in practice due to the nature of their service. Others have not always embraced change positively, as was noted by Brocklehurst in 2004, reported that while most health visitors believed that practice had to change, many noted that they lacked skills in public health work including 'community development, partnership working, project management, team leadership, research and evaluation' (p. 215). Support and development programmes are therefore required to enable change to occur and for practitioners to work with the community to meet identified needs.

According to Forester (2004) the move from individual interventions to the acquisition of a community development approach to practise requires organisational support, strong leadership, effective team working, partnership working with communities and other agencies and the ability to work with multiple agendas. Expecting practitioners to work at a community level as well as to provide expert family support may be unrealistic, although some services, such as that provided in Stockport have tackled this problem effectively. The Stockport model of health visiting has developed over many years with three distinct components: generic primary care health visiting, first parent visitor programme and community development workers. This tripartite model has been strengthened as part of the modernisation programme (Swann & Brocklehurst 2004) and the findings arising from Swann & Brocklehurst's research study remain are as relevant now as in 2004. They include:

- The need for consistent and visionary leadership
- Consultation with all concerned in the change process

- Strong support from management
- Support with appropriate training to provide high-quality family support and leadership in community development
- Close partnership working between the NHS, local authority and voluntary sector

Future directions

There is an urgent need for public health nurses to re-evaluate their contribution to the public health agenda and to seek out new ways of working that more effectively support collective as well as individual approaches to health care. The government has clearly identified that all nurses, midwives and health visitors are required to change existing practice and plan services, with others (DH 2002, 2007a). Services of the future are to be based on need with service users and the public being central to the planning and development process. Working in isolation, as identified by Smith (2004), is no longer a viable option. While geographical constraints or unsuitable premises have in the past inhibited collaborative working, changes to commissioning and investment in the provision of children's centres provide opportunities for more collaborative integrated ways of working.

Developing skills in partnership with the wider public health workforce and using opportunities to lead and influence change are essential components of specialist community public health practice. Health visitors, school nurses and occupational health nurses need to have the confidence to value their expertise and contribution to supporting clients, families, mothers and children, and see themselves as team players.

Public health nursing practice requires a high level of skill and one of its strengths is its ability to respond to policy change and adapt accordingly. SCPHNs have always been proud of their level of autonomy in practice, however, in the current political climate they need to adapt and function effectively as team leaders, leading and managing multi-skilled teams of community staff nurses, nursery nurses, children's workers, mental health workers and administrative

officers, among others. Yet at the same time they are required to work collaboratively with consultants in public health medicine, general practitioners, midwives, mental health service workers, social workers, community development workers, health promotion specialists, benefits advisers, nursery school workers and others from the state, voluntary and private sectors. Their role will be to lead a universal service that builds relationships with clients, supporting families in a proactive way in order to promote health, prevent ill-health and reduce inequalities in health (Lowenhoff 2004). The provision of innovative, accessible services that promote positive parenting, engaging communities as well as individuals, is vital to address public health priorities. In order to do so health visitors and school nurses must stretch their skills to accurately assess and identify health need and delegate to appropriately trained and competent teams. The development of children's trusts that bring health, social and education services together to secure integrated commissioning of services has been designed to facilitate this process (DH 2004).

The future for occupational health nursing is also potentially very exciting, for example, those who work in the Health and Safety Executive have a very specialised and defined role which uses their public health skills to optimum effect. However, for others who work in the wider field of occupational practice their skills are also in great demand, in assessing and enabling people to return to work. A number of initiatives from the Department of Work and Pensions across the UK have identified the potential for occupational health nurses to assist them in addressing this issue (DWP 2007). This will require occupational health nurses to work with partners outside of their place of employment, including housing, benefits agencies, primary care teams, among others. All nurses working in public health need also to develop their leadership role, embracing opportunities to influence service change and development on a strategic level and acting on ideas based on best available evidence that meet the needs of local people (DH 2002).

Conclusion

This chapter has explored the need for SCPHNs to participate proactively in public health provision at the individual, family and community level, working collaboratively with public, private and non-statutory agencies to promote health and prevent ill-health across all age ranges in different settings. Valuing health and treating it as a positive resource has always been central to practice. The requirement to modernise practice has been clearly identified in government policy. SCPHNs must value their knowledge and skills, confront the dilemmas they face in practice, and have the confidence to seek opportunities to plan, develop and lead new intervention approaches with the public by working with those families with the most challenging and complex need. To enable this process, supportive management and organisational structures need to be developed that facilitate advancing practice.

Equally importantly, new ways of measuring the effectiveness of specialist community public health nursing practice must be found, based on a realisation that public health activities can produce both short- and long-term benefits to society. Failure to engage in outcome measurement has the potential to exclude opportunities for developing imaginative and strategic public health approaches, identified as essential for promoting the health of society. As the Office for Public Management (2000, p. 40) advised, health visiting must be 'measured not by the activity it undertakes but by the difference it makes'.

Public health nurses have the ability to respond and adapt to political and professional change (Brocklehurst 2004a) if they are prepared to delegate some of their practice and work more strategically with our partners in education and social care. The way forward requires practitioners to recognise and accept the opportunities available to them and to form strategic alliances with other agencies and support local communities to identify and develop their own services (Brocklehurst 2004b). By working with seldom seen, seldom heard, families the service can help to reduce health inequalities and provide them with the opportunities to implement services required to support the population they serve.

References

Acheson, D. (1998) *Independent Inquiry into Inequalities in Health Report*. The Stationery Office, London.

Barlow, J., Kirkpatrick, S., Wood, D., Ball, M., Stewart-Brown, S. (2007) *National Evaluation Summary. Family and Parenting Support in Sure Start Local Programmes*. Department for Education and Skills Publications, London.

Brocklehurst, N. (2004a) The new health visiting: thriving at the edge of chaos. *Community Practitioner*, **77**, 135–139.

Brocklehurst, N. (2004b) Is health visiting 'fully engaged' in its own future well-being? *Community Practitioner*, **77**, 214–218.

Canoy, D. & Buchan, I. (2007) Challenges in obesity epidemiology. Short science review. Foresight tackling obesities: future choices. *Obesity Reviews*, **8**: 1–11. Available at: www.foresight.gov.uk.

Community Practitioners and Health Visitors Association (2006) *The Principles of Health Visiting: Opening the Door to Public Health Practice in the 21st century*. Ten Alps Publishing, London.

Council Education and Training Health Visitors (1977) *An Investigation into the Principles of Health Visiting*. Council for the Education and Training of Health Visitors, London.

Department for Children, Schools and Families (2007) *The Children's Plan: Building Brighter Futures*. The Stationery Office, London.

Department for Children, Schools and Families (2008) *Staying Safe: Action Plan*. Department for Children, Schools and Families, London.

Department for Children, Schools and Families/Department of Health (2008) *Healthy Weight, Healthy Lives: A Cross-Government Strategy for England*. Published by COI for the Department of Health, London.

Department for Education and Skills (2005) *The Common Core of Skills and Knowledge for the Children's Workforce*. Department for Education and Skills Publications, London.

Department for Education and Skills (2006) *Children's Workforce Strategy: Building a World Class Workforce for Children, Young People and Families. The Government's Response to the Consultation*. Department for Education and Skills, London.

Department for Education and Skills/Department of Health (2006) *Looking for a School Nurse?* DfES Publications, London.

Department for Education and Skills/HM Treasury (2007) *Aiming High for Children: Supporting Families*. HM Treasury Publications, London.

Department of Health (1997) *The New NHS: Modern, Dependable*. Department of Health, London.

Department of Health (1999a) *Saving Lives: Our Healthier Nation*. Department of Health, London.

Department of Health (1999b) *Making a Difference: A Strategy for Nursing, Midwifery and Health Visiting*. Department of Health, London.

Department of Health (2000) *The NHS Plan*. Department of Health, London.

Department of Health (2001) *Health Visitor Development Resource Pack*. Department of Health, London.

Department of Health (2002) *Liberating the Talents Helping Primary Care Trusts and Nurses to Deliver the NHS Plan*. Department of Health, London.

Department of Health (2004) *Every Child Matters: Next Steps*. Department of Health, London.

Department of Health (2005) *Choosing Health: Making Healthy Choices Easier*. Department of Health, London.

Department of Health (2006) *Our Health, Our Care, Our Say*. Department of Health, London.

Department of Health (2007a) *Facing the Future: A Review of the Role of Health Visitors*. Department of Health, London.

Department of Health (2007b) *World Class Commissioning: Vision*. Department of Health, London.

Department of Health (2008) *High Quality Care for All: NHS Next Stage Review. Final Report – Lord Ara Darzi*. Cm7432. Department of Health, London.

Department of Health/Department for Children, Schools and Families (2007) *Implementation Plan for Reducing Health Inequalities in Infant Mortality: A Good Practice Guide*. COI for Department of Health, London.

Department of Health/Department for Education and Skills (2004) *National Service Framework for Children, Young People and Maternity Services: Core standards*. The Stationery Office, London.

Department of Health, Social Services and Patient Safety Northern Ireland (2004) *The Review of the Public Health Function in Northern Ireland*. Department of Health, Social Services and Patient Safety Northern Ireland, Belfast.

Department of Health, Social Services and Patient Safety Northern Ireland (2005) *A Healthier Future: A Twenty Year Vision for Health and Well -being in Northern Ireland 2005–2025*. Department of Health, Social Services and Patient Safety Northern Ireland, Belfast.

Department of Health, Department of Health, Social Services and Patient Safety Northern Ireland, Scottish Executive Health Department, Welsh Assembly Government (2006) *Modernising Nursing Careers: Setting the Direction*. Department of Health, London.

Department for Work and Pensions (2007) *In Work, Better Off: Next Steps to Full Employment*. Department for Work and Pension, London.

Ellefsen, B. (2001) Changes in health visitors' work. *Journal of Advanced Nursing*, **34**, 346–355.

Forester, S. (2004) Adopting community development approaches. *Community Practitioner*, **77**, 140–145.

Government Office for Science (2007) *Foresight. Tackling Obesities: Future Choices – Modelling Future Trends in Obesity and Their Impact on Health*. Department of Innovation, Universities and Skills.

Home Office (1998) *Supporting Families*. The Stationery Office, London.

HM Treasury (2007) *PSA Target 18: Promote Better Health and Wellbeing for All*. HM Treasury, London.

Hunter, D.J. (2003) The Wanless Report and public health. *British Medical Journal*, **327**, 573.

Institute of Medicine (1988) *The Future of Pubic Health and Institute of Medicine*. Available at www.nap.edu (accessed 21 February 2008).

Keys, M. (1997) Health visitors reactions to implementing skill mix. *Nursing Standard*, **11**, 34–38.

Lobstein, T. & Jackson, L. (2007) *International Comparisons of Obesity Trends, Determinants and Responses. Evidence Review. Foresight. Tackling Obesities: Future Choices*. Available at: www.foresight.gov.uk (accessed 2 December 2008).

Lowe, R. (2007) *Facing the Future: Review of Health Visiting*. Department of Health, London.

Lowenhoff, C. (2004) Have talents: need liberating. *Community Practitioner*, **77**, 23–25.

Maher, J. & McFarlane, A. (2004) Inequalities in the outcome of pregnancy implications for policy. *Health Statistics Quarterly*, **23**, 34–42.

Mason, C. (1995) Towards public health nursing. In: *Community Health Care Nursing*, 3rd edition (ed. D. Sines). Blackwell Science, Oxford.

McPherson, K., Marsh, T. & Brown, M. (2007) *Modelling Future Trends in Obesity and the Impact on health. Foresight. Tackling Obesities: Future Choices*. Available at: www.foresight.gov.uk (accessed 2 December 2008).

Ministry of Health (1956) *An Inquiry into Health Visiting (The Jameson Committee)*. HMSO, London.

NMC (2002) *Code of Professional Conduct*. Nursing and Midwifery Council, London.

NMC (2004) *Standards of Proficiency for Specialist Community Public Health Nurses*. Nursing and Midwifery Council, London.

Office for Public Management (2000) *Leading the Future*. TG Scott, London.

Olds, D. (2006) The nurse–family partnership: an evidence based preventive intervention. *Infant Mental Health Journal*, **27**, 5–25.

Queen's Nursing Institute (2006) *Visions and Values*. Queen's Nursing Institute, London.

Scottish Executive Health Department (2003) *Partnership for Care*. Scottish Executive, Edinburgh.

Scottish Executive Health Department (2005) *Delivering for Health*. Scottish Executive, Edinburgh.

Scottish Executive Health Department (2006a) *Visible, Accessible and Integrated Care: Report of the Review of Nursing in the Community in Scotland*. Scottish Executive, Edinburgh.

Scottish Executive Health Department (2006b) *Delivering Care, Enabling Health*. Scottish Executive, Edinburgh.

Skills for Health and Public Health Resource Unit (2008) *Public Health Skills and Career Framework: Multi-disciplinary/Multi-agency/Multi-professional*. Skills for Health and Public Health Resource Unit, Bristol and Oxford.

Smith, M. (2004) Health visiting: the public health role. *Journal of Advanced Nursing*, **45**, 17–25.

Stoto, M., Abel, C. & Dievler, A. (eds) (1996) *Healthy Communities – New Partnerships for the Future of Public Health*. Available at: www.nap.edu (accessed 2 December 2008).

Swann, B. & Brocklehurst, N. (2004) Three in one: the Stockport model of health visiting. *Community Practitioner*, **77**, 251–256.

United Kingdom Central Council (2001) *Standards for Specialist Education and Practice*. United Kingdom Central Council for Nursing, Midwifery and Health Visiting, London.

Wanless, D. (2004) *Securing Good Health for the Whole Population*. HM Treasury, London.

Welsh Assembly Government (2005) *Designed For Life: Creating World Class Health and Social Care for Wales in the 21st Century*. Welsh Assembly, Cardiff.

Chapter 20 Modernisation of Primary Care: Innovation, Leadership and Enterprise Within the Workforce

Karen-Stubbs and Janice Forbes-Burford

Introduction

Since the implementation of *The NHS Plan* (Department of Health [DH] 2000) health reforms have moved at a rapid pace, imposing significant impact and changes on organisations, staff and professional groups working within the primary, secondary and social care sectors. One of the current challenges for the National Health Service (NHS), and for primary care in particular, is the implementation of the government's agenda to commission services that are:

- Responsive to patient needs and choice
- Delivered by a plurality of providers, including primary care trust (PCT) direct care provision, private/public sector partnerships, social enterprise and third sector organisations

The role and function of nurses working in both primary and community care nursing is central to the successful implementation of these changes. The reformed model of care delivery is characterised by a move away from services that are dominated by the secondary care sector delivered in outpatient clinics, towards local services delivered by a range of health professionals and practitioners with specialist skills and interests, working in the community within the new service delivery models which include walk-in centres and proposed polyclinics. The aim of the new services will be to deliver tailor-made care packages of personal care closer to the patient. The former Labour Prime Minster Tony Blair stated:

> 'our aim is to reshape the NHS… so that it is not just a national service, but also a personal health service for every patient.'

The *NHS Improvement Plan* (DH 2004a) (which outlined delivery imperatives to implement *The NHS Plan*) stipulated that more power will be devolved to the local level. PCTs were advised that they would control 80% of the future NHS budget, thus enabling them, through the use of the mechanisms of practice-based commissioning (PBC), to secure the best possible outcomes for individual patients.

Building on the *NHS Improvement Plan*, the publication of *Creating a Patient Led NHS* (DH 2005a) (which links into wider public sector government reform), described the creation of an NHS that is truly responsive to patients needs and wishes. The *Improvement Plan* emphasised the need to enhance patient choice, and ensure that patients have the necessary information to make decisions about their care. *Our Health, Our Care, Our Say* (DH 2006c) also reflects the emphasis on patient choice. The White Paper (a declaration of the government's intention for the future) sets out a vision of providing people with good quality social care and NHS service delivery in the communities where they live. The document proposes a radical shift in the way that services are delivered, ensuring that services are more personalised and that can be more easily accommodated within the schedule of peoples' busy lives. *Commissioning a Patient Led NHS* (DH 2007a) identified the necessary steps towards changing the way services are commissioned by frontline staff to reflect patient choice.

More specifically the DH, in its publication *Our Health, Our Care, Our Say* (DH 2006c), noted that there were four main goals that underwrote the future of comprehensive community health care services:

- Providing better prevention services with earlier intervention
- Supporting people with long-term needs
- Giving people more choice and a louder voice
- Tackling inequalities and improving access to community services

While the main theme of the paper aims to give patients more control and to make services more responsive to their needs it also provided operational guidelines on how the four main aims would be achieved:

- Giving general practitioners (GPs) more responsibility for local health budgets through PBC (DH 2008f).
- Shifting resources into prevention and health promotion closer to where people need it most
- Undertaking more care outside of hospitals and in the home. Introducing a new generation of community hospitals and facilities with strong ties to social care
- Better joining up of local services at the local level
- Encouraging innovation
- Allowing different service providers to compete for services, including removing barriers to entry for the third sector as service providers for primary care (DH 2006e)

The implementation of expert commissioning, which is led by recent NHS policy, requires a high level of engagement with a range of new third sector and private sector providers, weaving and integrating provision of services into the NHS as co-partners; as NHS-registered care providers. The aim is intended to drive up quality within the NHS, and ensure that services are commissioned from the most appropriate provider, irrespective of whether the organisation is an acute trust, foundation trust, independent sector or third sector provider. These matters were expounded in the *NHS Next Stage Review* vision for primary and community care (DH 2008f), which outlined proposals for world-class

commissioning in primary care, for the enhancement of user choice and for the differentiation of provider and commissioner services.

This supports the government's vision for the evolution of patient choice in an NHS market governed by transparent monitoring and accountability frameworks. This currently involves the Health Care Commission, legally known as the Commission for Healthcare Audit and Inspection (CHAI), the Commission for Social Care Inspection (CSCI) and the Mental Health Act Commission (MHAC). However, it is planned to amalgamate these into one body to be known as the Care Quality Commission in 2009 (DH 2006d). It should be noted however that the responsibility for CSCI functions relating to children were adopted by the Office for Standards in Education, Children's Services and Skills (Ofsted) in April 2007.

The NHS believes that supplier diversity will encourage innovation as suppliers compete with each other to provide better services for patients. The direction of travel is therefore set as the NHS moves from a supply-drive organisation to becoming a demand-led commissioner and provider of health and social care services for local patient populations. However, it is important to recognise that the NHS protects fiercely its public service ethos – of ensuring care is provided on the basis on need and not on the ability to pay. Future services must be designed for the convenience of the patient, not the professionals providing them. Obviously this echoes a long-established philosophy of patient-centred care within nursing. However, as a profession we must re-examine the degree of success that has been achieved in this context. Can patients, for example, access 24-hour care from community nursing services across the country?

What this chapter provides

This chapter provides a summary of current NHS reforms; this includes the high focus that the government now places on services being delivered for the needs of the patient and the community and the importance of commissioning role to achieve this aim. The overarching role of commissioning within the NHS is described together with the principles and functions under-pinning the delivery of world-class commissioning and PBC. The key reforms outlined as a result of the review of NHS services implemented by Lord Darzi are also presented (DH 2008a), to assist nurses to understand the changes that are being transacted and to recognise the complexity and depth, and impact and challenges for the workforce as these changes are implemented in the 'reformed' NHS (DH 2008e). The specific role that primary and community nurses and health visitors will be expected to make to the reformed primary care agenda have been set out in a specific policy document relating to the implementation of primary care in England (DH 2008g).

The range of skills and competencies that are required to enable the workforce to optimise the opportunities that are now available through new and existing organisations and models for service delivery to patients are highlighted. The tensions and challenges involved for nurses in moving forward from a centralised leadership approach to an entrepreneurial culture in primary care are discussed. Case studies are presented as examples of implementation of these changes.

Commissioning

Commissioning is a very broad and complex concept. By way of background and context the *Oxford English Dictionary* gives the following definition to the term 'commissioning':

> 'something entrusted to be done, delegated authority, body entrusted with some special duty.'

While PCTs are entrusted to lead the commissioning process described within *Commissioning a Patient Led NHS*, this responsibility is delegated to clinicians and frontline staff via PBC processes (DH 2004b). The 'special duty' that lies at the heart of commissioning is therefore entrusted to the staff and professionals who deliver services within primary care. It is anticipated that this shift in emphasis will make it

easier and more effective to commission services that are of direct relevance to the patient experience and which are embedded within their local communities, and led and implemented by the clinical staff who know them best.

However, the issue of developing capacity around the commissioning and contracting process, and engaging clinical staff at the level required to drive reforms forward create a challenging tension. The lack of a level playing field for new providers, the issue of short-term contracts, memory of the past failure of the internal market, together with a lack of business acumen within both provider and commissioning organisations have delayed, and slowed implementation, in particular in relation to PBC.

The role of commissioning in the NHS

Commissioning is a central part of the government's health reform agenda (Figure 20.1), and one that has a major impact on the way services will be delivered in the future. Overall commissioning reforms aim to create an NHS that (DH 2006a):

- Improves quality, responsiveness, effectiveness and efficiency
- Knows the quality of services and rewards excellence
- Listens to users and designs services to suit their needs and choices
- Develops and empowers organisations and staff
- Works with light touch monitoring and robust safeguards

The combination of system management reforms (procurement and tendering), with the introduction of a plurality of providers (which challenge the monopoly of the NHS) will result in a wider choice of providers from which commissions can be purchased (taking into account patient need and choice). The implementation of the commissioning process will ensure that money follows the patient, and that high-quality services are commissioned by the best and most efficient providers. The current government policy requires PCTs to evidence achievement against world-class commissioning standards in order to

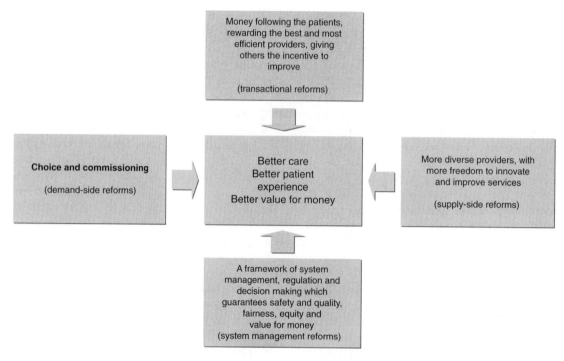

Figure 20.1 Commissioning – part of a comprehensive health reform programme. *Health Reform in England: Update and Commissioning Framework.* Department of Health (2006a), p. 6. Reproduced under the terms of the Click-Use Licence.

Box 20.1 Vision for world-class commissioning

- People will live healthier and longer lives
- Health inequalities will be significantly reduced
- Services will be evidence based and of the best quality
- People will have choice and control over the services that they use so that they become more personalised
- Investment decisions will be made in an informed and considered way ensuring that improvements are delivered from within available resources

World Class Commissioning (DH 2007b).

---

create services that will deliver better health and well-being for all (Box 20.1).

Commissioning – a definition

Commissioning has been defined by the DH as: 'The means by which we secure the best value

for patients & taxpayers. By "best value" we mean:

- The best possible health outcomes, including reduced inequalities
- The best possible health care
- Within the resources made available by the taxpayer'

'At the heart of commissioning are the millions of individual decisions of patients and clinicians that lead to the provision of care and the commitment of resources. Behind these clinical decisions lies a range of separate but related processes that collectively make up commissioning . . . a commissioning cycle'.

(DH 2006)

The processes and tasks described in the commissioning cycle (Figure 20.2) are strategic in nature and must be identified at a local level, and reflected in the PCTs local delivery plans and commissioning strategies. This needs, in

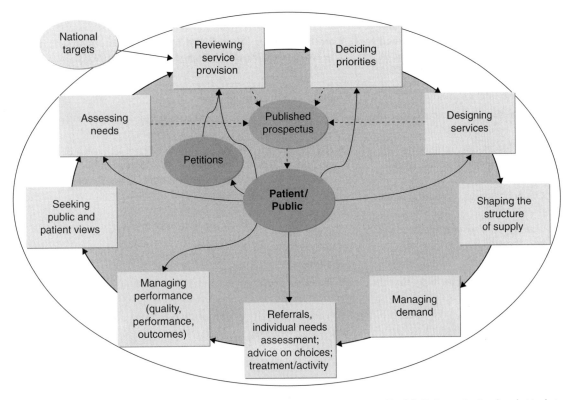

Figure 20.2   The commissioning cycle for health services -- DH. From *Health Reform in England: Update and Commissioning Framework – Annex: The Commissioning Framework*. (DH 2006a -- Annex p. 6). Reproduced under the terms of the Click-Use Licence.

turn, to reflect national and local population priorities and must enable the achievement of national health improvement targets.

Commissioning and fundholding: the past and the present

Many community nurses, particularly those who have worked in fundholding practices, will recognise some of the principles of the commissioning process that have been adopted by the Labour Government in *The NHS Plan*. Many of the principles contained therein emanated from the Thatcher era, which emphasised the importance of the internal market.

During the Thatcher and Major government administrations of the 1980s and 19990s market language was often used to drive the reform agenda, even though the influence of market philosophy was absent and weak. The use of

the term 'internal market' in the 1990s and the phrase 'money following the patient' described the desire to create a health care market that was responsive to patient choice. However, at that time the reforms were not radical enough and while they introduced transparency of costs and a contract mentality into the process of service purchasing, consumers were not given the power of choice. GP fundholders for example were subject to market incentives, but these were devised to engineer particular policy outcomes rather than to accrue real benefit for patients.

Market incentives do provide useful tools for central management and control, but a competitive market should not serve only as a political device for manipulating professionals to accept service change, but should act as a means of liberating the best services that people are able to

Table 20.1 The internal market versus commissioning

The internal market (introduced by the conservative government in *Working for Patients* [DH 1989])	Commissioning (introduced by Labour Government in *The New NHS, Modern, Dependable* [DH 1997])
Aims of the internal market:	Aims of commissioning:
• Contracting out services (more use of the private sector)	• The means by which we secure the best value for patients and taxpayers
• Value for money (improving management using skills from business.	• By 'best value' we mean: the best possible health outcomes, including reduced inequalities; the best possible health care; within the resources made available by the taxpayer
• Clinical budgets – knowing what things cost)	
• Quality (performance indicators and targets)	
Challenges:	Challenges:
• Two-tier system – inequity for patients	• Failure of internal market = lack of clinical engagement
• Short-term (1 year) contracts = high level of bureaucracy which was expensive	• Lack of capacity within primary care to undertake commissioning
• Government driven no professional representation	• Lack of commercial business skills in primary care
• Not mandatory – GPs could opt in and out	• Lack of robust data
	• Limited evidence about the effectiveness of services and treatments
	• Mandatory – 100% uptake required by government

provide. It is this element of Thatcher's internal market that was retained by Blair's Labour government and carried forward in *The NHS Plan*. The main feature, the separation between purchaser and provider (the internal market) has therefore been maintained through the current commissioning regimen that is being implemented at national level by the new NHS market (Table 20.1).

It is clear that the potential impact of the internal market mechanism has been harnessed within current reforms and the market concept integrated as a core strategic imperative for the modernisation of the NHS. The tension however, between the independent provider role of the GP, in tandem with their commissioning role as required via PBC presents a challenge to the

implementation of the commissioning agenda. In the internal market, savings made via commissioning were retained by the practice and acted as an incentive to practices to take on the extra work associated with the increased range of tasks involved. Therefore the benefits of fundholding to GPs were clear, many entrepreneurial GPs, nurses and primary care staff were enthusiastic and engaged during the fundholding era. They felt they were able to achieve real benefits for their patients, by commissioning patient services for their population and investing savings in developing their business. These same staff, under the new Labour Government, witnessed the dismantling of the internal market. This has made some practitioners wary of engaging further with the commissioning

Table 20.2   The commissioning function. (From Walsh, N. [2005] Developing nursing to transform primary care. Unpublished DH internal paper)

Element 1 – Commissioning Strategic design and development	Element 2 – Commissioning Operational and implement via contracting
Designing the scope and tender for services	Managing the provision of services
Understand current position (current activity, cost and quality)	Develop detailed service specification and tender pack
Establish future strategy (population need/public health/national targets)	Develop commissioning plan – outcomes drive (with social outcomes and clear outputs for service delivery)
Develop broad strategic specification for commissioning (including governance arrangements)	Performance and monitoring framework

agenda. This may explain the current low level of engagement with PBC in primary care, as some nurses and GPs feel that policy might change yet again if a new government is elected.

Currently all of the three major political parties include commissioning within their manifesto and it is clear that commissioning is here to stay, thus confidence is slowly starting to build again within the clinical community. The incentives for primary care organisations are now to focus on savings being reinvested in patient services for the benefit of the whole community rather than being allocated at practice level. Practices receive an 'indicative budget' intended to reflect the needs of their population. They agree a commissioning plan with the PCT. They are allowed to use a minimum of 70% of any freed up resources (savings) for reinvestment in patient care; agreement from the PCT is required for the proposed use of the remaining 30%. This is described more fully in the King's Fund paper *The Future of Primary Care: The Challenge of the New NHS Market* (Lewis & Dixon 2005).

The commissioning function

Commissioning may be described as the purchasing and contracting of health care services. In order to differentiate the concept of 'commissioning' from the previous terminology of 'purchasing' one might compare the order of a bespoke, made to measure suit, which fits the specific requirements of the buyer (commissioning) to buying an off-the-peg, readily available but standard fit (purchasing). Grant (2005) distinguishes between two levels of commissioning (Table 20.2). The first relates to service planning and design. This includes strategic work which involves identifying population need, determining priorities, understanding the market and defining where, how and by whom services should be purchased. The second focuses on the daily purchase of services, which involves the performance management of contracts and spending budgets.

PBC was always intended to be a multidisciplinary activity. Nurses have a unique relationship with patients and are therefore in an excellent position to advise on how services could be better provided. To achieve this, nurses working on the frontline in clinical practice should engage actively with the PBC process. However, in reality the majority of community nurses have yet to realise the importance of involvement with PBC.

One might argue therefore that frontline nurses are *not* proactive in engaging with the PBC agenda, but, based on the influence they could achieve on behalf of patients with respect to service quality, the question remains 'Why not?' Is this because nurses still see the focus of their role on service delivery? Does the issue of clinical hierarchy between doctors and nurses still play a significant role in the perceived merit of their acuity and therefore opinion with respect to influencing the commissioning agenda? Furthermore, have nursing staff been given the opportunity to learn and understand the concept, function and process of commissioning in any meaningful way? It appears that, in general, the current education portfolio for preregistration nursing programmes and continuing professional development (CPD) have limited content relating to the commercial and business skills required to facilitate effective engagement with this agenda. The education commissioning process, and the links between practice, policy and the process for commissioning education to support reforms, will need to become more integrated if true engagement of 'frontline' staff in PBC and policy implementation in general is to be achieved.

The role of the PCT in commissioning services

PCTs are at the centre of the modernisation of the NHS and are responsible for 80 percent of the total NHS budget. They are free-standing NHS organisation with their own governance boards, staff and budgets. PCTs are monitored by their local strategic health authority (SHA) and are ultimately accountable to the Secretary of State for Health. They work with other health and social care organisations and local authorities to make sure that the community's needs are met. PCTs may provide some care directly but their primary function is to commission the best services to meet the needs of their local population and in so doing may either provide services directly or commission them from others, such as general practitioners, dentists, pharmacists, and independent contractors, NHS acute trusts, voluntary groups, social enterprise organisations and private providers, with decisions on the selection of providers increasingly being informed on the basis of patient choice. PCTs as commissioning organisations are responsible for:

- Developing programmes dedicated to improving the health of the local community aligned to national and local performance indicators
- Deciding what health services the local population needs and ensuring they are provided

and are as accessible as possible. This includes hospital care, mental health services, GP practices, screening programmes, patient transport, NHS dentists, pharmacies, community advisory services, and opticians

- Bringing together health and social care, so that NHS organisations work with local authorities, social services, and voluntary organisations
- Ensuring the development of staff skills, capital investment in buildings, equipment and IT, so that the NHS locally is improved and modernised with the aim of continually deliver better services

The capacity and capability of PCTs to undertake commissioning at a local level is underpinned by two key initiatives designed to support the commissioning task and function within PCTs, and to develop the engagement of providers in the process. The first of the initiatives is defined in the *Commissioning Framework for Health and Well Being* (DH 2007a) and the second is described in *World Class Commissioning* (DH 2007b). It is obvious from the policy thrust contained in both documents that the government believes that strong market-based provision, coupled with providing people with greater choice and control over services and treatments, will result in improvements in overall patient care.

PCTs have also been involved in restructuring in order to divest themselves of provider functions that they previously held via the creation of 'arms length' provider organisations (as described by Havering PCT following the launch of the first Autonomous Provider Agency in London in June 2008 – unpublished paper). In essence, this further separates the PCT commissioner and provider functions, thus reducing the tension of both aspects operating within the same organisation. A step further is also witnessed in the establishment of autonomous provider organisations, which separate the business formally; such an example can be found within Havering PCT in North East London. This then enables the commissioning aspect of the PCT to engage with the concept of a plurality of providers, and the provider aspect of the organisation to compete in the market. However, for the majority of staff employed within service delivery, this philosophical shift may be difficult to embrace. In the main, the workforce still operates within a public sector paradigm and the notion of competing for contracts in an open market will not be familiar, unless previously involved in the days of GP fundholding. Indeed, some fundholding activity saw termination of established community nursing services contracts where GPs deemed them to be less than satisfactory for their needs, taking their business to providers outside their geographical patch. Where this occurred it caused major upheaval within community nursing teams and this negative experience has prevailed to influence the perception of those who were in clinical practice at the time, and could also go some way to explaining the lack of engagement with PBC.

Commissioning for health and well-being

In March 2006, the government published *Commissioning Framework for Health and Well-being* (initially a consultation document, now validated by the public), which argues that commissioners should concentrate on quality and outcomes when deciding their commissioning priorities. Eight steps were identified in this document for the provision of more effective commissioning (Box 20.2).

The publication of *Commissioning Framework for Health and Well-being* was driven by the fact that existing providers are sometime unwilling, or unable to provide new and innovative services themselves. Equally, the barriers that faced new entrants when they joined the provider market were high. The consultation therefore aimed to respond to some of these issues and aimed to create a fair playing field for existing and new providers by supporting the commissioning of services focused on transparent and measurable outcomes, promoting the development of strong and effective partnerships between commissioners and providers, introducing transparent and fair contract and procurement processes, and wherever possible engaging providers in needs assessment work.

Box 20.2   Health and well-being commissioning framework (DH 2006g)

Priorities

- Putting people at the centre of commissioning
- Understanding the needs of populations and individuals
- Sharing and using information more effectively
- Assuring high-quality providers for all services
- Recognising the interdependence between work, health and well-being
- Developing incentives for commissioning for health and well-being
- Strengthening local accountability
- Enhancing commissioners' capability and leadership

The shift towards commissioning and patient involvement in the process is further developed in the *NHS Next Stage Review; The NHS Operating Framework 2008 – 2009* (DH 2008b). This framework has health and well-bring as a true priority across the NHS and social care interface. PCTs will be required to work with local authorities and other partners to address how local delivery plans will achieve a series of national (and local) health and well-being priorities. Also key to implementing the framework for health and well-being and world-class commissioning is the need for infrastructure development for partnership between health and social care. In order to encourage this, the Local Government and Public Involvement in Health Act 2007 placed a new duty on both PCTs and local authorities to work together to conduct joint strategic needs assessments. An example of the process and outcomes that can be implemented and achieved through partnership is described in Box 20.3.

The example in Box 20.3 may be expanded further to demonstrate how strategic commissioning plans can be implemented at an operational level by practice nurses engaging in both the commissioning and the creation of innovative nurse-led services for patients with

> **Box 20.3   Setting up a chronic obstructive pulmonary disease (COPD) community service – Barking and Dagenham PCT**
>
> The PCT took part in the first PBC development programme delivered by the Improvement Foundation (IF). Leads from five GP practices, the PEC chair and the local medical committee representative were part of the team that attended all three IF workshops along with the PBC team at the PCT. This enabled the spread of good practice across the PCT and supported the development of business cases for service redesign.
>
> Through sharing ideas and making links with the other PBC sites, the team was able to start structuring the PBC agenda for Barking and Dagenham. Service redesign areas were developed from what was learned at the workshops about demographics, patient needs and demand for services.
>
> Working together, the team agreed the PBC framework for 2007–8, financial management and budgets, service redesign, local development plan priorities, and decided the level and quantity of patient level data that the PCT provided to practices on a monthly basis. In order to improve care for COPD patients, additional health professionals were recruited to the community team: a full-time consultant physician, a full-time clinical psychologist and a part-time nurse practitioner.
>
> In December 2007 the PCT reviewed the community COPD service and found the improvements had brought about a significant reduction in emergency admissions and outpatient flows into the acute hospital. It had also generated £298 000 of savings over six months.
>
> - Emergency admissions: Where COPD is the primary diagnosis, the total number of admissions in 2007–8 showed a percentage drop of 30.4% compared with 2005–6.
> - Admissions where COPD is mentioned, but is not the primary diagnosis, showed a drop of 13.8%.
> - Diversion of outpatient flows: The percentage reduction in general medical first outpatient appointments was 35.1% compared with 2005–6. The percentage reduction in general medical follow-up appointments was 12.1% compared with 2005–6.

chronic obstructive pulmonary disease (Box 20.4 and Figure 20.3).

World-class commissioning

'Adding years to life and life to years'

World-class commissioning will be the key vehicle for delivering a world-leading NHS, equipped to tackle the challenges of the twenty-first century. People are living longer, their lifestyles and health aspirations are changing, and the nature of public health and disease is evolving. By developing a more strategic, long-term and community focused approach to commissioning services, where commissioners and health and care professionals work together to deliver improved local health outcomes, world-class commissioning will enable the NHS to meet the changing needs of the population and deliver a service which is clinically driven, patient-centred and responsive to local needs (DH 2008f).

> **Box 20.4   COPD service for primary care patients**
>
> Central Surrey Health, which has set up a telephone based self-monitoring system for COPD patients. Patients call a dedicated number when they feel their symptoms have changed. Patients answer a personalised questionnaire using touchtone phone keys and a text alert is sent to the nurse, at their practice, if their condition has deteriorated. Hospital admissions have fallen 32% since the system was introduced and routine home visits and length of hospital stay have also dropped. This example highlights how practice-nurse-led initiatives can benefit in the main areas of focus for PBC. Practice nurses worked to identify patients, develop the new service model, and create the questionnaire and methodology. This project reduced referral rates, improved the management of long-term condition, and keeps people healthy working in partnership with the nurse team. Using an innovative method of communication to deliver the service was also well received by patients.

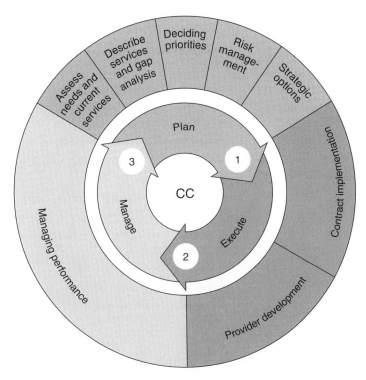

Figure 20.3 World-class commissioning: the commissioning cycle (National Association of Primary Care website (2007) webpage). Available at: www.napc.co.uk/pub-view.php?pubID=186. Reproduced under the terms of the Click-Use Licence.

December 2007 saw the announcement of a new statement of intent to develop world-class commissioning (DH 2007b). The statement describes a new vision for world-class commissioning and outlines a set of 11 organisational competencies that address how the commissioner capability will be developed. The statement also details how commissioning will be used as a key tool to shape the provision of health services and to create an effective demand-led market within the primary care sector.

As commissioning is the responsibility of PCTs, they will lead the drive to deliver service improvements. Aspiring towards becoming world class, and by adopting a more strategic approach to the commissioning of services, will result in the creation of a proactive, rather than reactive, health service. New competency frameworks will need to be developed to achieve this objective to ensure that staff possess the requisite skills and knowledge to work effectively across the commissioning and provider interface (Table 20.3).

Delivering a fair, personalised, effective and safe NHS

By placing greater emphasis on local needs assessment, and the priority of investments to deliver long-term improvements in health outcomes, world-class commissioning will be pivotal in reducing health inequalities. It is interesting to reflect on the past when considering the future. The Black Report on health inequalities was published by the Department of Health and Social Security (DHSS) in 1980. The political response did not embrace the report's findings; indeed, it was several years before the recommendations were openly discussed and accepted as valid. However, the issue of health inequalities remains a major issue in policy

Table 20.3 World-class commissioning competency framework and anticipated results (*World Class Commissioning Framework Competencies* [DH 2007b])

Competencies framework for world-class commissioners	Result in commissioners who:
Locally lead the NHS	Can assess population and patient need systematically
Work with local community partners	Listen to individuals and communities – especially those that are not often heard
Engage with public and patients	Commission for outcomes and outputs
Collaborate with clinicians	Understand and use the levers available to them:
Manage knowledge and assess needs	• Contracts
Prioritise investment	• Care resources and utilisation
Stimulate the market	• Incentives
Promote improvement and innovation	• Market development (i.e. third sector and social enterprise)
Secure procurement skills	Are capable and competent
Management the local health system	Are multi-disciplinary
Make sound financial investments	Can build effective partnerships

and challenges effective service delivery across the country, in spite of the rhetoric. Indeed, if one considers the focus of much policy in this context it would be easy to construe that these are the same issues wearing a new badge. Maxwell's six dimensions of health care quality (Maxwell 1984) have been a continuous central element of service improvement criteria: access, acceptability, appropriateness, equity, effectiveness and efficiency. These same issues have appeared as a recurring theme underpinning the change agenda in the NHS. Indeed, Chambers & Wakley (2005) have recently identified two further categories within Maxwell's quality framework: communication and continuity. It might be argued that all of these factors when combined describe the key determinants of health care quality, effectiveness and customer satisfaction.

One of the main differences with world-class commissioning is that it encourages patient engagement and greater clinical involvement of communities throughout the commissioning process. Increased clinical and patient input, combined with a more accurate assessment of longer-term local requirements, will ensure services are more closely designed to meet evolving patient needs, and fit within the DH quality framework. By encouraging the emergence of new services and providers, and promoting greater choice, world-class commissioning will open up new opportunities for the creation of innovative, local care solutions – all centred on the needs of the patient. In doing so, they will create an environment where innovation thrives and where safety and quality become prerequisites.

Innovation in commissioning

Several examples (Box 20.5) exist of innovative commissioning practice that have been designed to support the vision of an NHS that is fair, personalised, effective and safe, and which delivers the outcomes aspired to by NHS London (2007) in its publication *Healthcare for London: A Framework for Action: Consulting the Capital* and outlined in the *NHS Next Stage Review* (DH 2008a).

Nursing can play a significant role in addressing service deficits for the benefit of the population, but in order to do so, the profession must engage with the new NHS reform agenda. Community nurses should rise to the challenges presented by

---

Box 20.5 World-class commissioning examples

Heywood, Middleton and Rochdale PCT has joined forces with Sport England and the Big Lottery Fund to regenerate sports facilities in the community, supporting the long-term shift from diagnosis and treatment to prevention and the promotion of well-being. The PCT has also employed dedicated community workers to develop services that are of interest to the local population to encourage healthy lifestyles and improve public health.

Bournemouth and Poole PCT has, in partnership with its practice-based commissioners, established a new community-based palliative care service, that is improving end-of-life care for patients.

In Liverpool, the local PCT has set up a social inclusion team; the team members speak 13 different languages between them. The team will identify important health trends within different parts of the community and will help to widen health care access and compliance for people from ethnic minority groups.

In Birmingham, three PCTs have joined forces to improve male life expectancy, combating cardiovascular disease (CVD) in new and innovative ways. Having identified the patients most at risk of CVD, the PCT commissioned a pilot pharmacy screening service for the disease. The practical location of many of the participating pharmacies, along with their extended opening hours and 'drop in' approach, increased access for patients across Birmingham and, in particular, targeted deprived communities and those with lowest male life expectancy.

DH (2008h).

---

a changing landscape and ensure that their skills are developed and relevant to new service models. This will require a commitment to continuing professional development and engagement with the developing agenda for health and social care. It is clear that by further strengthening relationships between key local partners, such as PCTs and local authorities, world-class commissioning will ensure the formation of more effective links between different stages of the patient care journey, ensuring that overall care solutions remain highly personalised and effective.

This is an area of high expertise within the nursing community. Experienced community nursing staff are aware of the needs of their patients/clients and have always articulated a need for increased involvement in the design and development of services for patients. The opportunity for staff engagement in both PCT commissioning and provider functions has never been greater. There is, however, a significant difference between the skills required for clinical delivery and those needed for service development and innovation, and these are not meant to be necessarily mutually exclusive. Many nurses have developed increased skills in order to move into non-nursing, management roles in which their

transferable skills can be positively exploited, but apart from some nurse-led service provision enabled by GP contracting, nurses appear at present to remain at the periphery, rather than taking centre stage in developing new services.

Healthcare for London: A Framework for Action (incorporating the principles of world-class commissioning)

In his review, commissioned by the Secretary of State for Health in 2007, Lord Darzi (DH 2008a, 2008g) set out four overarching themes for the NHS over the next ten years. He described the vision of a health and care system that is fair, personalised, effective and safe. World-class commissioning will be central to achieving this vision.

The first published delivery plan, based on Lord Darzi's anticipated vision at the time related to NHS London. *Healthcare for London: A Framework for Action* (NHS London 2007) focuses on services directed and designed from a patients' point of view. The proposal and ideas contained within the framework (Box 20.6) formed part of a major stakeholder consultation exercise that yielded the following five princi-

---

Box 20.6   Health care for London: principles

- Services should be focused on individual needs and choices
- Services should be localised where possible or regionalised where that improves the quality of care
- There should be joined-up care and partnership working, maximising the contribution of the entire workforce
- Prevention is better than cure
- There must be a focus on reducing differences in health and health care across London

---

ples upon which the future of London's health care services will be focused in the future.

The NHS has made major improvements over the past 20 years, while science and medicine have developed in ways that could not have been foreseen. However further change and improvement is required if our NHS is to perform effectively in the future. There are eight major reasons why change is needed for London (and for other regions in the UK) (Box 20.7). Lord Darzi's *Next Stage Review* also focused on local changes (DH 2008c, 2008f) and reflected the views of patients. The results have been outlined in the next stage review, which sets out five pledges which PCTs should have regard to when creating their strategic vision and commissioning plans (Box 20.8).

Box 20.7   Reasons for change – health care for London 2007

- The need to improve Londoners' health
- The NHS is not meeting Londoners' expectations
- One city, but big inequalities in health and health care
- Hospital is not always the answer
- London should be at the cutting edge of medicine
- The need for more specialised care
- Workforce and buildings are not being used effectively
- The need to make best use of taxpayers' money

Box 20.8   *Next Stage Review: Leading Local Change* (DH 2008c)

Five pledges
- Change will always be to the benefit of patients. This means that they will improve the quality of care that patients receive whether in terms of clinical outcomes, experience or safety
- Change will be clinically driven. Change will be to the benefit of the patient by making sure that it is always led by clinicians and based on the best available clinical evidence
- All change will be locally-led. Meeting the challenge of being a universal service means the NHS must meet the different needs of everyone. Universal is not the same as uniform. Different places have different and changing needs – and local needs are best met by local solutions.
- You will be involved. The local NHS will involve patients, carers the public and other key partners. Those affected by proposed changes will have the chance to have their say and offer their contribution. NHS organisations will work openly and collaboratively.
- You will see the difference first. Existing services will not be withdrawn until new and better services are available to patients so that they can see the difference.

The five pledges shown in Box 20.8 aim to ensure that the right changes happen for the right reasons, based on what is clinically best for patients. It could be suggested that these pledges have a better alignment with the philosophy of nursing, and therefore may promote increased levels of engagement, particularly at a local level with both the commissioning and provider agenda.

Practice-based commissioning

PBC is the policy vehicle for ensuring clinical involvement occurs at a local level in the strategic level commissioning process. PBC has been heralded as a panacea for driving NHS reforms. The DH when launching the initiative in 2004 stated that PBC would bring 'greater involvement of front-line doctors and nurses in commissioning decisions'. We have discussed previously in this chapter some of the similarities of PBC to fundholding, and identified a range of factors that may have inhibited the pace of implementation of PBC.

Based on the principle that GPs and primary care teams are best placed to identify what their patients require, PBC is designed to improve the quality of patient services and ensure the effective use of NHS resources by involving GPs directly in the commissioning process. PBC aims to encourage GPs to identify, plan and deliver more efficient and effective care pathways for their patients. They will have a clear incentive to assess carefully the appropriateness, effectiveness and efficiency of services (particularly those provided within the acute sector) that they commission for their patients and to identify whether those services could be more appropriately provided within alternative settings, in particular in the primary care sector or at home (DH 2008f).

While PBC has received widespread support among the main political parties and key NHS stakeholders groups, implementation in primary care has been less visible. The King's Fund report (2007) states that although the NHS now boasts 'universal coverage' of PBC, this refers more accurately to the creation of an environment in which PBC could thrive, rather than one in which it is actually flourishing.

Aims of PBC

PBC refers to the process of devolution of commissioning roles from PCTs to general practice teams, which in turn will be expected to deliver services via indicative budgets that remain managed by their local PCT. The DH objectives outlined in its guide *Practice Based Commissioning, Practical Implementation* (DH 2004c), identified the following PBC outcome objectives:

- Greater variety of services
- Services delivered by a greater number of providers and in settings that are close to and convenient for patients
- More efficient use of services
- Greater involvement of frontline doctors and nurses in the commissioning decisions

Given that the principles of PBC were described and introduced in 1997, with implementation and

guidance following later in 2004 within the government's *NHS Plan* (DH 2000). It is fair to say that implementation has been slow. There are many reasons for this laboured journey, including:

- Reorganisation of PCTs (since 2005) as part of the NHS rationalisation process
- Priority emphasis to ensure financial balance
- Meeting national NHS delivery targets (18 week and access)

In many primary care organisations, PBC has been regarded as yet another task to be achieved among a range of other imperatives. Consequently some PCTs have yet to realise the benefits that PBC could yield. Indeed, PBC when managed effectively, and carried out in partnership, will impact on the design and delivery of a rich range of innovative provider services provided by a plurality of providers within the new NHS market. Perhaps the real success of PBC will be measured by the number of new and innovative services that emerge, which truly reflect the demographics and culture of local communities and neighbourhoods in the design and delivery of the services that are provided.

Table 20.4 presents a discussion point to illustrate the main barriers to PBC and why it is different to GP fundholding.

Central to the vision of health care delivery for the twenty-first century is the idea that a significant proportion of care currently delivered in an acute setting should be delivered in the community. National commissioning guidance outlined in Figure 20.4 indicate that services may be expected to fall into one of three groups which will largely determine the routes through which they might be procured.

- Services that are so closely linked to acute services that there is no practice alternative to them being delivered by the main local acute trust.
- Services where there is scope for a range of different providers to operate in a given area with activity being determined by patient choice rather than contracting arrangements.
- An intermediate category of services where plurality of provision is not appropriate but

Table 20.4 Barriers and differences: practice-based commissioning (PBC) and fundholding

Main barriers to PBC	Differences between PBC and fundholding. PBC is not fundholding because:
Lack of primary care trust (PCT) support/PCT turmoil	Procurement will be routine, rules based processing at a supra PCT/national level:
Financial constraints/short-term approach	• Standard prices/tariffs
Lack of quality data/information	• Standard format contracts
Lack of protected time	• Standard national targets
Lack of GP engagement and low morale	• Standard quality standards
Lack of knowledge about the process	Commissioning decisions will be about:
Insufficient incentives	• Volume and location of referrals
Lack of co-ordination	• Pattern of care
Lack of communication	• Greater partnership between clinicians and patients
Impact of PbR/unhelpful attitudes of secondary care colleagues	
Threat of competition	
Lack of space	
Poor quality facilities	
Lack of leadership	
Lack of knowledge about governance and legal issues	

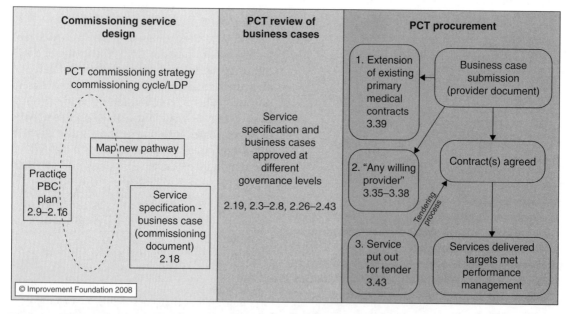

Figure 20.4 Practice-based commissioning. Commissioning and Procurement Overview (2008) (www.improvementfoundation.org/resource/dl/29). From Commissioning and Procurement Overview, Improvement Foundation.

which are not so linked to acute services that there is no practical alternative to their being delivered by the main local acute trust.

Understanding the relationship between commissioning vision and world-class commissioning and practice-based commissioning

The government commissioning agenda focuses on the procurement of a wide range of high-quality, personalised health and social care services. This has led to a concerted effort being made by PCTs to guarantee patient choice by diversifying the supplier base. Consequently new markets have been created in which a plurality of providers now compete to offer services to patients utilising a variety of contracts, and models of service provision.

Service providers

Within the NHS the model of primary care service delivery in England has remained fairly constant for many decades, centred on the general practice independent contractor (the local GP) providing general medical services to patients via an NHS negotiated central contract. Primary care and community nurses have been employed by either a GP, or the PCT. With the implementation of the NHS reform agenda, and in particular the commissioning reforms detailed above, the introduction of choice and contestability presents many new opportunities for the NHS provider workforce. Nurses no longer have to be employed by other organisations, there is greater flexibility and potential to work as a self-employed contractor, create new nurse-led organisations independently or work in equal partnership with other clinicians to create social enterprise or third sector organisations.

In an unpublished paper produced by the DH in 2005, Walsh identified ten potential models of nursing roles for the future (Box 20.9). Additional skills and competencies have now been defined for advanced nurse practitioner, nurse practitioner and nurse consultant roles, making it easier for them to define their contribution to new contractual processes and

---

> **Box 20.9   Nursing roles in service provision**
>
> - Nurse run practices
> - Co-located nursing services
> - Nurse-led primary care services (targeted at specific patient groups)
> - Integrated nursing team private limited companies
> - Multi-disciplinary professional partnerships
> - Limited liability partnerships
> - Limited companies
> - Nursing cooperatives
> - Multi-specialty teams
> - Nursing chambers
>
> (Walsh, N. [2005] Developing nursing to transform primary care. Unpublished DH internal paper.)

---

provider services. Many of these senior nurses are beginning to demonstrate their potential to secure contracts for the provision of a range of services and to become independent providers for health and social care services (see Chapter 15). Nevertheless, at this point in time, there is scarce evidence of the nursing profession embracing the opportunity to become entrepreneurial, or to lead on the development of new, innovative 'autonomous provider organisations'. It does therefore pose an important question for consideration: Why are nurses expected to be entrepreneurial in this world of policy change and opportunity?

The nursing population is but a reflection of the social and cultural milieu in which it exists. It is not separate from, but an integral part of society and its members belong to many different and varied categories within it. Would any other such sample of the population, other than those with a recognised interest and flair for business, demonstrate a predilection towards entrepreneurship? Conferences and workshops abound in an attempt to seduce the nursing fraternity to become entrepreneurs within health care provision but surely we should expect only the same percentage of interest to be generated among the profession as would be found in the rest of society.

Certainly, nursing has demonstrated an ability to adapt and develop in the recent past in the context of new roles and responsibilities, for example, the creation of clinical nurse specialist posts, nurse consultants, community matrons. Nursing has also led the way in the development of non-medical prescribing, which has without doubt changed the patient experience positively (see Chapter 18). What is clear, however, is that the NHS reform agenda rightly seeks to benefit patients first and foremost. Commissioners have the right to demand the best quality services for the population they serve, evidenced by the best clinical competence available (DH 2008f).

A new strategy published in June 2008 by the DH (2008d) provides patients and the public with an even stronger voice, enabling them to make informed decisions and have greater choice and control in managing their health and health care. *Our Vision for Primary and Community Care* (DH 2008d), published as part of the *Next Stage Review of the NHS*, sets out the future direction for primary and community care in England, where essential standards are ensured and excellence is rewarded. It focuses on personal and responsive health care – providing integrated care based around the person, rather than focusing on just their individual symptoms or care needs (DH 2008f).

The strategy underlines the central role primary and community care services play in keeping people healthy, preventing illness and promoting healthy life-styles as well as tackling regional variations in health and well-being. Within the NHS, primary and community care services are highly valued by patients and the public – for the personal continuity of care they provide and for their strong ties with local communities. The new vision for primary care will protect the highly popular and effective system of registering with a local GP, but give family doctors a stronger role in working with other clinicians, local authorities and other organisations to provide the right services, in the right place and at the right time to meet individual needs. The GP patient survey will be extended to encourage patient feedback and greater public accountability for staff working in primary care. Patients will be able to register online and

have a greater range of options for consulting with their GP (e.g. by telephone or email). Practice funding will be reformed to reward GPs who take on new patients to support greater patient choice. Other key issues within the strategy include:

- Personalised care plans for those with longer-term conditions, and for those with complex health needs – a care coordinator
- Individual health budgets will enable patients to have greater control over how NHS funding is used to support their care
- Creating a new secure web-based system called 'myhealthspace', allowing people to access and update their personal care record, to share information with their care team, and book appointments and order repeat prescriptions
- Faster and simpler access to a wider range of community-based services such as minor ailments services and health checks in high-street pharmacies, walk-in services, and self-referral to physiotherapy or podiatry services for example
- More online performance and quality information available on NHS Choices website to enable patients to compare GP and community health care services and view patient feedback
- Identifying those most at risk of ill-health and offering early interventions that help keep people healthy for longer, working with GPs to amend the Quality and Outcomes Framework to reflect this and providing stronger incentives for early intervention. High-performing GPs will have greater freedoms to develop new services for their patients, working with other primary and community clinicians by reinvigorating PBC
- Piloting more joined up services to help people who want to return to work but are struggling with back problems, stress, etc.
- Increasing access to 'healthy living services', making it easier for GP practices to refer or point people towards walk in services that best meet their needs such as exercise classes, stop smoking support or help in managing stress.

Contracts for providers

A provider is defined as an organisation that offers health or social care services under contract arrangements to a purchaser. A commissioner is a budget-holding body that buys health or social care services from a provider on behalf of its resident population. A commissioner can be a PCT or a PBC cluster or a patient (empowered to commission their own services under direct payments legislation). A range of contracting methods are already in use and available for deployment in primary care settings to support the provision of an eclectic range of local services (Rowe 2005; Walsh, N. [2005] Developing nursing to transform primary care. Unpublished DH internal paper.).

Personal Medical Services

Personal Medical Services (PMS) are NHS services that may, or may not include a GP as a partner. Examples include GP practices that focus on a specific service provision, such as the homeless, or nurse-run practices (Box 20.10).

Box 20.10 Example of use of PMS to improve primary care services

A practice in Lincolnshire had experienced problems recruiting a GP to fill a long-standing vacancy. This led to pressure on existing staff and appointment which impacted on access targets. The practice established a new system for dealing with requests for GP appointments. This involved each patient being triaged by a nurse practitioner and, where appropriate, being managed by the nurse or nurse practitioner rather than the GP.

The initiative resulted in more appropriate use of GP time, a consistent reduction in same-day appointments (62%) expansion of the nurse practitioner service. The project was funded under the practice's Personal Medical Service Agreement.

Alternative Provider Medical Services (APMS)

These services can be provided by commercial providers, not for profit organisations, third sector providers (voluntary sector, cooperatives), social enterprise organisations and others.

Specialist Personal Medical Services

These services are provided by the NHS to an unregistered population or a population with specific needs but they do not need to include the provision of essential services. Specialist Personal Medical Services are especially perceived as a route through which specific community nursing services are delivered but to date there have been few reported cases of their use (see Box 20.11 for an example).

Box 20.11 Tower Hamlets Homeless project – nurse-led case study of the homeless project Health E1

This innovative project provides a service for people who are homeless or in temporary or hostel accommodation or of no fixed abode. Patients are able to register with Health E1, a nurse-led service. This means that the patient's first point of contact is with a nurse. The nurses have undertaken specialist additional training and are able to look after many health needs that were previously only managed by a GP.

The team at Health E1 includes a nurse practitioner, a clinical nurse specialist in mental health, two clinical nurse specialists in substance misuse, a health care assistant, a receptionist and a practice Manager. Two GPs also provide sessional services to the project.

PCT Medical Services

These are services that are provided directly by a primary care organisation and where all the staff involved in the practice, including the GPs are employed by the PCT.

In addition to developing new contract mechanisms to create an increased market and freedom for service provider, new organisations founded on business principles have been created. These include foundation trusts, social enterprise organisations, polyclinics and community interest companies.

Foundation trusts

NHS foundation trusts are a new type of NHS organisation established as independent public benefit corporations that are free from central government control and from strategic health authority performance management. They act as providers of health care according to core NHS principles – free care, based on need, not ability to pay and are accountable to local people (who are able to become members and governors). In addition they are free to innovate for the benefit of their local community and patients and determine independently what capital investment is needed to improve their services through their ability to retain any financial surpluses that they generate and to borrow in order to support investment in service redesign and expansion.

NHS foundation trusts are embedded in the NHS culture as a fundamental part of the modernisation and reform programme. They reflect the move from a centrally managed service towards one that is managed locally and which is more responsive to patients. In line with the programme of reforms set out in *The NHS Plan*, The Health and Social Care (Community Health and Standards) Act 2003 established NHS foundation trusts as independent public benefit corporations modelled on cooperative and mutual traditions. They exist to provide and develop services for NHS patients according to NHS principles and standards and they are subject to NHS governance and inspection systems. The acquisition of foundation trust status enables the transfer of ownership and accountability from Whitehall to the local community, enabling local foundation trusts to tailor their services to best meet the needs of the local population and thereby tackle health inequalities more effectively.

The purpose of establishing NHS Foundation Trusts is to:

- Devolve more power and responsibility to local level so that hospitals are able to response to the needs of their local population
- To bring about improved access to higher quality services for NHS patients by incentivising innovation and entrepreneurialism
- Devolve accountability to local stakeholders including NHS patients and staff

- Operate governance arrangements that provide local stakeholders and the public with opportunities to influence the stewardship of the organisation and its strategic development
- Support patient choice by increasing the plurality and diversity of providers within the NHS

The first foundation trusts were established in April 2004, and by 2008 there were 96 NHS foundation trusts on the Public Register (www.regulator-nhsft.gov.uk/register_nhsft.php [Monitor 2008]). The creation of NHS foundation trusts has played a key role is sustaining the progress that the NHS has made in recent years in its quest to drive up quality and to engage the public in the governance of its local services. The government is committed to delivering an all foundation trust model for the NHS as soon as possible which includes ambulance and mental health trusts. However, not all NHS trusts are in a position to achieve foundation trust status immediately and may require active preparation and development to reach the standard required for foundation trust status approval.

Social enterprise and third sector providers

Our health, Our Care, Our Say (DH 2006c) introduced the concept of social enterprise models of service delivery in primary and community care and advised that such services can form part of a commissioning strategy and assist local providers to develop responsive services based on direct engagement with patients and members of the public. As already identified, the NHS is developing from an organisation that fitted people around services to one that is working to fit services around people. Indeed *Our Health, Our Care, Our Say* (DH 2006c) advised, as its sixth aim, a desire to encourage different service providers to compete for service provision and in so doing was explicit in its intention to attract more third sector organisation provider agencies. However, the policy paper also acknowledged that there are considerable barriers to entry into the NHS market. To address this issue, the Third Sector Commissioning Task Force was set up and a Social Enterprise Unit was established at the DH in 2005 (DH 2005b). Its role was to coordinate policies relating to third sector participation, aiming to enshrine the government's plan to create synergy between statutory health and social care services, local charities, local groups, voluntary organisations and social enterprises (DH 2008f).

Third sector organisations

This is a collective name for organisations which include charities, local groups, voluntary organisations and social enterprise organisations. Third sector organisations possess expertise in specific areas, and significant insight into the needs of the groups they represent. Social enterprise models offer the opportunity for a sound commercial relationship to be created between public sector commissioners of health and social care services and third sector providers of those services and provide expertise and understanding of the groups they represent.

Social enterprise 'a definition'

The government defines a social enterprise as 'a business with primarily social objectives whose surpluses are principally reinvested for that purpose in the business or in the community, rather than being driven by the need to maximise profit for stakeholders and owners' (DH 2006f). Well know examples of social enterprises include Jamie Oliver's restaurant Fifteen, The *Big Issue* magazine, John Lewis and fair-trade coffee company Café direct. Within the NHS the Expert Patient Programme and the Innovation Academy, which were previously centrally funded development projects, are now established as social enterprise organisations.

The integration of new organisations working with an emphasis on coordinating services across a range of organisations are a key plan of the government's public service reform agenda. The DH Social Enterprise Unit will be working with social enterprises to identify pathfinders that will lead the way in delivering innovative health and social care services.

Social Enterprise Action Plan: Scaling New Heights (DH 2006f) signalled continued government commitment to supporting social enterprise, not just to deliver public services but to help change society for the better. In April 2008 the Social Enterprise Investment Fund programme (SEIF) was launched to encourage social returns and stimulate the delivery of health and social care by social enterprise (DH 2007c). A fund of £1000 million over a four-year period is available to new and existing social enterprises to deliver innovative health and social care services.

Primary care responding to the modernisation agenda

To reflect the key issues identified within the modernisation agenda, of care designed and delivered for maximum benefit for the patient and the community, with a range of contracts and organisations through which services can be provided, the following new models of service have developed.

Treatment centres

NHS reforms also require the implementation of a new range of diagnostic and treatment centres, designed to offer fast, safe, pre-booked day and short-stay surgery and diagnostic procedures in areas that have traditionally had the longest waiting times, such as ophthalmology and orthopaedics. Treatment centres will play an important part in modernising the NHS and delivering a patient-centred health service. Whether they are NHS run or managed by companies in the independent sector, the additional capacity that they provide will be crucial in bringing down waiting times and giving patients more choice about when and where they are treated.

Independent sector treatment sectors (ISTCs)

Independent sector services are delivered by autonomous independent sector providers (independent companies) in accordance with the founding NHS principles of treatment free at the point of delivery and available according to clinical needs, rather than the ability to pay. They provide significant scope to introduce new and innovative ways of delivering health care to NHS patients by adapting traditional NHS models to suit local health care needs. They are managed via service level agreements with the NHS and patients can expect a standard of service that is at least the same as that provided by the NHS. GPs and/or local support services can give patients information about the choices and treatment centres that are available.

Private sector providers

An example of a private sector provider, Virgin Healthcare (VHC) has entered the market and is keen to work in partnership with GP practices to form new primary care health centres, such as those proposed by the Darzi review (DH 2008a,g). The Virgin offer is that GPs will run the practice clinical services and VHC will run the back office support services and health care centres. VHC will lease the properties, take on the VAT burden and the GPs will retain the General Medical Services income element. In this way, VHC will enable GPs to reduce time spent of management issues and provide more time for them to focus on the delivery of clinical health care services for their patients.

Polyclinics – integrated health care centres

Polyclinics, or GP-led health centres have become synonymous with one man – Health Minister, Lord Darzi. In his review of health services in London, (NHS 2007), he advised that he wanted to see a network of polyclinics to replace ageing GP services. His proposals called for 150 GP-led clinics to be set up across registered there.

Lord Darzi has noted that such new service configurations hold the key to creating an integrated and personalised NHS. His vision contains a quest for a range of services traditionally carried out in hospitals, alongside those of general practice, such as minor surgery, dermatology, diabetes care and diagnostic scans, to become available in these community centres. Medical

advances mean that the NHS can provide more and more specialised care, but if that is to be achieved, hospitals need to be freed from the daily grind of dealing with minor ailments. What is more, patients can often find themselves transferred between GPs and hospitals because of a lack of diagnostic testing facilities in the community. The equipping of polyclinics with magnetic resonance imaging (MRI) scanners, blood testing facilities and X-rays should resolve this.

Currently, these 'centres' have yet to be 'described', configured and established. However, they will clearly need to be assessed and evaluated in terms of success to determine whether or not they have delivered against the government's policy promise.

Urgent care provision

Each year millions of patients have short-term illnesses or health problems that are not life-threatening, such as a chest or bladder infection but for which they need quick and convenient treatment. Most people with an urgent care need (referring to care that is needed immediately or within the next day or two) will ring their GP practice for an appointment. Urgent care is provided by a range of service providers which include:

- GP practices
- Out-of-hours GP services
- Pharmacists
- Dentists
- NHS Direct
- Walk-in centres
- Ambulance services
- Local emergency departments

GP practices

The local GP surgery offers a wide range of services, including advice on health problems, physical examinations, diagnosis of symptoms and prescribing medication and other treatments. The doctor will usually be supported by a team of nurses, health visitors and midwives, as well as other specialists, including physiotherapists and occupational therapists. Patients should expect to see a doctor within 48 hours or another professional within 24 hours.

Out-of-hours services

All practices are covered by a local the GP out-of-hours service. The service operates every day, from 18.30 p.m. to 8.00 a.m. and all hours during weekends and bank holidays. Initial contact is made by telephone and this may be followed advice over the phone (62% of cases), a face-to-face consultation (30%) or a home visit (8%). The service also receives calls for the on-call district nursing team and access to community services.

Pharmacists

Pharmacists can offer advice and treatment for many conditions, including ear infections, coughs, colds, diarrhoea and headaches. They are your 'health experts on the high street'; patients do not need an appointment to see them, nor do they need to be registered with a GP. They provide free advice and if appropriate will supply patients with medicines, although referral to a GP may be needed in certain circumstances before medicines can be dispensed. Pharmacy First is an example of a primary care scheme which enables people to receive medical advice and medication from a pharmacist on conditions such as sore throat, diarrhoea, heartburn, back pain and coughs. Patients are able to access the service from their local GP surgery. The private sector has been quick to identify the potential for citing pharmacy services within super-markets and all the major chains (Tesco, Sainsbury's, etc.) now have in-house pharmacies in some cases provided by Boots the Chemist. Nurse prescribers can feature successfully in such developments (DH 2008g).

NHS Direct

NHS Direct is a phone service staffed by nurses and professional advisers, giving confidential health care advice and information 24 hours a day. The service covers what to do if you or a family member feels ill and information on particular health conditions and local health services (such as GPs, dentists and out-of-hours pharmacies or self-help and support organisations. Over two million people access NHS Direct every month. It has also launched the NHS Direct digital TV service which has become one of the largest interactive services in the UK.

Walk-in centres

Walk-in centres are staffed by nurses and GPs who offer easy access for those who need help for a wide range of minor injuries and illnesses. The services complement those provided ordinarily at the local general practice. No appointments are necessary. In major cities privately run commuter centres are sited within or close by to mainline stations to provide services to commuters before and after work.

It is clear that nurses play a central and essential role in designing and implementing the service models outlined above. At the highest level, consultant nurses and advanced nurse practitioners are competent to deliver diagnostic services safely and can, and do become equal partners in general practice and with other organisations. However, for many practitioners the prospect of leaving the NHS may be daunting but there are certainly good reasons for staff branching out on their own. For example, it may provide staff with the opportunity to use their personal talents and skills more effectively or provide a way back into work following early retirement or redundancy.

Leadership

Leadership is all about creating value for customers and citizens and making work worthwhile for staff. It requires courage, resilience and commitment. It is clear that bold leadership from within organisations, and from key individuals is required if we are to meet the growing expectations of patients, and to deliver the challenging reform agenda for modernising the NHS (DH 2008g). Along with most public services, the NHS is part way through a journey of improvement. David Nicholson, a former Chief Executive Officer of the NHS, has described the journey like this (*Guardian* 2006):

'In 2000 the first step was to build capacity in the service, building new hospitals, and recruiting additional staff. The second step was to make the health service more responsive to patients and providers.'

While these reforms have considerably increased patient choice, the language was very technical. Using terms such as contestability, PBC and competition made it sound like the health care was being industrialised, and some felt the public sector values were pushed into the background. This was far from the case, but the government decided that these perceptions should be challenged and confidence restored in the original NHS values. This has being taken forward through the *NHS Next Stage Review*, led by Lord Darzi, (DH 2008a). In his report a new clinical vision of excellence has been unveiled, which when combined with the power of the cherished NHS ethos will deliver a potent and heady recipe for success. In order to realise this vision a new system of leadership will be required to enable the workforce to move forward positively within this backdrop of constant change. In order to do this leadership styles will need to change at a system, organisational and personal level. To support this change the NHS has developed the *NHS Leadership Qualities Framework* (DH 2006b) specifically for the NHS and sets the standard for outstanding leadership in the service. It describes the qualities expected of existing and aspiring leaders both now and in the future. The framework can be used across the NHS to underpin leadership development, for individuals, teams and organisations. The *NHS Leadership Qualities Framework* provides a foundation for:

- Setting the standard for leadership across the NHS at all levels
- Assessing and developing the performance in leadership by individual and organisational assessment
- Integrating leadership across the service, systems and related agencies
- Adapting leadership to suit changing context

The framework describes the key characteristics and attitudes and behaviours which leaders in the NHS should aspire to. The framework has a number of applications which include:

- Personal development
- Board level development
- Leadership profiling for recruitment and selection
- Career mapping
- Succession planning
- Connecting leadership capability
- Performance management

It describes the qualities expected of NHS leaders now and in the future.

It could be suggested that policy development is about leadership. Covey (1989, p. 101) asserts that leadership deals with the top line (What are the things I want to accomplish?) and that management is a bottom line focus (How can I best accomplish certain things?) He continues in this vein offering the insight 'management is efficiency in climbing the ladder of success, leadership determines whether the ladder is leaning against the right wall'.

The role of leadership is to ensure that we are travelling in the right direction. Much time, effort and attention has been paid to leadership development in nursing services. The Leading an Empowered Organisation programme provides one such example and has been delivered to over 40 000 frontline managers and has been evaluated positively (Jones 2005). Certainly, different leadership skills are required at different organisational levels: nursing roles are established within all of these levels, from direct patient contact, ward management to board-based strategic planning. Continuing the focus on leadership development within the profession is therefore central to the success of the NHS reform agenda.

Professional roles and development opportunities

The implications for clinical practitioners will include a range of opportunities to deliver services for patients in alternative ways and to develop their own skills and knowledge. This could extend opportunities for users to access nurse and allied health professional (AHP)-led services (DH 2008g).

The result of the changes in commissioning and contracting over the past three years provides opportunity for the nursing profession to lead on the development and delivery of future services for patients as never before. Decentralisation and devolution of power to frontline clinical staff is a key principle of the modernisation reforms. Changes to structures, contracts, governance and performance are being introduced with the aim of achieving a more responsive, locally accountable service. These changes are complex and costly (both in terms of financial and human investment) and the impact on workforce needs to be measured and understood. At a national level the immediate task will be to increase the number of 'entrepreneurial' nurses to begin to move forward towards implementation and establishment of services using new contract opportunities. The most significant motivator for many nurses adopting new roles, and working in new ways, (many of whom will be based in primary care) is that of securing greater autonomy within which to work, develop and extend their practice (DH 2008g).

Other motivating factors include greater flexibility and increased control for an efficient work–life balance. Traditionally nurses have valued the flexibility of community nursing services and part-time work in GP practices. Some are also attracted to working for themselves in small organisations where they are able to directly make a difference to patient care, but will the number of innovative and entrepreneurial individuals who make this shift be able to demonstrate and apply sufficient leadership skills and abilities to achieve the sweeping, wholesale changes that the government is seeking?

There is also a need for a paradigm shift, from a model of care that focuses on health care maintenance to one which is outcome driven and co-designed and co-delivered with clients and users. The development of Patient and Public Involvement strategies is now a prerequisite which supports the above notion and clearly identifies the service user as an equal partner in their care.

Conclusion

Lord Darzi's final report of the NHS Next Stage Review, *High Quality Care for All*, sets out wide-ranging proposals that place quality of care at the heart of everything the NHS does (DH 2008a). The overall purpose of the review has been to help local patients, staff and the public in making the changes they need and want for their local NHS. Applied to the family of nursing within primary, secondary and tertiary care services, this key policy development acts as a positive lever to strengthen and promote the patient centred philosophy of professional nursing.

Specialist community public health nurses, working in both health visiting and school nursing will be expected to play a pivotal role in child and family health, preventative services and public health. Indeed there will be support for careers and new educational opportunities in health promotion. Practice nurses, district nurses and community nursing teams will have a significant contribution to make in supporting people at home with long-term conditions and helping people to stay healthy. Indeed, the review's ambition 'is to ensure that the NHS delivers high quality care in all aspects – an ambition that is impossible to achieve without high quality nursing' (DH 2008a, p.17).

The vision for the future for nurses, midwives, and health visitors is clearly described by Lord Darzi in his new vision for primary care and community care. His strategy responds to the message contained in this chapter for increasing education investment to support service delivery by investing in new programmes of clinical leadership, innovation and high-quality training and giving primary care clinicians more control over budgets and personnel decisions. Community health services will be transformed to unlock the talents of the 250 000 nurses, health visitors, allied health professionals and other staff who play such a crucial role in providing personal care for children and families, older people and those with complex care needs. This will include adoption of new metrics which will allow community staff to demonstrate quality, and to base their clinical performance on the best available research evidence. Lord Darzi also announced that a new national board, which includes leading community nurses, has been established to implement a Transforming Community Services Programme that will reduce variations in care and health practice and outcomes and promote service excellence.

Clearly, while the above embraces the contribution of all relevant professions there are significant opportunities for nursing throughout the clinical spectrum. In terms of developing the workforce, the Darzi review identified the following core principles to underpin a quality focus for the reformed NHS: patient centred; clinically driven; flexible; valuing people; promoting lifelong learning. These principles align robustly with the central tenets of the nursing profession and can thus be embraced in developing and innovating the services we provide to patients. The tenets and principles outlined in this chapter support Lord Darzi's vision and promote the contribution that nurses can make to the reform agenda:

'Nurses play a vital role in the NHS, they will always be at the heart of shaping patient experience and delivering care'

Lord Darzi (DH 2008a, p. 17)

References

Chambers, R. & Wakley, G. (2005) *Clinical Audit in Primary Care: Demonstrating Quality and Outcomes*. Radcliffe, Oxford.

Covey, S. (1989) *The 7 Habits of Highly Effective People*. Simon and Schuster Ltd., New York.

Department of Health (1989) *Working for Patients*. The Stationery Office, London.

Department of Health (1997) *The New NHS, Modern, Dependable*. The Stationery Office, London.

Department of Health (2000) *The NHS Plan, A Plan for Investment. A Plan for Reform*. The Stationery Office, London.

Department of Health (2004a) *The NHS Improvement Plan*. The Stationery Office, London.

Department of Health (2004b) *Practice Based Commissioning: Engaging Practices in the Commissioning Process*. The Stationery Office, London.

Department of Health (2004c) *Practice Based Commissioning, Practical Implementation*. The Stationery Office, London.

Department of Health (2005a) *Creation of a Patient Led NHS*. The Stationary Office, London.

Department of Health (2005b) *Welcoming Social Enterprise into Health and Social Care: A Resource Pack for Social Enterprise Providers and Commissioners*. The Social Enterprise Action Plan, London.

Department of Health (2006a) *Health Reform in England: Update and Commissioning Framework: Annex – the Commissioning Framework*.

Department of Health (2006b) *NHS Leadership Qualities Framework*.

Department of Health (2006c) *Our Health, Our Care, Our Say: A New Direction for Community Services*. The Stationery Office, London.

Department of Health (2006d) *The Future Regulation of Health and Adult Social Care in England*. The Stationery Office, London.

Department of Health (2006e) *No Excuses. Embrace Partnership Now. Step towards Change! Report of the Third Sector Commissioning Taskforce*. The Stationary Office, London.

Department of Health (2006f) *The Social Enterprise Action Plan: Scaling New Heights Investment Fund – 2007/2008*. The Stationery Office, London. Available at: www.cabinetoffice.gov.uk/third_sector/social_enterprise/action_plan.aspx (accessed 2 December 2008).

Department of Health (2006g) *Commissioning Framework*. The Stationery Office, London.

Department of Health (2007a) *Commissioning a Patient Led NHS*. The Stationery Office, London.

Department of Health (2007b) *World Class Commissioning Competencies*. The Stationery Office, London.

Department of Health (2007c) *The Social Enterprise Investment Fund – 2007/2008*. The Stationery Office, London.

Department of Health (2008a) *High Quality Care for All. NHS Next Stage Review. Final Report*. The Stationery Office, London. Available at: www.dh.gov.uk/en/Healthcare/OurNHSourfuture/index.htm (accessed 2 December 2008).

Department of Health (2008b) *NHS Next Stage Review: The NHS Operating Framework*. The Stationary Office, London.

Department of Health (2008c) *NHS Next Stage Review: Leading Local Change*. The Stationery Office, London.

Department of Health (2008d) *NHS Next Stage Review; Our Vision for Primary and Community Care.* The Stationery Office, London. Available at: www.dh. gov.uk/en/Publicationsandstatistics/Publications/ PublicationsPolicyAndGuidance/DH_085937 (accessed 2 December 2008).

Department of Health (2008e) *NHS Next Stage Review: A High Quality Workforce.* The Stationary Office, London.

Department of Health (2008f) *NHS Next Stage Review: Our Vision for Primary and Community Care.* Gateway reference 10096. The Stationary Office, London.

Department of Health (2008g) *NHS Next Stage Review: Our Vision for Primary and Community Care: What it Means for Nurses, Midwives, Health Visitors and AHPs.* Gateway reference 10096. The Stationary Office, London.

Department of Health (2008h) *World Class Commissioning and the Darzi Review.* Gateway reference 9565. Available at: www.dh.gov.uk/en/Manag ingyourorganisation/Commissioning/Worldclass commissioning/DH_083197 (accessed 2 December 2008).

Department of Health and Social Security (1980) *Inequalities in Health: Report of a Working Group.* Black Report. Department of Health and Social Securit, London.

Grant, J. (2005) *Incentives for Reform in the NHS.* King's Fund, London.

Guardian (2006) *David Nicholson Interviewed by John Carvel.* September 2006.

Improvement Foundation (2008) *Practice Based Commissioning. Commissioning and Procurement Overview.* Available at: www.improvementfoundation. org/resource/dl/29 (accessed 2 December 2008).

Jones, K. (2005) *British Journal of Community Nursing,* **10**, 92–96.

King's Fund (2007) *Practice Based Commissioning from Good Idea to Effective Practice.* King's Fund, London.

Lewis, R. & Dixon, J. (2005) *The Future of Primary Care. Meeting the Challenge of the New NHS Market.* King's Fund, London.

Maxwell, R. (1984) Quality assessment in health. *British Medical Journal,* **299**, 1470–1472.

National Association of Primary Care (2007) *Commissioning Framework for Health and Social Care.* National Association of Primary Care, London.

National Health Service (2007) *Healthcare for London: A Framework for Action: Consulting the Capital.* National Health Service, London.

Parliament (2003) *The Health and Social Care (Community Health and Standards) Act.* London.

Parliament (2007) *The Local Government and Public Involvement in Health Act.* London.

Rowe, A. (2005) *Alternative Models for the Provision of Current Primary Care Trust Managed Community Nursing.* A Paper outlining possible options. Northamptonshire and Rutland Strategic Health Authority, Leicester.

Chapter 21 Inter-Professional Practice Teaching and Learning

Keiron Spires

Introduction

The concept of practice-based learning and teaching is not new, nor is the concept of practice-based teachers. Indeed nursing started as a 'taught in practice' profession, and over time it has evolved into the mix of practice- and classroom-based learning and teaching found today. Over this time there have been different teaching and supervision roles, such as sister tutors, clinical teachers, nurse tutors, lecturer practitioners, practice facilitators, fieldwork teachers and practice educators, and lecturers. All of these roles came about in response to changes in the profession, and have manifested themselves in the way that those wishing to enter the profession have been prepared for their roles.

The need for support while students are in practice has been the subject of much debate over the years, and in particular many have commented on a seeming 'theory–practice' gap (Lathlean 1997). In the community setting, the role of the practice teacher has been very important to ensure that the actual practice of community nursing and health visiting is underpinned by both applied knowledge and tacit experience, although there have been long standing concerns regarding the lack of standards of community practice teachers (Hudson 2000). The National Health Service (NHS) trusts, including primary care trusts (PCTs) have recognised the need to support learners at all levels and have frequently employed staff in various practice teaching roles, or have developed joint appointments with education providers. This process has been haphazard, with varying levels of support offered to learners, and with staff having different preparation for these roles. As is always the case, this is driven by budgetary constraints and staffing levels, as well as by the learning and teaching requirements of the learner, the professional regulator (the Nursing and Midwifery Council [NMC]) and the employer.

Moreover, there has been a move towards the application of work-based learning and work-based assessments (Flanagan *et al.* 2000), as well as a general recognition of the need to provide a workplace environment consistent with the philosophy of adult and lifelong nursing. This in turn has increased the need for staff based in practice to develop their competencies and capabilities to become proficient to support the needs of a wide range of learners. The adoption of more open ways of learning has led to a need for new strategies for facilitating and assessing within the practice environment. Staff supporting students in practice settings, need to have both practice expertise and educational knowledge. This will allow them to work in partnership with colleagues in higher education institutions (HEI) and with clinical colleagues, providing a seamless and coherent framework of practice based learning and teaching. Those in new practice education roles, both in acute and community settings, will have the ability to influence curriculum and course development, as well as offering specialist advice and support to colleagues involved in supporting students and more importantly will be integral to assessing and assuring that learners are fit to practise.

The position of those supporting students in all areas of practice was formalised by the NMC in 2006 when it published *Standards to Support Learning and Assessment in Practice*. This publication set out the mandatory requirements for all types of students wishing to register or record their teaching and practice learning qualifications with the NMC. The NMC's new policy framework for learning, teaching and assessment replaced all other existing published professional standards for learning and assessment in practice. These standards affect all nurses and midwives who work with students, and in turn influence all practice areas that have students working within them.

This chapter presents the NMC's standards for learning, teaching and assessment in practice, and discusses their application to contemporary community health care nursing (and specialist community public health nursing). The chapter then considers a range of theoretical perspectives that underpin practice learning, teaching and assessment and provides examples of their practical application.[1]

NMC standards to support learning and assessment in practice

In 2006, the NMC devised a single developmental framework to support learning and teaching in practice. The framework sets out what knowledge and skills nurses and midwives need to apply when supporting students undertaking NMC approved programmes leading to registration or a recordable qualification. Outcomes are identified for each level of responsibility so that there is clear accountability for the decisions made that lead to entry to the register. The framework sets out four stages of development and responsibility. It is possible to enter and exit the framework at any level with credit being awarded for prior learning in a previous stage.

- Stage 1 covers all registrants. All registrants have a duty to facilitate students of nursing and midwifery as set out in the code of professional conduct (NMC 2008).
- Stage 2 identifies the standards for mentors. Mentor qualifications are recorded on local registers held by placement providers.

- Stage 3 identifies the standards for practice teachers for nursing or specialist community public health nurses. These qualifications are also held on local registers.
- Stage 4 identifies the standard for a teacher of nurses, midwives or specialist community public health nurses. This qualification may be recorded on the NMC register.

There is a clear expectation that support for learning and teaching will be given based on five principles:

(1) Those making judgements about a student must be on the same part of the register as that which the student is intending to enter
(2) They must have developed their own knowledge, skills and competency beyond that of registration by continuing professional development
(3) They should hold professional qualifications equal to or at a higher level than the students they are supporting and assessing
(4) They should have been prepared for their role to support and assess learning and met the appropriate NMC defined outcomes
(5) Those intending to record their teaching qualifications must have completed an NMC-approved teacher preparation programme within an approved institution (e.g. a university)

The framework contains eight domains, each of which relates to the four stages of development outlined above. Each has outcomes set out under the following domains:

Establishing effective working relationships: 'Demonstrating effective relationship building skills, sufficient to support learning as part of a wider interprofessional team, for a range of students in both practice and academic environments' (NMC 2006, p. 48).

Facilitation of learning: 'Facilitate learning for a range of students, within a particular area of

---

[1] The latter sections of this chapter have been adapted from Anne Robotham (2005) Assessment of competence to practise and the new NMC teaching standards. In: *Community Health Care Nursing*, 3rd edition. (eds D. Sines, F. Appleby & M. Frost). Blackwell Science, Oxford.

practice where appropriate, encouraging self-management of learning opportunities and providing support to maximise individual potential' (NMC 2006, p. 49).

Assessment and accountability: 'Assess learning in order to make judgements related to the NMC standards of proficiency for entry to the register or for recording a qualification at a level above initial registration' (NMC 2006, p. 50).

Evaluation of learning: 'Determine strategies for evaluating learning in practice and academic settings to ensure that the NMC standards of proficiency for entry to the register or for recording a qualification at a level above initial registration' (NMC 2006, p. 52).

Creating an environment for learning: 'Create an environment for learning, where practice is valued and developed, that provides appropriate professional and interprofessional learning opportunities and support for learning to maximise achievement for individuals' (NMC 2006, p. 53).

Context of practice: 'Support learning within a context of practice that reflects health care and educational polices, managing change to ensure that particular professional needs are met within a learning environment that also supports practice development' (NMC 2006, p. 54).

Evidence-based practice: 'Apply evidence-based practice to their own work and contribute to the further development of such a knowledge and practice evidence base' (NMC 2006, p. 55).

Leadership: 'Demonstrate leadership skills for education within practice and academic settings' (NMC 2006, p. 56).

These outcomes are set out in detail in *Standards to Support Learning and Assessment in Practice* (NMC 2006), and it these standards that inform the design, delivery and outcomes assessment of mentorship and teaching courses and study days provided by approved institutions. The standards are updated regularly by the NMC and published in its 'Registrar Circular Letters', which provide a valuable reference tool for students, educators, commissioners and employers.

Putting the standards into practice

It is important to recognise that these standards and expectations apply to all nurses and midwives commencing at the point at which they register their initial qualification. The NMC regards the framework as a natural part of continuous professional development and as such creates an expectation that nurses and midwives will undergo development to enable them to become mentors, 'sign off' mentors, practice teachers and teachers depending on their role and the type of students they are supporting.

The NMC requires the nursing and midwifery professions to provide a regular supply of appropriately educated and supported mentors and practice teachers who are capable of providing support and guidance to learners, assisting them to gain new skills or applying new knowledge to improve their practice and the quality of patient care. Mentors and practice teachers should also be competent and able to offer reassurance and facilitate learning and professional growth. They manage the students' learning in order to protect the public by observing the students' practice and assessing the student's level of proficiency in the acquisition of new knowledge, skills and values to ensure that NMC-defined outcomes and competencies are met. Mentors provide a similar standard of support to pre-registration nursing and midwifery students to initial registration. For midwifery students support is provided by 'sign off' mentors. For students studying as specialist community public health nurses (SCPHN) and community health care nurses practice learning support is provided by practice teachers. These roles are both rewarding and challenging and demand a significant level of commitment and motivation to practice learning and its contingent responsibilities of facilitating and providing effective learning, teaching and assessment in practice. Their workload should be adjusted to reflect this.

All students are required to evidence the outcomes of their learning through possession of an 'ongoing achievement record' (or a variation of a student passport), including comments from mentors, 'sign off' mentors and practice teachers. The 'record' is designed to follow students from placement to placement enabling judgements to be made about their progress on the basis of continuity. Those involved in making decisions about students' performance must record their judgements clearly, supported by evidence of performance, informed by an assessment of the student's application of skills and knowledge in practice and the demonstration of appropriate values.

The NMC framework has been designed so that each level of practice learning support can, in turn provide mentorship support to those practice 'learning/teaching' staff who have achieved NMC competence at the level below their own standard of skill acquisition. In this way, for example, mentors should seek support from 'sign off' mentors when they are working with students who are not performing at the expected level. In the same way employers (e.g. PCTs) should consider appointing a nurse with a formal NMC recorded 'teacher' qualification to provide support for their 'practice teachers' to support them in their work with community health care nursing or SCPHN students, or alternatively make formal arrangements with an approved HEI for an approved 'teacher' to provide 'long-arm' support within the trust.

The NMC needs to be assured that all students have been assessed and 'signed off' as capable of safe and effective practice at the end of their programme. This involves reviewing and 'validating' the student's passport as well as working closely with the student during their last summative placement. The NMC have recognised that this requires additional 'mentorship' skills, and has introduced a higher standard of mentorship to be undertaken by appropriately prepared 'sign off' mentors for pre-registration nurses and midwives, and by practice teachers for community health care nursing and SCPHN students.

The design of suitable educational programmes is the responsibility of teachers, who will work in tandem with clinical colleagues to ensure that programmes are fit for purpose. In the past the role of teacher has been seen as regarded specifically as a university-based lecturer; however, this is changing rapidly with an increasing number of teachers qualifying as

NMC-recorded 'teachers' working in the practice setting. These roles are most commonly associated with the support of pre-registration students and are found mainly in the acute trusts (although some PCTs are also employing practice-based teaching staff). These staff are often practice educators or practice facilitators and should not be confused with the practice/fieldwork teachers working in community settings. Those nurses working as joint appointees as lecturer practitioners are also likely to have the NMC-approved teaching qualification.

The role of practice education and assessment crosses a range of practice areas too. For example, pre-registration students undertaking community placements can be mentored by community nurses who hold a mentor, sign-off mentor or practice teacher qualification providing they have the same initial registration as that which the student is studying for. However, the NMC requires that a registered nurse must sign off a nursing student, and a registered midwife must sign off a midwifery student. Although this might appear complex, the NMC framework is flexible in application to a range of settings and student groups. However, the framework is designed to ensure that students, while in the practice area, are adequately supported, supervised and assessed by appropriately qualified nurses and midwives who have attained specific learning, teaching and assessment standards prescribed by the council. The framework also shifts some of the responsibility and accountability for student learning to the practice area, which is right and proper, considering the time spent in practice and its importance to the overall preparation of students and their requirement to evidence both fitness for practice and proficiency in care delivery.

Mentorship in community practice

Changes in the NHS towards a more primary-care-led service require that all students understand the partnerships between primary, secondary and specialist services. Students need to appreciate that the majority of admissions to hospital start and finish in the community setting. Cook (cited in Young & Curzio 2007) suggested that the number of district nurses was falling, in contrast with the overall growth in the number of nurses working in the community, which reflected the growth in community nursing in new and different ways. This means that community placement providers have to find suitable placements for pre-registration nursing, post-registration nursing and students from other related disciplines. This in turn requires placement providers to have an adequate supply of appropriately qualified and prepared practice teachers and mentors in place to support these students.

Historically, mentoring has been seen as an informal process between a mentor and his or her protégé. Now it is seen to encapsulate a hierarchy of roles, those of teacher, counsellor, negotiator, supervisor, entertainer and coach (Gray 1994). This represents a change to a role focused more on structure and process. Davies *et al.* (1994) writing from a nursing perspective regarded a mentor to possess good communication skills, with a motivation to teach and support students able to demonstrate enthusiasm, friendliness, patience, a sense of humour, and professionalism, while having realistic expectations and an ability to give suitable feedback to the student.

Community nurses feel that the standard of mentor required to support specialist community health care nurses and SCPHNs is different because of the knowledge and skills required to support students in a wide range of complex and demanding placements (Young & Curzio 2007). It is clear then, that mentors, sign-off mentors and practice teachers need to be well prepared for their roles, and that students entering these placements must also be prepared to take advantage of a range of learning opportunities within a safe practice environment.

Although the NMC has stated that all registrants should be mentors once preceptorship has ended there is no compulsion to do so, or to continue to develop towards becoming a practice teacher. Nursing and midwifery still relies on volunteers to come forward for mentorship training. Mentoring is something special. It involves a close one-to-one working relationship and involves far more than just the transfer of knowledge and skills by acting as a role model. Demands are placed on mentors and practice teachers and they need to be prepared for this. Many of the issues seen in establishing the mentor/practice teacher workface are not new. Phillips-Jones in 1989, for example highlighted the commonest problems in mentoring programmes as being:

- The assumption that mentoring is obvious and anyone can do it
- Insufficient numbers of qualified mentors
- Inadequately prepared participants

Preparation of practice teachers

The preparation of mentors and 'sign-off' mentors is the same for community placement providers as it is for those providing acute and hospital based placements. What sets the community placement providers apart is the need to have staff qualified to undertake the community practice teacher role. The NMC has set out principles for the preparation of community practice teachers, which are utilised by HEIs to design and implement community practice teaching courses. Since most professions have similar requirements it is likely that courses will be offered as interprofessional learning and teaching programmes – something that is encouraged by professional bodies.

Programmes to prepare community practice teachers should be offered at a minimum of level H (Honours level BA/BSc), although most seem to be at M (master's) level in recognition of the experience and the continuing professional development (CPD) needs of those undertaking these courses. The course must include 30 days protected teaching time – to include both academic and practice settings, and include relevant work-based learning.

Preparation should build on the NMC standards and requirements for mentors and 'sign-off' mentors and so by default a community practice teacher is also qualified to function in these roles. Any courses offered by HEIs should be completed within six months, and should provide the foundation for undertaking an NMC-approved teacher preparation programme.

Many community practice teaching courses are integrated within a teacher training programme so that students are able to 'step off' at the practice teacher level, or continue ('step back in') to complete a formal teacher qualification.

Nurses wishing to become community practice teachers should be able to use Assessment of Prior (Experiential) Learning (AP(E)L) to offset attendance on a course. Attendance at previous mentor courses should attract AP(E)L accreditation. Most universities allow students to transfer an H level mentor course into an M level practice teacher/teacher programme. Once qualified as a community practice teacher and recorded as such with their PCT, nurses are required by the NMC to update and maintain their knowledge and skills. Annual CPD updating should be undertaken by all mentors and community practice teachers. Details of all such CPD updating should be recorded on the employer's (PCT's) live mentorship database/register.

Community placement providers should use evidence of annual updating as part of the triennial review of all their staff. As well as performing the roles and responsibilities of mentor/'sign-off' mentor for pre-registration students, they also have a particular role with SCPHN/community health care nursing students. They should only support one SCPHN student at a time, and are responsible and accountable for making the final sign-off in practice confirming that a student has successfully completed all practice requirements for a SCPHN qualification. In summary, the criteria for recognition as a community practice teacher are:

- They will have previously been qualified to fulfil the role of a mentor and will have progressed to undertake further preparation to meet the NMC standards
- They must be registered on the same part or sub-part of the register as the students they are assessing
- They should have developed their own skills and knowledge beyond that of initial registration and possess a specialist practice qualification

- They should have the capability to design, deliver and assess programmes of learning in practice settings, supporting a range of students
- They should be able to support learning in an inter-professional setting
- They should be able to make judgements about the competence (or deficiencies) of students and be accountable to the NMC for such decisions (keeping records/evidence that enable them to do this)
- They should provide leadership to all those involved in supporting learning and assessment in practice

Registrants who undertook their educational programmes to prepare them to become community practice teachers before the new NMC regulations came into force (and after 2002) can map their experience and qualifications against the 2006 NMC standards. If the PCT endorses the mentor of community practice teacher's ability to practise their teaching, learning and assessment skills proficiently then their name can be added to its 'live register' of updated 'mentors and teachers'.

Learning, teaching and assessment in practice

The competencies and skills needed to support learning teaching and assessment in practice have been outlined above. What follows is an overview of the knowledge required to be an effective mentor or community practice teacher. The theoretical underpinning for learning, teaching and assessment in practice is based on these four themes:

- Knowledge in practice
- Action in practice
- Competence
- Proficiency

Knowledge in practice
In an analysis of the conceptual and syntactical structure of nursing knowledge (Carper 1978) identified four patterns of knowing:

(1) Empirics, the science of nursing
(2) Aesthetics, the art of nursing

(3) The component of a personal knowledge in nursing

(4) Ethics, the component of moral knowledge in nursing

Carper (1978) argues for empathy as an important mode in the pattern of aesthetic knowing and the more skilled a nurse becomes in the perception and empathy in the lives of others, the more knowledge and understanding is gained. In particular, the argument is carried into the recognition that what is done in part must be related to the whole. In other words, decision-making in relation to what is appropriate and effective for the client must be chosen and guided to suit their circumstances. This requires the health care practitioner to interpret the felt experience of others and identify patterns and rhythms of lived life, in order to create a repertoire of choices for the client, based on the aesthetic. Personal knowledge, Carper argues, is about knowing self and is based on the interpersonal transactions between professional and client. Carper argues for reciprocity in client – professional relationships, and sees this as personal knowing which extends not only to other people but also to relations with oneself.

Knowledge in the moral component is what Carper (1978) considers to be the ethical dimension of modern health care. In community health care nursing, where the basis of intervention by practitioners is concerned with education, empowerment and partnership, difficulties arise where health care is impeded by deprivation, both psychosocial and economic-educative. Community nurses and SCPHNs may plan health care pathways with clients in the full knowledge of the socio-economic inequity which may temper the choices available. In this sense the primary care practitioner is forced down a moral pathway which, although embodying the concept of equality of service provision to people and the respect for human life, nevertheless is aware of the dilemmas involved in offering support in a range of circumstances, some of which may give cause to be of poorer quality.

In using patterns of knowing, Carper considers that each 'pattern of knowing' must be conceived as necessary for achieving mastery in the nursing discipline. However, she also comments that none alone should be considered sufficient, nor are they mutually exclusive. Each of these separate but interrelated and independent fundamental patterns of knowing should be taught and understood according to its distinctive logic.

Schön (1983) proposes that the professions are bound by a form of professional knowledge that fails to take into account the indeterminacy of practice. Schön argues that the dominant epistemology (a branch of science which deals with the nature and validity of knowledge) of practice is technical rationality which relies on the assumption that empirical science (based on positive facts and observable phenomena) is the only source of objective knowledge about the world. Schön suggests that there is an area in professional practice where practitioners can make use of research-based theory and technique, but equally there are other areas where there are uncertainties and value conflicts that are incapable of technical solution. Benner (1984) also makes the point that not all knowledge embedded in expertise can be captured in theoretical propositions, or in analytical strategies that depend on identifying all the elements that go into a clinical decision.

Action in practice

An assumption can be made that action in practice is based on the use of knowledge. However, such is the nature of practice that situational factors may cause the practitioner to perform in a manner which may, seemingly, be divorced from a knowledge base. Schutz (1972) posited an idea of meaningful social action that he said was an adequate description of professional practice. Jarvis (1992) carried this idea further by suggesting that one had to understand action, and especially the sort of action that is not 'hands-on', such as community health care practice, in order to realise a theory of professional practice. Jarvis (1992) considered action to be dependent on levels of conscious planning, conscious monitoring and conscious retrospection (reflection). Jarvis advises that professional practice consists of several categories of action occurring at any one time, all of which may have varying levels of conscious planning, monitoring and retrospection. This is because experimental action is dependent on the practitioner modifying practice, using all his or her theoretical knowledge and intuitive experience in the context of the situation (transferable skills). Experimental action is exciting and creative but so also is repetitive action when carried out with high conscious levels of monitoring, planning and retrospection. In many ways repetitive action can be considered as 'doing the job', but doing a 'good' job. It is underpinned with theory, but this is tempered to meet the demands of the situation. Advising a mother, for example how to cope with demanding toddler behaviour, requires SCPHNs to adapt the advice given to the contextual situation. It is important that in the conscious practitioner thinking processes, high levels of planning, monitoring and reflection are achieved. The practice teacher plays a significant part in assisting the 'novice' practitioner to challenge prior assumptions and to adapt her practice to meet the specific needs of the client and the presenting situation.

Competence

In the nursing profession, Benner (1984) has applied the Dreyfus model of skill acquisition by chess players and airline pilots, to show how a student passes through five levels of proficiency: novice, advanced beginner, competent, proficient and expert. She argued that the different levels reflect changes in three general aspects of skilled performance. One is a movement from reliance on abstract principles to the use of past concrete experience as paradigms. The second is a change in the learner's perception of the demand situation, in which the situation is seen less and less as a compilation of equally relevant bits, and more and more as a complete whole in which only certain parts are relevant. The third is a passage from detached observer to involved performer engaged in the situation. The methodology used was a consensus approach using expert nurses to identify situations and the interpretative strategy was based on Heideggerian (1962) phenomenology

which fits the description of constant comparative method (Glaser & Strauss 1967), to identify meanings and content. Eraut (1994) applauds Benner's use of the Dreyfus model of skill acquisition but challenges the assumption that how clinical decisions are made by experts is also how clinical decisions ought to be made.

Cameron-Jones (1988) uses Medley's (1984) work in attempting to determine competency in the teaching profession. Medley used four terms as basic clarification – competency, competence, performance and effectiveness. He defined competency as a single knowledge, skill or professional value that a teacher might be said to possess: competence as the repertoire of competencies that a teacher possesses and which is regarded as sufficient in principle for the teacher to practise safely; performance as what the teacher does on the job; and effectiveness as the effect the teacher's performance has on the learners. Medley's work is important in that it begins to worry at what a competent profession might show, and it is interesting that Medley considered the last characteristic – that of effectiveness – as the bottom line. Cameron-Jones then raised the question of whether the most competent professional is the one with the greater collection of competencies or the one who is most effective in terms of performance outcomes.

The two approaches outlined above in the teaching and nursing professions illustrate early approaches and attempts to articulate the concept of competency. Cameron-Jones (1988) comments that Medley's work was the result of a paper written at a time when there was a crisis of confidence among the public at large as to education's productivity and its claim to the status of professionalism. Benner's work was a remarkable piece of research using a methodology that had little to do with the nursing profession but demonstrated the value of critical incident analysis to articulate clinical excellence in nursing. The approaches differ considerably because Medley looked at the teacher and the abilities possessed whereas Benner was more concerned about the experience-in-context of the nurse. Interestingly, neither author looked to the outcome as an expression of competence.

The problem with some of Medley's early thinking is that if a practitioner possesses a competency or competencies, then it is likely that these will be task-based or behaviourist. Gonczi (1994, p. 28) points out that the possession of individual competencies can be seen as

'positivist, reductionist, ignores underlying attributes, ignores group processes and their effect on performance, is conservative, atheoretical, ignores the complexity of performance in the real world and ignores the role of professional judgement in intelligent performance.'

Gonczi suggests that this model of competence was originally adopted by training programmes with specified competency standards based on behaviours or tasks. Indeed the NVQ system developed by Jessup (1991), appears to have the first two levels following a behaviourist/task based pattern. Gonczi puts together the complex combinations of attributes such as knowledge, attitudes, values and skills, and sees the practitioner using them within a specific situation, using professional judgement. He argues that these show that competence is relational, bringing together disparate things, such as the abilities (attributes) of individuals, the appropriate professional situation and the need for intelligent performance.

Returning to Medley's (1984) suggestions of four basics of competence, there arises an interesting question about a guarantee of competence rather than a guarantee of effectiveness or a guarantee of performance. Medley points out that professionals are not expected to guarantee results, rather they offer the best effort to use competence in the best interests of clients/patients. He, therefore, sees effectiveness and performance as being lesser than competencies (attributes). Miller *et al.* (1988) suggested two senses in which competence can be defined: competence equating to performance, referring descriptively to an activity, and competence as a quality or state of being of an individual. Girot (1993) linked the suggestion of a state of being with Runciman's (1990) work which also considered competence as a state of being,

but Runciman struggled with the difficulty in observing this 'state of being' and decided that it would be seen as competent performance. Thus competence and performance united in this way returns the thinking to Medley's (1984) basic characteristics of competence – competency, competence, performance and effectiveness.

McMullan *et al.* (2003) in examining the literature on assessing competence looked at three approaches, behavioural, generic and holistic, and the assessment of these. The behavioural approach suggested that simple, objective levels of competence are distinguishable. Successful performance demonstrates underlying knowledge and understanding, but competencies are fragmented and non-transferable and ignore the context. In the generic approach assessment incorporates underlying knowledge, understanding and skills but there is the assumption that competencies are transferable and then assessment becomes difficult. In the holistic approach this incorporates context, ethics, and the need for reflective practice and is therefore difficult to assess.

Proficiency

In its various publications the NMC (2002, 2003, 2004, 2006) has concentrated on proposals for standards using principles, domains and competencies. The discussion above has highlighted the difficulty writers had in articulating competence as a measurable phenomenon. In the light of the statement above it is therefore necessary to consider whether the mechanisms for assessing proficiency differ from assessing competence. Returning to Benner's (1984) original work, she made some interesting statements in her descriptor of proficient (p. 27) as related to nurses in practice in the acute field:

'Characteristically, the proficient performer perceives situations as wholes rather than in terms of aspects, and performance is guided by maxims. Perception is a key word here. The perspective is not thought out but presents itself based upon experience and recent events. Proficient nurses understand the situation as a whole because they perceive its meaning in terms of long-term goals.'

Benner makes useful recommendations on teaching a proficient performer by suggesting teaching by case studies and that proficiency is enhanced if the student is required to cite experience and exemplars for perspective. Eraut (1994) approves Benner's use of the Dreyfus model and recognises that proficiency takes quite a different approach to the job: normal behaviour is not just routinised but semi-automatic; situations are apprehended more deeply and the abnormal is quickly spotted and given attention. Thus progress beyond competence depends on a more holistic approach to situational understanding. Girot (1993) considers that in assessing competence a holistic approach is likely to be more valid than an individual fragmented competencies approach, and thus this would appear to be closer to the descriptor of a proficient performer: 'perceives situations as wholes rather than in terms of aspects'.

It would seem, therefore, that if it is possible to gain an accurate assessment of practitioner proficiency, a method of assessing reflection must be part of the process. In developing a theory of reflection and teacher education Goodman (1984) was concerned that the meaning of the term reflection is clarified and his argument focuses on the need to recognise that reflection is not just a quiet rumination. If reflection is to be a worthwhile goal within teacher education then our notion of it must be comprehensive. First, reflection suggests a need to focus on the substantive, rather than utilitarian concerns. Second, a theory of reflection must be legitimate and integrate both intuitive and rational thinking. Finally, certain underlying attitudes are necessary in order to be truly reflective.

Dewey (1933) referred to routine thought, which is a process of thinking, and may lead to problem solving, but is in direct opposition to that of reflection. Routine thought is about how we confront, manage and deal with immediate situations, it does not allow time to reflect because it lacks the patience necessary to work through one's doubts and perplexity. Goodman (1984) identifies rational thought, which is clearly distinguishable from routine thought, and which some observers equate to reflection.

However, Goodman argues that rational thought does not encompass intuitive thought, which is associated with the spark of creative ideas, insight and empathy. He thus posits reflective thinking as occurring with the integration of rational and intuitive thought processes. Drawing again on Dewey (1933), Goodman identifies three attitudes as prerequisites for reflective teaching:

- *Open-mindedness* – an active desire to listen to more sides than one
- *Responsibility* – there must be a desire to synthesise ideas, to make sense out of nonsense and to apply information in an aspired direction. This attitude fosters consideration of the consequences and implications beyond questions of immediate utility
- *Wholeheartedness* – the internal strength necessary for genuine reflection and the ability to work through fears and insecurities

Goodman's (1984) levels of reflection are:

- 1st level – *reflection to reach given objectives:* criteria for reflection are limited to technocratic issues of efficiency, effectiveness and accountability
- 2nd level – *reflection on the relationship between principles and practice:* there is an assessment of the implications and consequences of actions and beliefs as well as the underlying rationale for practice
- 3rd level – *reflection that besides the above incorporates ethical and political concerns:* issues of justice and emancipation enter deliberations over the value of professional goals and practice and the practitioner makes links between the setting of everyday practice and broader social structure and forces

Tools for assessment of proficiency in practice

Reflective journal analysis

Assessors may use a student's reflective journal to gain some insight into the maturing processes of reflection shown by the student when gaining practice experience. Johns (1994) suggested the following guidelines for keeping a reflective journal:

(1) Use an A4 notebook.
(2) Split each page.
(3) Write up diary events on left side.
(4) Use right hand side for further reflection.
(5) Write up experience the same day if possible.
(6) Use actual dialogue wherever possible to capture the situation.
(7) Make a habit of writing up at least one experience per day.
(8) Balance problematic experiences with a satisfying experience.
(9) Challenge yourself at least once a day about something that you normally do without thought/take for granted – ask yourself – 'Why did I do that?' (i.e. make the normal problematic).
(10) Always endeavour to be open and honest with yourself – find the 'authentic you' to do the writing.

The community practice teacher plays an important part in unpacking the reflective journal jointly with the student. Language and metaphor use in the journal requires exploration and checking back with student conceptualisation of the experience articulated. Initially, of course, this process is a shared process during the period of shadowing of the community practice teacher by the student. However, later, when the student is practising alone and articulating the content of the practice intervention, it is essential to explore the meaning of language and metaphor used. This entire process should be normalised to the extent that it becomes totally integrated into the student's subsequent qualified practice. Good community health care nursing practice should always be managed in such a way that the practitioner deliberately allows time for reflection.

Portfolio
The second type of tool to enable the assessment of practice proficiency is a portfolio which, in nurse education, is used for both professional and personal development. In the UK, portfolios have been part of nursing for many years, particularly as an assessment strategy to integrate theory and practice. Students acquire knowledge and skills, such as problem-solving and critical thinking from academics, however, they acquire and develop equally important practical skills and experiences from clinicians.

The content of a portfolio should contain carefully selected examples of the achievements of learning outcomes. The selection depends on the proficiency and creativity level of the student, applicability of past experiences, depth of self-reflection and purpose of the portfolio. Reflective processes have to be used, in the sense that the student needs to reflect on how the item selected will demonstrate to the assessor theory–practice integration and development. For example, a student may have been asked to prepare a discussion session for a new group. The session plan could be used subsequently for the portfolio with an attached rationale for the content items selected for the session, as well as evidence of the effectiveness of the project. Box 21.1 provides a model for the provision of structured supervision.

Too much information in a portfolio creates an unwieldy collection of documents with possibly too fine an analysis of learning; too little information is a sterile exercise. It is important that a portfolio is not just a collection of items in a folder, but that it shows how reflection on these items by the student demonstrates learning (McMullan *et al.* 2003). In reality, it is difficult to grade the contents of a portfolio as a sole example of practice grading, but the portfolio and the reflective journal can be part of the total practice grading process.

Practice assessment documentation
Discussion in the preceding sections on competence and proficiency suggests that in both instances there is an indeterminacy of true definition and possible assessment. Nevertheless it is possible to build on previous approaches to practice assessment. In time, and with sufficient data an interpretive strategy based on Heideggerian (1962) phenomenology which fits the description of constant comparative method

---

Box 21.1   A model of structured reflection (Carper 1978; Johns 1994)

(1) *Description of the experience*
   - Phenomenon – describe the here and now experience
   - Causal – what essential factors contributed to the experience
   - Context – what/who are the significant background actors to the experience
   - Clarifying – what are the key processes (for reflection) in this experience

(2) *Reflection*
   - What was I trying to achieve?
   - Why did I intervene as I did?
   - What are the consequences of my action for:
     — Myself
     — The client/family
     — The people I work with?
   - How did I feel about this experience when it was happening?
   - How did the client feel about it?
   - How do I know how the client felt about it?

(3) *Influencing factors*
   - What internal factors influenced my decision-making?
   - What external factors influenced my decision-making?
   - What sources of knowledge did/should have influence my decision-making?

(4) *Could I have dealt better with the situation?*
   - What other choices did I have?
   - What would be the consequences of those choices?

(5) *Learning*
   - How do I now feel about this experience?
   - How have I made sense of this experience in the light of past experience and future practices?
   - How has this experience changed my ways of knowing?
     — Empirics
     — Aesthetics
     — Ethics
     — Personal

---

by Glaser & Strauss (Glaser 1978; Glaser & Strauss 1967), it can be proved that practice can be effectively assessed. This was shown to be possible by Robotham (2001).

Unpublished work by Robotham (1994) suggested that professional practitioners work with two general capabilities – a technical capability and a knowledge-based capability. A technical capability consists of the personal professional resources, skills and strategies used by a practitioner, e.g. listening skills, good articulation, true empathy, ability to challenge, assertiveness and so forth. Knowledge capability is the cognition skill to use valid knowledge to underpin practice, conceptualise links between complexities of practice and a multiplicity of theories, and see the boundaries between professionalism and the broader social structure. Assessment of fieldwork practice can become an emotionally charged activity where there is resistance and challenge in terms of subjectivity or objectivity.

The position of the community practice teacher as assessor becomes fraught with difficulties when set within the above contexts. In gaining his or her own experience, a community practice teacher will have developed a personal set of skills that will work most effectively in the situations of giving and receiving, negotiating and compromising. Indeed it may take several years to become experienced and effective, and yet the community practice teacher assessor is making a judgement on the abilities of a student to show effectiveness in the early days of practice.

Subjectivity, in the light of the above, would seem to be about the values and beliefs of the assessor and could lead to prejudging of issues within the intervention process between student and client which do not fit the community practice teacher's expectations of how the intervention should be performed. Jarvis & Gibson (1985) make the important observation that the emotion of subjectivity is considerably reduced where it is made very clear that it is the practice that is being commented on, and not the practitioner as an individual. Nevertheless, Jarvis & Gibson also show how (Rowntree 1992) use of the term descriptive assessment, which is objective assessment, viz. the student implemented an interaction with the client in a specific way, must be coupled with a judgement on the effectiveness of the intervention. This intervention may not have been carried out in a way that the community practice teacher might have used, but if the outcome was effective then the subjectivity becomes softened towards objectivity bound up in the outcome observed.

The practice assessment document should be designed in order to allow the student to provide evidence to satisfy the learning outcomes of major aspects of their fieldwork experience. At least two examples should be given for each outcome.

Conclusion

It can be seen that there is a long history of support for learning and teaching in community practice areas, and that community placement providers have always tried to provide proficient staff to carry out this role. However, some employers have not always provided a systematic programme of support or preparation for their community practice teachers. The NMC framework is very clear about what is required in terms of student support, and also specifies what preparation staff require in order to provide this support. Crucially the NMC has made it clear that supporting students is the function of all registered nurses and midwives, and that taking on mentorship and higher roles should be seen as part of CPD. The NMC framework sets out the particular requirements for community placement providers to ensure that they possess an adequate number of appropriately qualified community practice teachers in order to support, mentor and sign-off community and specialist nursing students. The NMC recognises the increasing complexity of community placements (sponsored by a variety of providers) and the variety of students passing through them.

Community practice teachers and mentors may need to act as mentors and 'sign-off' mentors for pre-registration students as well as community and specialist students, and may also be required to offer support to students from other disciplines. Nurses and midwives undertaking these roles need sound preparation and the time and space to develop the necessary knowledge and skills. With the shift in responsibility and accountability they need to be aware of their professional role as well as their educational role, and be prepared to account for their decisions. They should be involved in the design of practice assessment so that they are fully engaged in the whole process from start to finish. This in turn requires that they have the underpinning understanding of assessment of competency and proficiency in practice.

Well-prepared students and well-prepared mentors and community practice teachers will combine to create fulfilling and worthwhile practice experiences, and will ensure that those seeking registration on whichever part of the register are fit to practise.

References

Benner, P. (1984) *From Novice to Expert. Excellence and Power in Clinical Nursing Practice*. Addison-Wesley, California.

Cameron-Jones, M. (1988) Looking for quality and competence in teaching. In: *Professional Competence and Quality Assurance in the Caring Professions* (ed. R. Ellis). Chapman and Hall, London.

Carper, B. (1978) Fundamental ways of knowing in nursing. *Advances in Nursing Science*, **11**, 13–23.

Davies, B., Neary, M. & Phillips, R. (1994) *The Practitioner Teacher: A Study in the Introduction of Mentors in the Pre-Registration Nurse Education Programme in Wales.* Welsh Office.

Dewey, J. (1933) How we think. In: *Reflective Practice in Nursing: The Growth of the Professional Practitioner* (1994) (eds A. Palmer, S. Burns & C. Bulman). Blackwell Science, Oxford.

Eraut, M. (1994) *Developing Professional Knowledge and Competence.* Falmer Press, London.

Flanagan J., Baldwin S. & Clarke D. (2000) Work-based learning as a means of developing and assessing nursing competence. *Journal of Clinical Nursing*, **9**, 360–368.

Girot, E.A. (1993) Assessment of competence in clinical practice: a phenomenological approach. *Journal of Advanced Nursing* **18**, 114–119.

Glaser, B.G. (1978) *Theoretical Sensitivity. Advances in the Methodology of Grounded Theory.* Sociology Press, Mill Valley CA.

Glaser, B.G. & Strauss, A. (1967) *The Discovery of Grounded Theory.* Aldine Publishing Company, Chicago.

Gonczi, A. (1994) Competency based assessment in the professions in Australia. *Assessment in Education*, **1**, 27–43.

Goodman, J. (1984) *Reflection and Teacher Education: A Case Study and Theoretical Analysis.* Interchange 15/3. The Ontario Institute for Studies in Education, Ontario.

Gray, B. (1994) What is mentoring? *Education and Training*, **36**, 4–7.

Heidegger, M. (1962) *Being and Time.* Harper and Row, New York.

Hudson, R. (2000) *Professional Briefing. Practice Educators. Preparing for New Roles in the NHS.* CPHVA, London.

Jarvis, P. (1992) Reflective practice and nursing. *Nurse Education Today*, **12**, 174–181.

Jarvis, P. & Gibson, S. (1985) *The Teacher Practitioner in Nursing, Midwifery and Health Visiting.* Croom Helm, London.

Jessup, G. (1991) *Outcomes: NVQs and the Emerging Model of Education and Training.* Falmer Press, London.

Johns, C. (1994) Guided reflection. In: *Reflective Practice in Nursing* (eds A. Palmer, S. Burns & C. Bulman). Blackwell Science, Oxford.

Lathlean, J. (1997) *Lecturer Practitioners in Action.* Butterworth Heinemann, Oxford.

McMullan, M., Endacott, R., Gray, M., Jasper, M., Miller, C.M.L., Scholes, J. & Webb, C. (2003) Portfolios and assessment of competence: a review of the literature. *Journal of Advanced Nursing*, **41**, 283–294.

Medley, D. (1984) Teacher competency testing and the teacher educator. In: *Advances in Teacher Education* (eds L.G. Katz & J.D. Raths). Ablex, New Jersey.

Miller, C., Hoggan, J., Pringle, S. & West, G. (1988) *Credit Where Credit's Due.* The Report of the Accreditation of Work-Based Learning. Scottish Vocational Educational Council, Glasgow.

Nursing and Midwifery Council (2002) *Requirements for Pre-Registration Health Visitor Programmes.* The Nursing and Midwifery Council, London.

Nursing and Midwifery Council (2003) *Third Part of the Register: Specialist Community Public Health Nursing. Proposed Competency Framework Consultation Document.* The Nursing and Midwifery Council, London.

Nursing and Midwifery Council (2004) *NMC News.* Nursing and Midwifery Council, London.

Nursing and Midwifery Council (2006) *Standards To Support Learning And Assessment In Practice.* Nursing and Midwifery Council, London.

Nursing and Midwifery Council (2008) *The Code: Standards of Conduct, Performance and Ethics for Nurses and Midwives.* Nursing and Midwifery Council, London.

Phillips-Jones L, (1989) *The Mentee's Guide; The Mentor's Guide; The Mentoring Program Coordinator's Guide; Mentoring Program Materials Kit.* Coalition of Counselling Centers, Grass Valley, CA.

Robotham, A. (1994) *Are Academic Levels in Health Visiting Theory Discernible in Practice?* Unpublished dissertation for Master's in Education, University of Wolverhampton, Wolverhampton.

Robotham, A. (2001) *The Grading of Health Visitor Fieldwork Practice.* Unpublished thesis, University of Wolverhampton, Wolverhampton.

Rowntree, D. (1992) *Assessing Students: How Shall We Know Them,* 2nd edition. Kogan Page, London.

Runciman, P. (1990) *Competence-Based Education and the Assessment and Accreditation of Work-Based Learning in the Context of P2000, Programmes of Nurse Education, A Literature Review.* National Board for Nursing, Midwifery and Health Visiting for Scotland, Edinburgh.

Schön, D.A. (1983) *The Reflective Practitioner.* Basic Books, New York.

Schutz, A. (1972) *The Phenomenology of the Social World.* Heinemann, London.

Young, A. & Curzio, J. (2007) Preparing students for primary care. *Journal of Community Nursing*, **21**, 4–8.

Chapter 22 User Involvement: The Involved and Involving Community Health Care Nurse

Professor Bob Sang

Introduction and overview

The twenty-first century can be the era when community health care nursing comes into its own, working in partnership with patients, their families and communities. My contribution rests on the proposition that, for very good reasons, twenty-first century community health care nursing will be holistic and relational, whereby individual practitioners, working as members of the multi-disciplinary teams, will 'co-produce' health improvement, working and learning with patients/users, their families and friends, informed by the newly legislated patient and public involvement (PPI) system.

> 'Realising our vision for a world class NHS means working differently.... We need to empower patients and given health and social care staff greater flexibility to respond and lead'

> Lord Ara Darzi (*Our NHS, Our Future*, Department of Health [DH] 2007a)

The first part of the chapter focuses on the theme of 'Involvement', exploring the policy context of the past ten years leading to the current legislative agenda and the major service reviews led by Lord Darzi (DH 2007a, 2008a), reflecting on the growing significance of 'Involvement' for aspiring practitioners, and the possibility 'Involvement' offers for clinicians and health care practitioners to change their practices and relationships. The second part explores the drivers of twenty-first century health care from the point of view of an informed, active citizen and service user with an expectation of 'holistic care'. Finally, it reflects on the importance of relationship-based care and the

implications for community nurses as practitioners and entrepreneurs in the complex, rapidly changing, world of local health care.

However, before we go any further, let me put to rest the time-wasteful and meaningless debate about the concept of 'Involvement'. Academics and legislators alike love this debate, as do the growing numbers of consultants who work in this field: from well-known brands, such as Mori the pollsters, to *ad hoc* agencies such as the NHS' National Centre for Involvement. In this chapter I am much more interested in another 'I': the 'I' of *improvement* that arises naturally out of properly conducted involvement. Community nurses have a key role to play in the health improvement of people and communities; in improving the experiences of patients/users when they need direct care services, and in the planning and investing in the improved design of local services. As a result, community nursing can contribute to our wider understanding of how to humanise and to localise health care services at the very time when these are coming under increasing demographic pressure. Let us now look at how this might be the case.

The very word 'patient' or 'user' in social care means that a person is involved. A diagnosis, or assessment – formal or informal; 'lay' or professional – means that something is happening that is a risk to health and well-being. But, equally, people are not only 'patients' or 'users': they have complex, changing personal circumstances and relationships and, crucially, they have to address (or ignore!) their rights and responsibilities as citizens. Consider the triangulation of roles as shown in Figure 22.1.

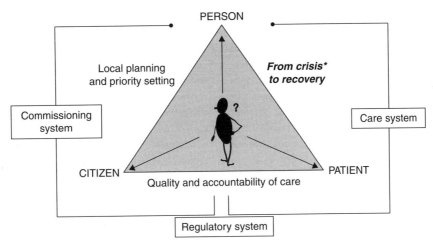

Figure 22.1   Triangulation of roles. *Where most people believe patient involvement begins and ends.

Patient and public involvement in health (PPIH) has extended to all three domains: the delivery of care, its quality assurance, and longer-term planning and funding (so-called 'commissioning'). This analysis is fundamental to understanding the desire to prioritise the development of community services:

> 'From the outset it needs to be clear that the rationale for providing care closer to home is based on the better use of highly specialist skills – not the dilution of them. We want to see specialists fully engaged as partners in designing new patient pathways.'
>
> (DH 2006)

The impact of this will be that community services, especially community nursing, will become crucial to the sustainable development of local care, and in this community nurses have a key role, as they work together with patients/citizens in the design, development, and delivery of modern health care: *involving to improve*. So, how has involvement with local people become such an important requirement of modern health care: both in principle and in practice?

The modern 'PPI' system

Aneurin Bevan's vision for the National Health Service (NHS) encompassed much more than health services. He foresaw the potentially democratising effect of an institution that encapsulated the very best of public endeavour, scientific advances and a ubiquitous local presence: a national body, valued and 'owned' by every local community. The vision has never been fully realised, principally because powerful vested and political interests have contrived to dominate the NHS, keeping its structures and systems away from direct local accountability and control (creating a profound 'democratic deficit' in health). In essence, a system has evolved over almost 60 years that has been grounded in a paternalistic and centralist 'culture of dependency', whereby all decisions – from individual decisions about treatment and care, to major decisions about the nature and location of services – have been shaped and/or determined by those at the centre who are in the habit of 'doing good' to and for others. This culture is reflected within the very language of 'patient involvement' and in the structures and practices which, as currently deployed, ensure that the involvement of 'lay' people in the NHS remains on the terms dictated by those within the management system and at the political centre of the NHS. Consequently we still risk tokenism on a grand scale if this structural and paternalistic legacy of the health sector remains unchallenged, compromising Lord Darzi's promising vision (DH 2007a, 2008a).

The latest reforms (see below) do offer the potential of *co-determination* – a mature inter-dependent relationship between local citizens and the NHS and its service partners, especially local clinical practitioners: thus it is at a local level that the real potential for involvement is emerging. However, if the reforms promoting community-based services are to work in practice, then, as stated above, basic assumptions need to be continually monitored and challenged to ensure that policy-makers and their local supporters understand the paradigmatic difference.

For example, I recently observed an earnest well-intentioned discussion where a mix of local activists (PPI forum members, service users, advocates, community development workers), and NHS managers and clinical professionals debated the potential structure of their new local involvement networks (LINks – see below). While they had acknowledged the interim nature of their thinking (as the relevant legislation was then going through the committee stage in Parliament) they failed to reflect on the assumptions underpinning their discussions, i.e. the assumption that *it was their role to speak for patients' interests and not to enable patients to speak for themselves.*

There was a consequent bias in both the substance *and* in the process. For example, two women working with asylum seekers and ethnic minority groups struggled to be heard because authority was conceded – by default – to those arguing forcefully about the representativeness of the LINks and how existing vested interests could be reconciled. They did not hear what the women had to say. Indeed, they were modelling the very behaviour (i.e. the traditional paternal-ist-centralist model of involvement in health care) that will continue to undermine the new policy intentions and leave us with a paradigm of involvement that is inequitable, non-inclusive and anti-participatory. So, what does this 'lesson' imply for community nurses, who spend much of their time with vulnerable and unheard people?

From a bottom-up community development perspective an alternative model has been growing from some time – a pluralist model of citizen participation, grounded in values of active informed citizenship, human rights and responsibilities, and robust implementation of the principles and practices of sound equalities work (see below). Such experience influenced the latest PPI reforms that introduced LINks and can now result in genuinely democratic innovation quite unlike what has gone before – a paradigm shift from the models of patient and public involvement previously experienced in the UK, whereby interest groups vie for influence with local officials. LINks offer the potential to be genuinely independent, socially inclusive and effective in enabling patients and citizens to speak to their own experiences and aspirations. However, for this model to take hold, we would do well to learn from recent history.

There have been several attempts to reform PPI and its value to the NHS; and two parliamentary inquiries. In 1974, community health councils (CHCs) were established as arms-length appointed bodies managed through the then regional offices of the NHS. In 2003, they were replaced by Patient and Public Involvement Forums (PPIFs), principally because they were seen as inconsistent in their performance and unrepresentative of local people. PPIFs, supported by a national commission, failed to meet expectations: indeed, they appeared to provoke the same criticisms as did their predecessors, the CHCs (House of Commons 2007). As I write, PPIFs are being replaced by the LINks, which will have the remit to cover health and social care under the Local Government and Public Involvement in Health Act 2007.

LINks are intended to differ in three crucial respects from either CHCs or PPIFs: they will be contracted through local government and not the NHS; they have a specific brief to be socially inclusive; and their role is to report, assiduously, on patients', users' and carers' experiences, providing useful and reliable data to trusts, local authorities, and the health and social care regulators. Their role is not representative, but enabling and informing, supported by organisations called HOSTs, drawn by competitive tender from the voluntary and community sector in each local authority area (Fig. 22.2).

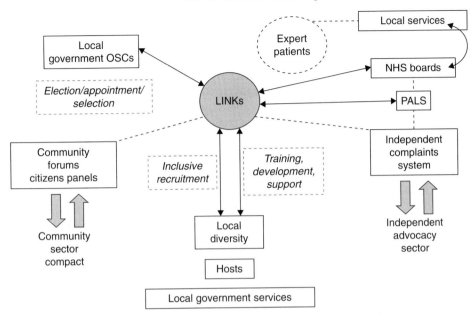

Figure 22.2   The emerging framework.

Effective and appropriate patient and public involvement at a local level will depend on how quickly we all, as colleagues and as fellow citizens, learn to adopt and engage with LINks and take advantage of the new roles and modes of participation that local people have been developing in communities during the past 30 years, enabled by Human Rights legislation and community development practice (see Table 22.1). In addition to these evolving roles and modes, there is growing recognition that they can been applied to a new set of priorities, which have arisen as a direct response to the key historic failings of the NHS, addressing the new purposes of a modern health service, thus:

- *Challenging health inequalities*: depends on effective cooperation between civic and social entrepreneurs, with services developments led by nurse entrepreneurs (e.g. Secure Health; Open Door; Central Surrey Health)
- *Robust, transparent decision-making*: results from increasing community governance capacity, allied to open corporate governance and scrutiny processes and, where appropriate,

deployment of inclusive, consensual methods of widening public participation
- *Continuous services improvement*: characterised by:
  — Networked PALS (Patient Advice and Liaison Services), accessible and responsive across the whole system – appreciating the patient experience as the catalyst for change, working with lay advocates
  — 'Expert patient' participation in clinical governance and service reviews
  — Accessible lay advocacy, working in mental health, learning disabilities and elderly care services
  — Transparent independent communications within local forums and scrutiny processes, enhanced by multi-cultural support services
- *Personalised and integrated care*: based on inter-agency collaboration, multi-disciplinary working, and informed patient choice

Whether these priorities are best addressed through a consumerist market-orientated system and/or through maintaining a strong public service ethos and management system is the

Table 22.1 Democratic and participatory roles

Civic entrepreneurs: public servants who work as internal change agents and as valued partners with local people and their organisations, fostering an open participatory culture within the system, e.g. patient and public involvement managers

Social entrepreneurs: local people who facilitate capacity-building, active citizenship and engagement in social-democratic and service enterprise

Expert patients: people with long-term conditions (disabilities and chronic disease – mental and physical) who learn to manage their own health journeys and, in so doing, work in partnership with service teams and services' management on services development and improvement

Independent lay advocates: local citizens and independent practitioners who support marginalised and excluded people in participating in decisions that affect their lives

Community governance: independent means of ensuring effective, inclusive local democratic participation in decision-making: a necessary complement to corporate citizenship (e.g. neighbourhood groups)

Nurse entrepreneurs: practitioners who lead new service and commissioning developments, working in active partnership with local people and patients

---

focus of an underlying political debate, which has polarised opinion about the way forward for health and social care. An alternative perspective is emerging, as described above, based on a social partnership between patients and professionals, and between communities and the agencies of health and social care.

This twenty-first century agenda, now being pursued through Lord Darzi's reviews (DH 2007a, 2008a), raises important questions for the devolving NHS, wherein primary care trusts (PCTs), in partnership with their co-terminous local authorities, are positioned to become the critical local structure fulfilling their new commissioning role. Principally:

- What are the complementary cultural and practical implications for management, professionals and employees?
- What is the PCTs' role in supporting local capacity building: especially in relation to health improvement?
- How will this change the nature of governance and decision-making: i.e. especially in relation to major service changes?
- How do we nurture/grow/recognise the importance of the role of the civic/social entrepreneurs?

The above questions and tensions are also are also reflected in the recently launched programme for 'World Class Commissioning' (DH 2008b), which will become increasingly important to local people as patients and as citizens. It is here that there will be major challenges for community nursing leaders as they take on the new and influential roles, both in service development and in commissioning, building on their local knowledge, relationships, and insight into what really works for vulnerable people and their families and communities.

The new lexicon: the structural challenge of roles, skills and responsibilities

The new policy proposals lead us to consider the following points. *Public involvement in health* is concerned with achieving active, responsible citizenship through extending people's participation in the following:

- Independent monitoring and scrutiny of health system performance and decision-making
- Acting as volunteer advocates with local complaints and independent advocacy schemes, ensuring fellow citizens are included in the decision-making that affects their lives
- Engagement in the regeneration and renewal activities that foster health improvement and reduced health inequalities at a local levels

The above are complementary roles requiring considerable investment in the development of citizenship and social entrepreneurship.

Citizen participation entails the fair and inclusive involvement of local people in all the levels of health decision-making. Community governance is enhanced by properly recruited citizens' panels and citizens' juries, and by independent community forums: crucial to the new requirement for PCTs to involve local people in planning, commissioning, and decision-making. Patient involvement in health is concerned with ensuring that patients and potential patients can engage in mutually respectful, properly informed dialogues about their journeys towards better health outcomes.

Thus, the patient experience becomes the principal catalyst for improvement.

The implications are profound for clinicians who work with patients/users day-in and day-out:

- Diagnosis/assessment is a mutually informing process, inter-relating patients' experiences and insights with objective clinical data and the exercise of clinical judgement and sensitivity
- The planning and execution of clinical interventions is communicated, and, where possible, negotiated – taking account of the accessibility of care, the appropriateness of available resources and patients' circumstances
- Ongoing recovery and normalisation represents a 'handover' of the balance of responsibility from the clinical team to the individual and their carers/supporters

The two, complementary, processes of public and patient involvement described above come together in four formal processes, informed by the work of the local LINks:

- *Local government overview and scrutiny committees* (OSCs): working transparently and cooperatively with local politicians and local government officers to ensure robust scrutiny of health decision-making and services' provision

- *Corporate governance*: taking part in boards and decision-making processes, as *appointed* members
- *Clinical governance*: contributing to the monitoring and assessment of clinical services and to educational and standard setting processes with clinical teams (i.e. The 'Expert Patient' model, see below)
- *inclusive services' management*: ensuring that patient/carer/relative experience is integral to services' facilities and process improvement – including assuring information, communications, and referrals processes (the key role of PALS)

Figure 22.2 demonstrates how the above structures are intended to sit together as a single system, reflecting the triangulation of roles introduced in Figure 22.1. But, there formalities represent only part of the 'PPI' picture. In a society where the future sustainability of health and social well-being of local communities depends on the successful delivery of new service models (see above), partnership with local professionals will be the crucial ingredient of the new system of involvement. Above all, from a patient/user perspective, the effectiveness and sustainability of the new service models that are emerging through the current reforms, depends on the adoption and delivery of holistic principles and practices. I shall endeavour to explain what this means, from my independent patient's perspective, in the next section, which also explores potential impact on twenty-first century community nursing.

A patient's perspective: developing a holistic approach

Much of my own learning and development has been experiential and reflective, often building on dialogues with the practitioners I have met through my own health journey. However, setting that experience aside, I have also found myself confronting and challenging embedded practice and the systemic abuse of patients in 'mainstream' services: first as a 'whistle blower' and then through establishing the original lay advocacy schemes in the UK following a series of widely reported scandals (Sang & O'Brien 1984). It was a matter of public record at that time that tens of thousands of vulnerable people living in long-term 'care' were experiencing appalling levels of neglect, physical and sexual abuse, and denial of basic human rights, let alone deprivation of access to much-needed services such as physiotherapy, good general medicine, speech therapy and so on. Many of the people I met were not clinically 'sick' but had still been detained in these 'clinical' environments for over 40 years, because they were not believed by clinical 'experts' to be capable of living full, integrated lives.

Much has changed in the 30 or so years since the inquiry reports on these scandals (Martin 1984), however many of the underlying institutional assumptions and professional expectations have remained, as stated in the first part of this chapter. Despite the rhetoric of 'community care' and 'integrated seamless services', holism, as I understand it, has not been achieved and is not being achieved for growing numbers of our fellow citizens: especially those with long-term conditions and disabilities. Compare the systemic neglect and abuse of the 1970s and 1980s with the findings from the evaluation of a therapeutic community-based mental health service:

'Patients (identified) what factors were most beneficial in improving their sense of wellbeing: the relaxing and calming nature of the therapy sessions; the time spent with patients as individuals, being pampered and touched, on a one-to-one basis; talking; sharing problems and being listened to'.

(Collins & Edwards 2007)

While this nurse-led initiative was, and is, being funded within the NHS, its longer-term future remains in doubt, despite the aspirations and expectations of growing numbers of our fellow citizens. So, what can be done, by whom?

In 1997, I was commissioned, on the occasion of the fiftieth anniversary celebrations of the NHS, to clarify the UK's citizens' aspirations for the next 50 years of development of that revered institution. One of the most powerful statements arising from the event was: 'We want to be treated as whole people with whole lives, and we want to be involved'. These aspirations reflect what I continue to hear from local people everywhere: a real desire for the NHS to become more holistic: designing and developing services in ways that reflect their lives, their responsibilities, and their aspirations, recognising that they have a legitimate part to play – as citizens. My report was launched concurrently with the White Paper that underwrote the New Labour reforms, building on *The NHS Plan* (DH 2007b). Since that time the reform programme has continued unabated and, despite significant investment in 'PPI' and the two attempts described above to reform the PPI system (Health Select Committee [HSC] 2007). As outlined in the first part to this chapter, it appears that New Labour's 'patient-centred' programme initiated over ten years ago remains incapable of delivering an across the board sustainable, truly holistic care system and culture, hence the appointment of Lord Darzi for a further review of NHS services (DH 2007a, 2008a).

A respected commentator on the NHS, Andy Cowper, recently took a stock-take of the NHS: 'We do know that there's a net surplus of a couple of billion pounds and that activity continues positively towards the 18 week "referral to treatment" target. Healthcare acquired infections appear to be coming down...' (Cowper 2008). Interestingly, Cowper later in his article also hints at a change to come: greater emphasis on patient self management; personal budgeting; a greater emphasis on community-based services; and a new more inclusive system of local involvement, which may be regarded as emergent 'holism'.

Behind the scenes of this period of growth and reform has been the emergence of a more considered economic analysis, commissioned by the Treasury and led by Sir Derek Wanless (2002, 2004). As it becomes increasingly apparent that the reforms, while doubling investment in the NHS, have had a limited beneficial impact on health and well-being, so government will be forced to revisit Wanless' important analyses. (Remember, the Wanless reports were commissioned by Gordon Brown, the current Prime Minister (see below), during his time as Chancellor of the Exchequer.) And, indeed, a more holistic, preventive policy *is* emerging, offering a longer-term, more collaborative, approach.

With the recent change of Labour leadership has there begun a change in the rhetoric, confirming Cowper's helpful analysis:

'The next phase of Reform is targeted to keeping you healthy and fit, and puts you far more in control of your own health and your own life. And in the long run a preventive service personal to your needs is beneficial not just to individuals but to all of us as we reduce the costs of disease.

Choice between providers has been among the forces for changes that have meant hospitals, GPs and others have been thinking about how they offer the kind of personal service we all expect. But real empowerment of patients will come from going further – the driving force: higher patient aspirations, more patient expertise, more trust between clinicians and patient, patients becoming fuller participants and partners in health and health care.

In this way the nature of NHS provision will and must change – to be based not just on what it can do for you but what, empowered with new advice, support and information, you can do for yourself and your family.

So if in the last generation the big medical advance was the doctor administering antibiotics, in the coming generation it will be patients working with doctors and NHS staff to improve our own health and manage our own conditions.

And this means health professionals building on the plethora of good evidence-based practice that exists already – and becoming champions and advocates of more empowered patients: the doctor not just physician but adviser; the nurse not just carer but trainer; patients more than consumers – partners.'

(Brown 2008)

In other words, a fundamental change in roles and relationships, on all sides. How will these reinforced policy intentions be achieved? Given the growing prevalence of long-term conditions, surely community nurses will be at the forefront of these changes.

Alongside the re-emergence of talk about partnership with patients, consumers and citizens, there is an explicit shift towards empowerment and localism, building on the reforms described in the previous section. The next phase of reform includes locality-based commissioning (planning and prioritising NHS resources) and, more significantly for the longer term, 'patients' themselves are challenging and changing the discourse. Initiatives such as the Expert Patient Programme in long-term conditions, the Wellbeing and Recovery Action Planning in mental health, 'In Control' in Learning Disabilities, are connecting with learning from lay advocacy and the independent living movement – reinforced by the Human Rights legislation – to promote active engagement and, crucially, a more holistic approach to reform that recognises the inherent complexities of people's lives. In recent months I have begun to meet community nurses acting as champions and facilitators for these developments, often working in impoverished and culturally diverse communities, engaging with the daily complexity of people's lives, their physical and mental health, and their challenging circumstances.

I learned a long time ago as a scientist that any system that contains more than three interacting variables is hard to measure and hence predict. Further, the introduction of new agents, such as medication, has a further complicating effect. As biological beings, we are subject to multiple variables: from our genetics and biochemistry and skeletal and nervous systems, to our little understood sense and consciousness. We are also emotional and intellectual beings, with feelings and beliefs, habits, and attitudes. And then, things change – constantly – in our daily lives and circumstances. All of this impacts on our health, well-being, and functioning. When someone does get sick or injured, then clinical practitioners, especially community nurses, necessarily become involved with this dynamic complexity.

For example, accurate diagnosis and treatment have limited long-term value for people who have low confidence, exacerbated by poor housing and worklessness. Solutions, and hence long-term improvement, means engaging with people in the context of whole lives: listening, facilitating their active participation and working in multi-disciplinary, inter-agency partnerships. In recent months I have met community nurses who are developing their roles to engage with such complexity as link workers, care coordinators, social entrepreneurs and a director of care employed jointly by the PCT and the local authority. Above all, they are learning to work facilitatively and collaboratively with patients themselves. And, for these developments to grow, we, patients, must also learn and grow.

Stepping out and up: 'patients' no more

Compare the following two quotes from mental health service users, showing how different interventions give rise to very different experiences.

'I very quickly became institutionalized myself. I was scared to come out because I was in this enclosed world where I knew what was going to happen. There were routines, mealtimes, getting up times, medication times, OT [occupational therapy] times. There were routines and I had no responsibilities'.

(Ridge & Ziebland 2006)

'...but I hadn't actually realized I'd been in recovery. I had to go to a recovery conference to kind of realize I was in recovery [laugh]. It means that life is changing. It is not changed. It's a constant thing, its always changing. It changes every day and I notice things that I didn't, that I haven't noticed for years. I can listen to music and appreciate it in a different way... it can move me now'.

(Ridge & Ziebland 2006)

More recently, from the field of cancer, my colleague Jan Alcoe expands on these insights:

'Surprisingly, illness presents us with unexpected moments of fun, happiness, peace, and fulfilment which arise from a growing ability to live in the moment. We discover personal strengths and qualities we didn't know we had. These can help us to cope in positive ways with change and the challenges we face, and to find a new sense of balance and well-being'.

(Janki Foundation 2008)

Essentially, while the NHS Reforms have (at least until now) been based on the exploitation, regulation, and marketisation of curative and interventionist 'acute' medicine and so-called 'patient choice', it has been patients themselves who, together with holistic practitioners, have been developing an alternative view. This emerging paradigm shift is one of the keys to the co-creation of a sustainable system, as apparently recognised by Gordon Brown: provided that 'we', the patients, and 'you', the practitioners, learn to work together to promote a model of service that both engages and empowers us in the mutual endeavour of health improvement. In this respect 'holism' is central to Wanless' 'fully engaged' scenario and hence the sustainability of the NHS and social care.

The potential for common ground is significant and real:

'Even doctors who thought of themselves as compassionate, recognise they can do better once they experience life as a patient.'

(*New York Times* 2008)

The deep, shared challenge, is to move away from models of treatment and care that focus solely on 'sick role' and hence interventionist care. Medicine is about much more than that, as holistic practice demonstrates in its many forms and traditions. 'Patients' are much more than that also: 'Label Jars, Not People', as the 'three-dimensional framework' in Figure 22.3 illustrates.

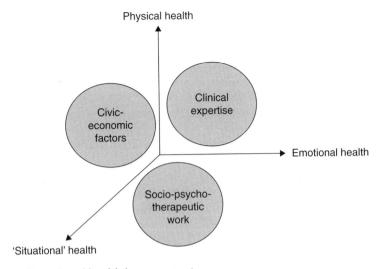

Figure 22.3 Three-dimensional health improvement.

The corporate sector – public and private – relies on labelling to sustain sick role and the over-medicalisation of care:

'A deep, taken for granted assumption in our culture is that if you have a "problem" or a "need" you get a label: "patient", "user", "client", "sick", "disabled", "handicapped". One consequence of such labelling is the separation of citizens into categories and groups defined by the service models that have been constructed to "meet this need/problem". Very powerfully, at the point of diagnosis/analysis, individuals are defined only by their "special needs" and/or their dysfunctioning, thus excluding their many purposes, roles, capabilities, aspirations and so forth, as parents, partners, entrepreneurs, and citizens. We cease to be seen as active players in the economy and culture, and become defined not only by provider categories ("special need", "asthmatics", "depressives"…) but also, crucially, by powerful provider interests. Thus in the proposed quasi-market, "the money will follow the patient" becomes a threat to liberty, not an opportunity to choose.'

(Sang 2007)

By removing their 'labels' and engaging fully as themselves, thousands and thousands of people with genetic and long-term conditions and disabilities are transcending the sick role and inspiring the co-creation of a new twenty-first century paradigm, based on mutuality, dialogue and a fresh narrative about health care. Yet, we do of course get sick, and often this is complex, resulting from the co-morbidities that arise from living with long-term conditions. The 'modern' response has been to attempt to standardise medicine and regulate practice against 'evidence-based guidance'. But, this increasingly managerial approach to medicine flies in the face of everything we – patients and practitioners – know from a holistic perspective. Thus:

'Managing care one person at a time is especially important. The notion of the "average" patient is virtually meaningless in healthcare, even more so with people with chronic conditions. The application of standardised treatment protocols almost invariably leads to under-treating some portion of patients and over-treating the others. Complications increase, outcomes suffer, and healthcare costs rise'.

(Pollak 2005)

Dr Pollak and his colleagues have now demonstrated the crucial importance of achieving and using entirely personalised, patient-centric, data, working with renal patients in New York (Pollak & Lorch 2007). Their renal patients live 35% longer than the 'norm' for people with such a complex, co-morbid condition and, more importantly, they are in a position to manage their lives and their well-being collaboratively with the multi-disciplinary team: holism-in-action. Crucially, the community nursing practitioners share the data and, as full team members, they work with patients to fulfil all aspects of living.

Yet, Drs Pollak and Lorch work within the constraints and rigours of the US market system. 'Their' patients are living with end-stage renal disease and are uninsurable. The data provided by their shared record system supports a day-to-day informed dialogue with the whole clinical team. Their work was first introduced to me in the late 1990s (Sang 1999), and as the 2007 results demonstrate, they have achieved successful, shared management of complex long-term conditions, working with people who may be experiencing multiple co-morbidities and continuous risk to life and well-being. Is there a useful link between Pollak and Lorch's applied science and holistic practice – between our bio-medical selves, our conscious selves, and our active, engaged selves?

If holism enriches the emotional being, can we begin to connect to our beliefs and choices about 'what works' and harness learning from science and experience; from reason and deep emotion? How will community nurses harness the theoretical and practical guidance and resources, contained in the other chapters of this book, reflect on their growing experiences of patients and their circumstances, and take an appropriate leadership role in developing and delivery services that are safe and locally sustainable? Clinicians, entrepreneurs *and* facilitators of learning, involvement, and improvement!

Conclusion: co-creating health care improvement

Essentially, I am arguing for a much more 'bottom-up' approach to health care reform, based on a working partnership between citizens

and professionals, enabled by the new system of PPI. The policy drivers 'talk the talk' of engagement and empowerment, but it is at a local level where creative practitioners are beginning to make a real difference to both the commissioning and provision of care, based on their empathy and ability to work collaboratively with other professionals and with 'clients/service users'. The Darzi reviews (DH 2007a, 2008a) are beginning to model this co-creative approach, illustrating that the sustainable improvement in health called for by Wanless (2002), can indeed by achieved.

Remember: 'We want to be treated as whole people with whole lives' (Sang 1998). More importantly the above frameworks demonstrate the inherent complexity of human living and the inter-dependence of the factors that impinge on health and well-being, positively and negatively. Far too complex for the rigid rationality of marketised, evidence-based medicine. Community nurses are positioned betwixt and between the uncertainly and unpredictability of peoples lives, especially those living with long-term conditions and disabilities, and the politicised managerial system that increasingly relies on the mantra of evidence-based choice. In this modern context, relationships with patients themselves provide the best data for clinical practice and for influencing decision-making.

Patient involvement is all starting to come together from a policy perspective. However, policy will only get us so far when the legacy culture is acting against us. So, my question is: 'How can *we* develop a strategy to support the development of a system that promotes health and well-being, drawing more heavily on the social model introduced above, when biomedicine is the cultural model that consistently pulls in the opposite direction?'. I would also add a rider, or supplementary question 'How can holistic nurse practitioners contribute to implementing such a strategy?' (see Figure 22.3). My colleague, Dr Alf Collins, and I have begun to clarify the importance of dialogue and relationships in sustaining a productive, adult-to-adult (i.e. inter-dependent) relationship between citizens who learn by experience and those who

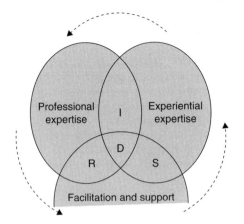

Figure 22.4 Developing therapeutic dialogues. I = Information (personal and clinically rich); R = Reflective practice; S = Self-management; D = Dialogue.

learn through professional development (see Figure 22.4; with thanks and appreciation to Dr Alf Collins, Chair of the Joint Board on SelfCare).

Clearly, the model shown in Figure 22.4 can be developed and deployed iteratively, enabling practitioners and citizens to learn together, co-creating solutions: from personal well-being and recovery planning, to sharing tough choices about the planning of services and, ultimately, their redesign on *stochastic* principles (i.e. the whole PPI agenda described earlier). The stochastic nature of medicine has been recognised since the time of Aristotle, and has been conveniently forgotten as medicine has become merchandised (Lerodiakonou 1993). As noted above, the inherent complexity addressed by every citizen, as they learn to engage with disease or injury, creates the need for an integrated, dialogic response:

> 'Science and narrative, the quantitative and the qualitative, are not competitors, but represent a complementary duality. Narrative preserves individuality, distinctiveness, and context, whereas quantitative methods and evidence-based guidelines offer a solid foundation for what is reliably and generally correct'.

> (Roberts 2000)

The challenge to holistic community nursing practitioners is *both* to develop their evidence-base *and* to change the basis of the narrative. Much of this chapter has been inspired by my work with therapeutic practitioners such as Collins, Roberts, Lorch and Pollak and also, as well as with patients, often facilitated by community nurses who are already shifting the culture of practice and taking on the new roles and opportunities described above. By bringing our learning from applying the civic (rights and responsibilities) and social models (our diversity and complexity) of improvement, we can now engage with the scientific and stochastic roots of clinical practice in pursuance of its continuing reform. That reform can now focus on the sustainability of health and health care, ensuring that community nursing has an integral and efficacious part to play in partnership with patients themselves.

References

Brown, G. (2008) Speech on the National Health Service, King's College London. Gordon Brown, 8 January 2008.

Collins, J. & Edwards, M. (2007) Treating the whole person. *Mental Health Today*, 30–32.

Cowper, A. (2008) Editorial. *British Journal of Healthcare Management*, **14**, 136.

Department of Health (2006) *Our Health, Our Care, Our Say: A New Direction for Community Services*. Department of Health, London, para 6.6, 130.

Department of Health (2007a) *Our NHS Our Future: NHS Next Stage Review – Interim Report* . Lord Ara Darzi. Available at www.dh.gov.uk/en/Publicationsandstatistics/Publications/PublicationsPolicyAndGuidance/dh_079077 (accessed 1 December 2008).

Department of Health (2007b) *The New NHS: Modern, Dependable*. Department of Health, London.

Department of Health (2008a) *High Quality Care for All: NHS Next Stage Review*. Final Report – Lord Ara Darzi. Cm7432. Department of Health, London.

Department of Health (2008b) *World Class Commissioning*. Department of Health, London.

Health Select Committee (2007) Inquiry into patient and public involvement in health. House of Commons HC 278-1, April 2007.

Janki Foundation (2008) *Lifting Your Spirits*. Janki Foundation, London, p. 5.

Lerodiakonou, K. (1993) Medicine as a stochastic art. *Lancet*, **341**, 542.

Martin, J.P. (1984) *Hospitals in Trouble*. Martin Robertson & Co, London.

New York Times (2008) *Interview with Dr Robert Klitzman, 'When Doctors Become Patients'*. Tara Parker-Pope, *New York Times*.

Pollak, V.E. & Lorch, J.A. (2007) Effect of electronic patient record use on mortality in end stage renal disease, a model chronic disease: retrospective analysis of 9 years of prospectively collected data. *BMC Medical Informatics and Decision-Making* **7**, 1–15.

Pollak, S. (2005) *The Benefits of Integrated Health Records Systems: Report to the Department of Health*, December 2005.

Ridge, D. & Ziebland, S. (2006) 'The old me could never have done that': how people give meaning to recovery following depression. *Qualitative Health Research*, **16**, 1038–1053.

Roberts, G. (2000) Narrative and severe mental illness: what place do stories have in an evidence-based world. *Advances in Psychiatric Treatment*, **6**, 432–441.

Sang, B. (1998) Introduction. In: *Citizens' Voices*. King's Fund Report to the NHS 50th Anniversary Conference. King's Fund, London.

Sang, B. (1999) Modernising renal services. *British Journal of Renal Medicine*, **4**.

Sang, B. (2007) A citizen-led coalition for integrated care. *Journal of Integrated Care*, **15**, 41–51.

Sang, B, & O'Brien, J. (1984) *Advocacy in the UK*. King's Fund, London.

Wanless, D. (2002) *Securing Our Future Health: Taking a Long-Term View*. HM Treasury, London.

Wanless, D. (2004) *Securing Good Health for the Whole Population: Population Health Trends*. HMSO, Norwich.

Index